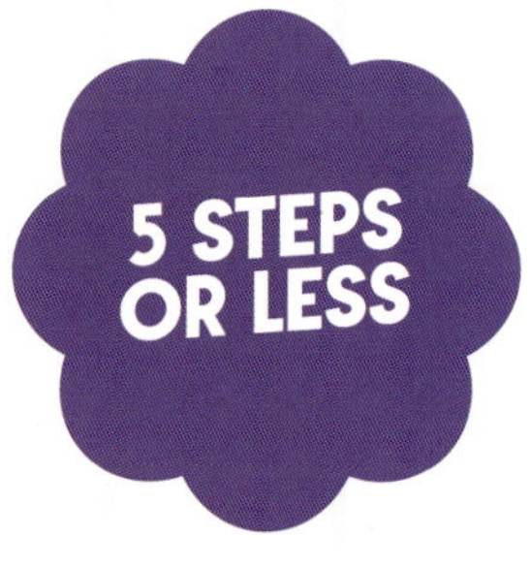

Making cooking simple.

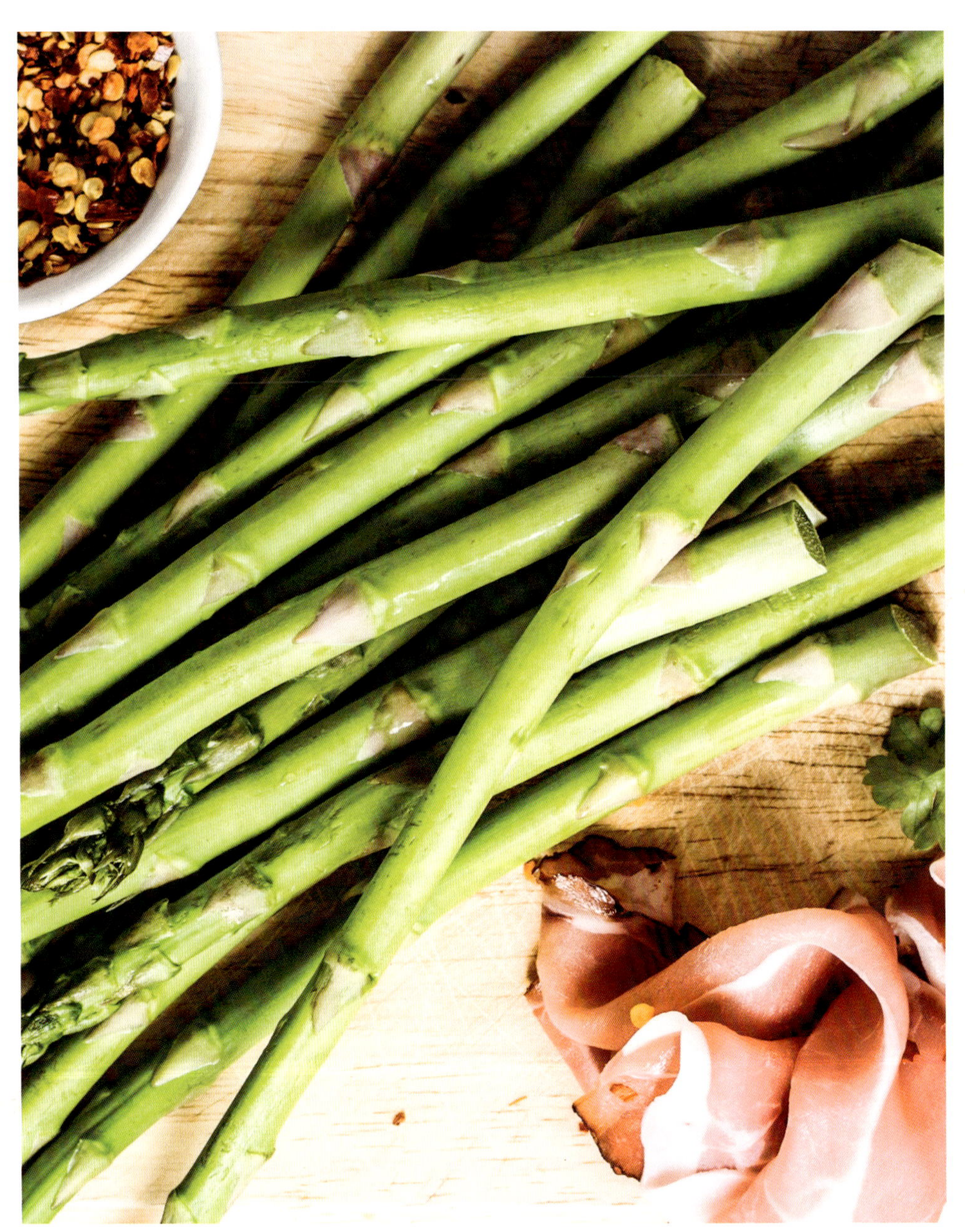

Love your low-carb life with the beautiful and easy recipes in this cookbook. You'll feel good, look good and can enjoy the proven health benefits, all while eating delicious meals that can be shared with friends and family.

You'll find heaps of options for every meal of the day here, and there's no need to miss out on sweets and treats either. This is low-carb as it should be: irresistibly tasty, sociably shareable and just too easy.

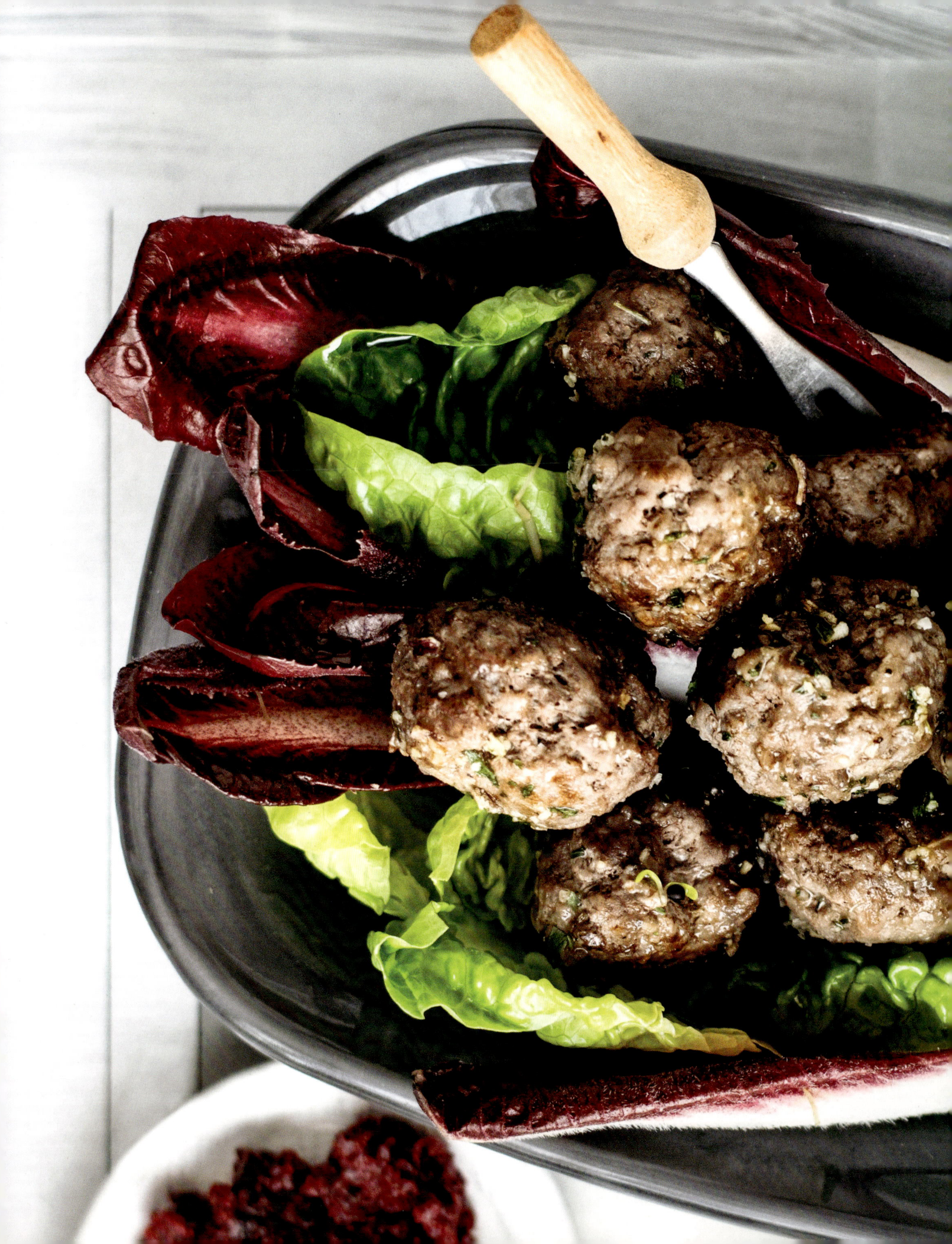

EAT EASY

Low-Carb

HERRON

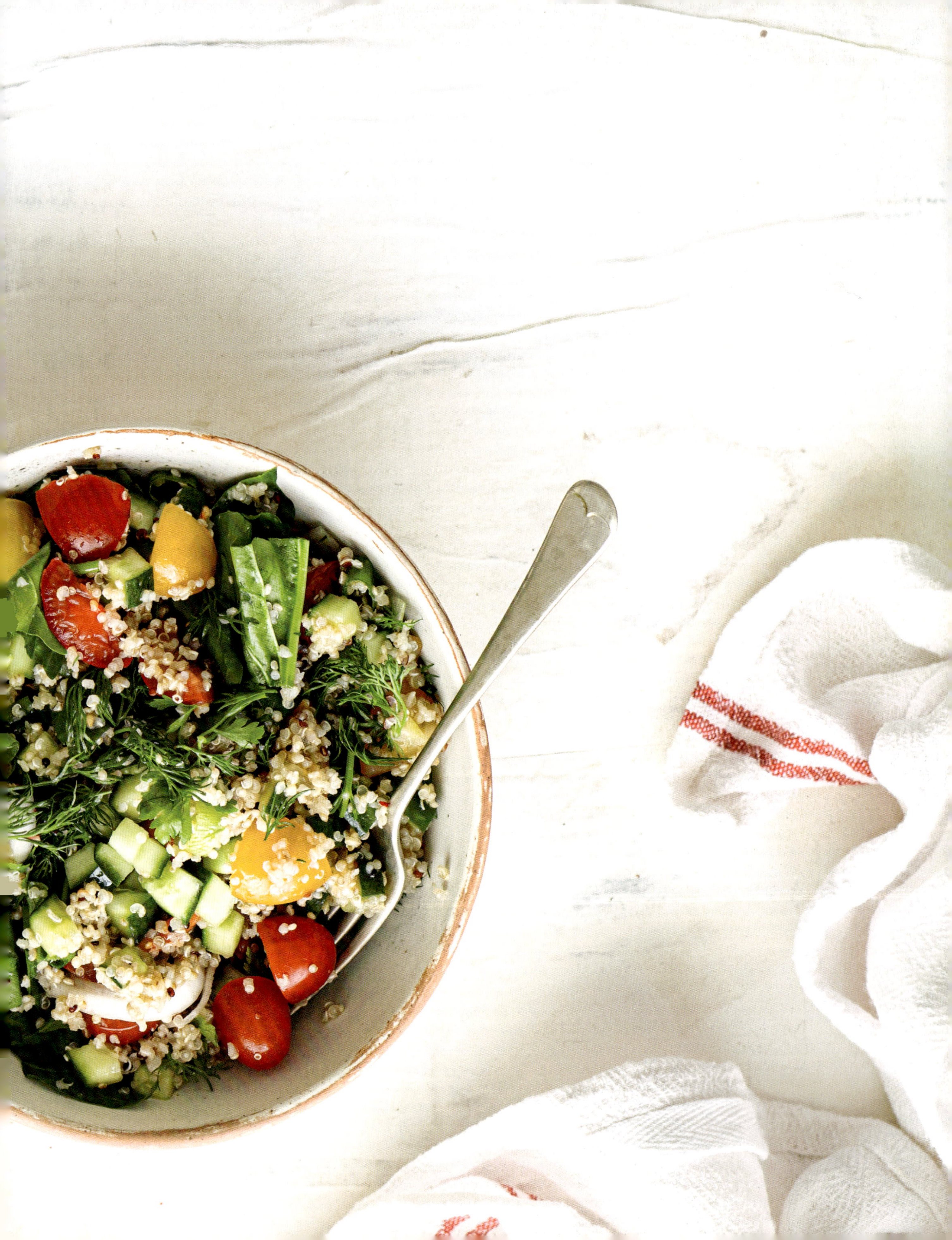

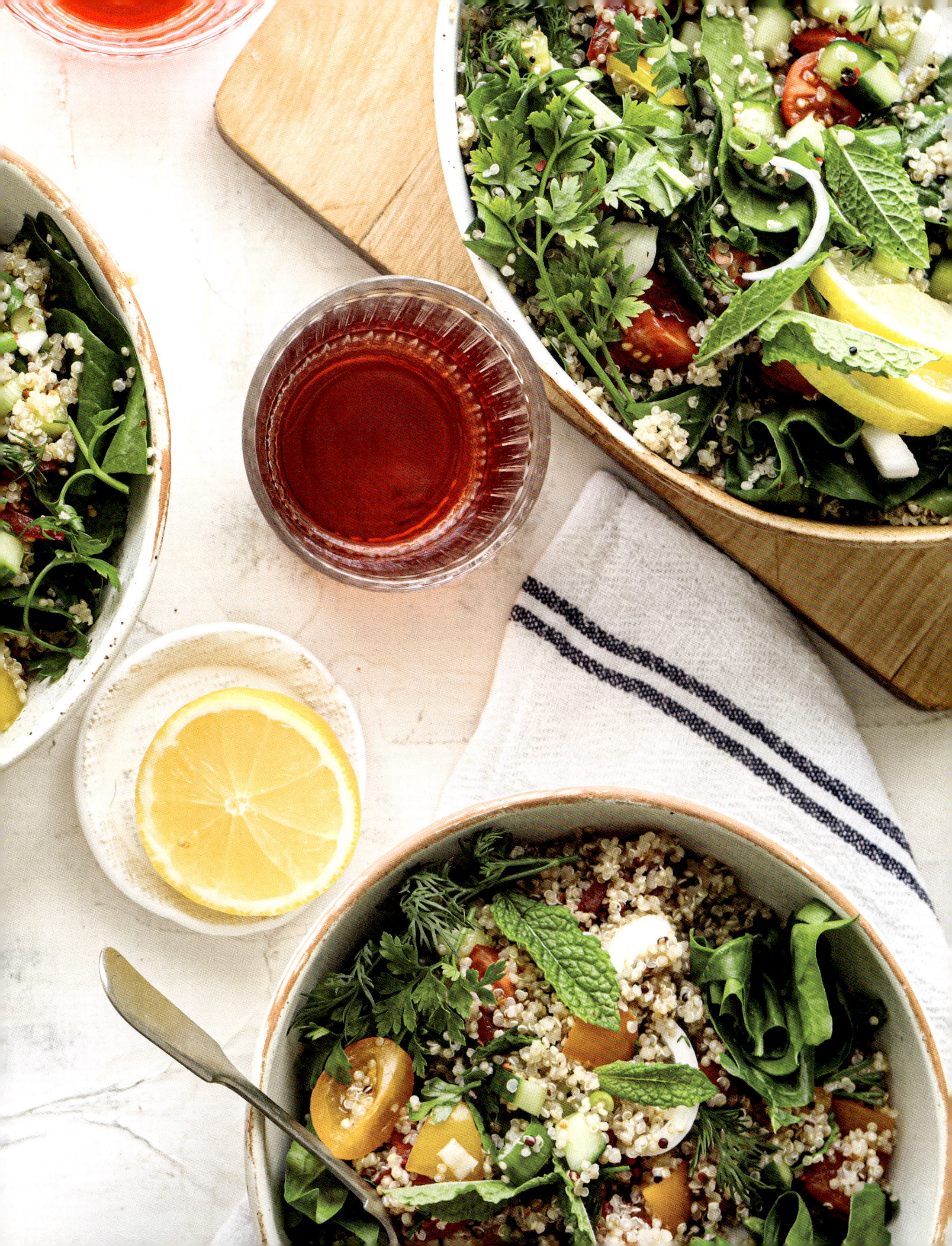

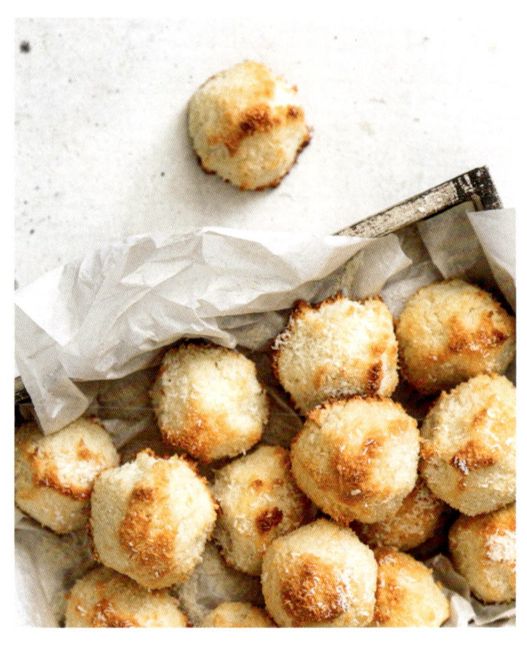
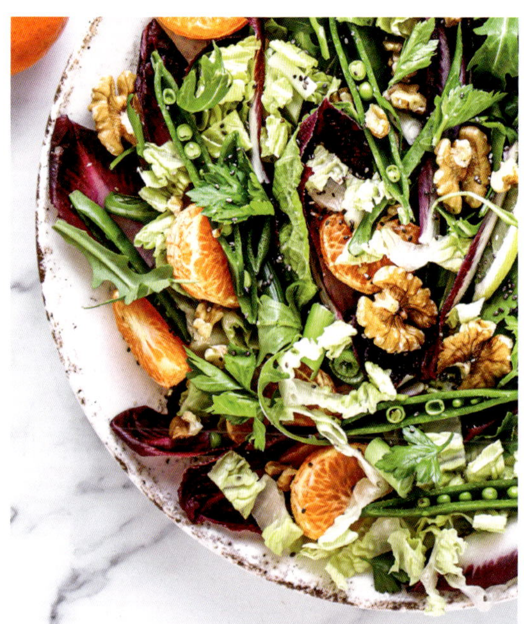
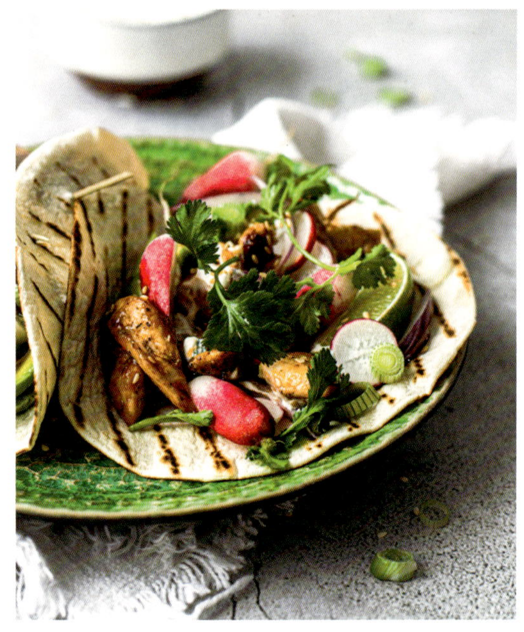
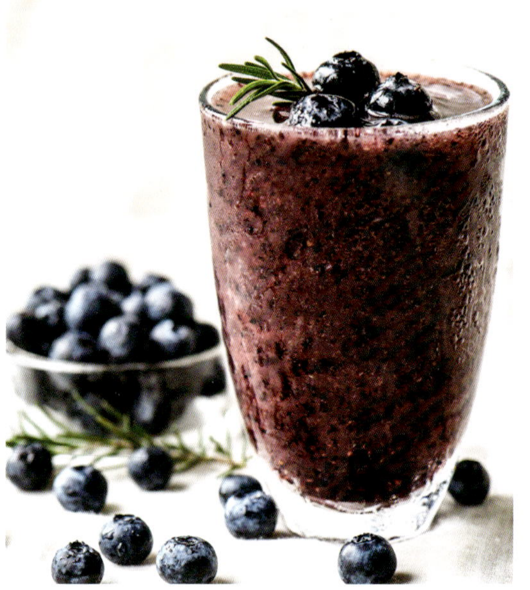

CONTENTS

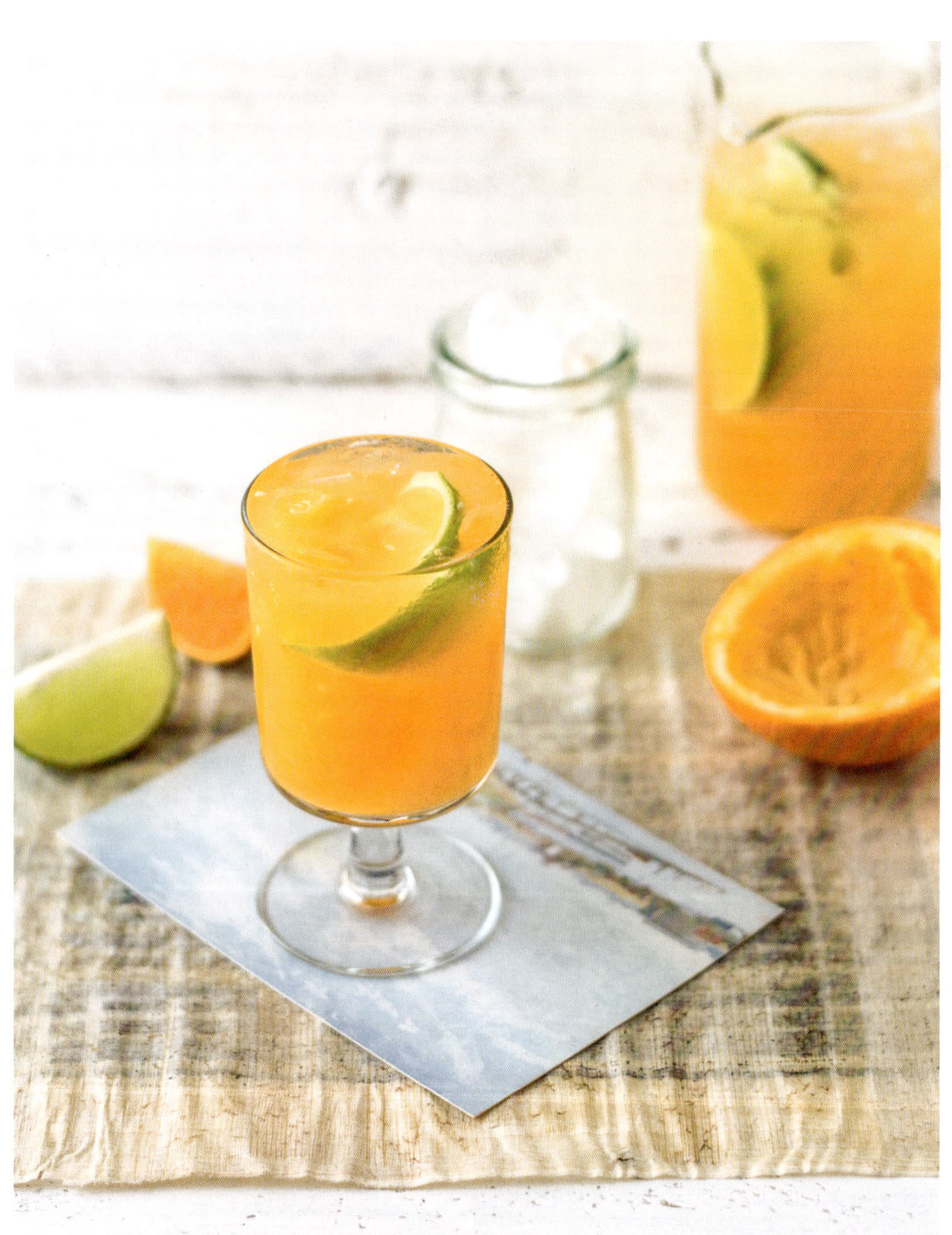

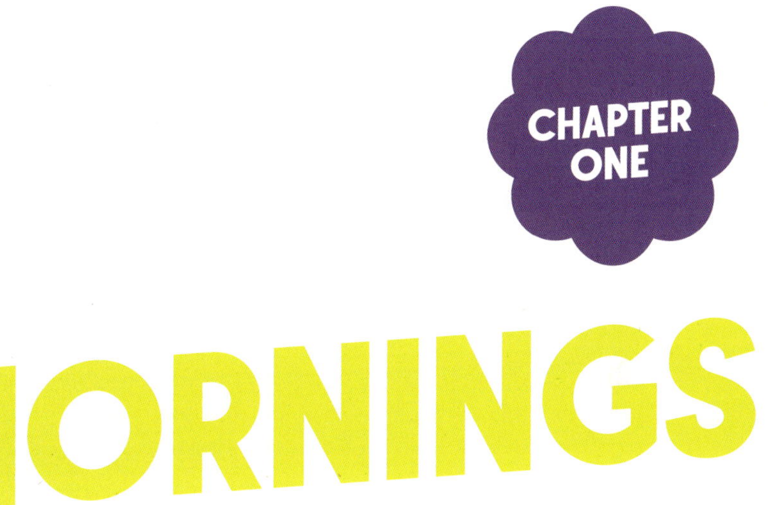

CHAPTER ONE

MORNINGS

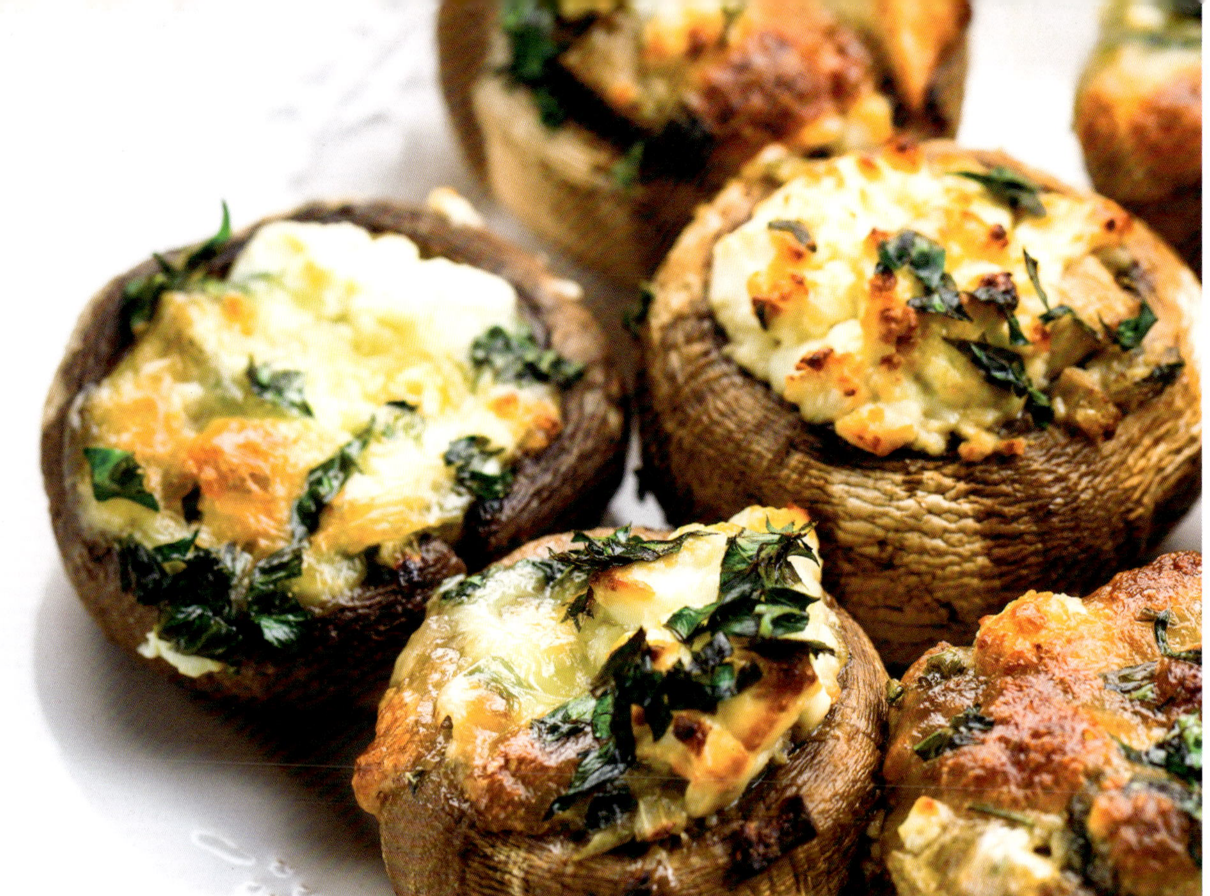

STUFFED MUSHROOMS

- 2 tbsps olive oil
- 1 small onion, finely chopped
- 1 clove garlic, crushed
- 8 large button mushrooms, wiped and stems removed and finely chopped
- 120g feta cheese
- 120g cream cheese
- ¼ cup (10g) parsley, finely chopped
- Salt and pepper to taste
- ¾ cup (100g) grated tasty cheese

STEPS

Preheat oven to 180°C.

1. In a small frying pan, heat the olive oil over medium heat. Fry the onion, garlic and chopped mushroom stems for 5 minutes until onion is softened. Remove from heat and set aside.
2. In a medium bowl, combine the feta and cream cheese, half the parsley and the onion mixture. Season to taste.
3. Spoon the cheese mixture evenly into the mushroom caps and place on a lined baking tray.
4. Sprinkle each mushroom with the grated tasty cheese and bake for 20 minutes or until browned on top.
5. Serve warm garnished with the rest of the parsley.

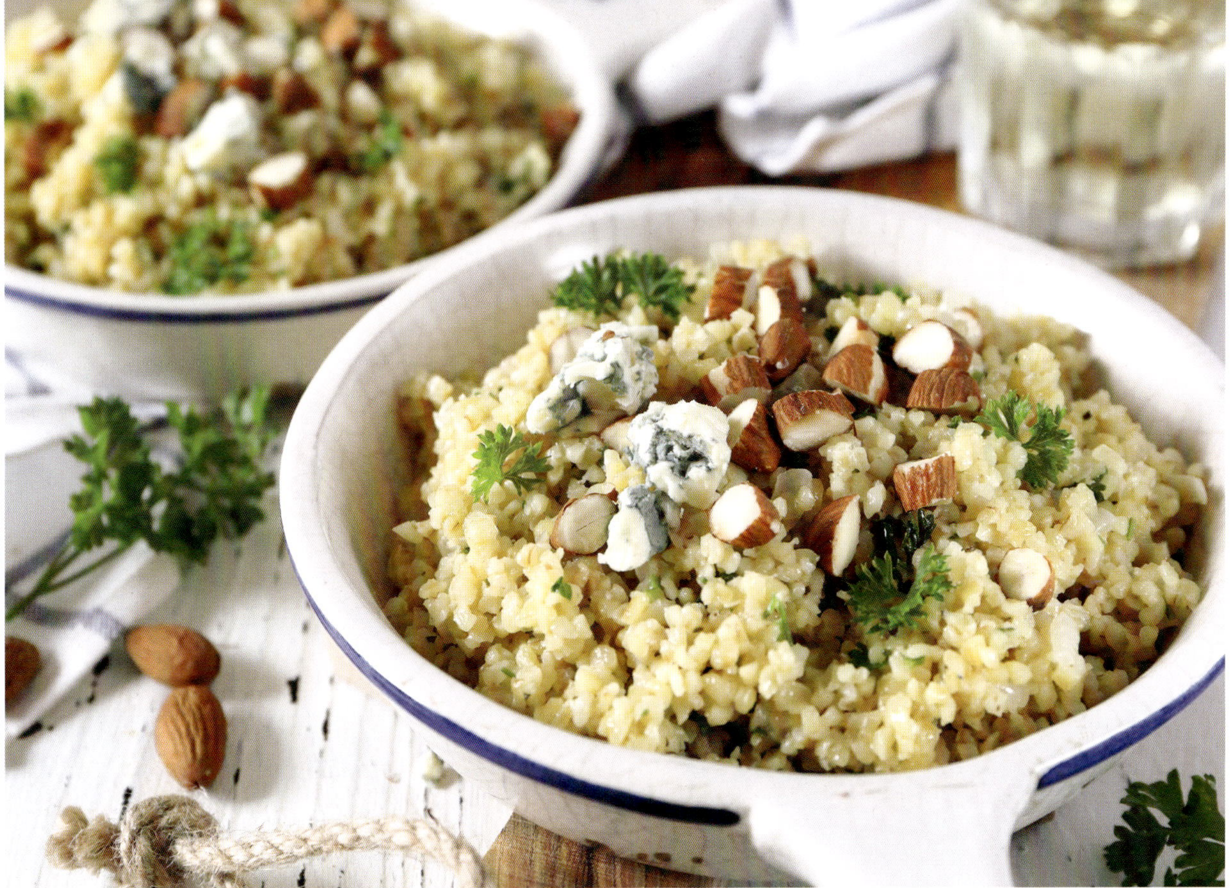

SERVES 2 | PREP + COOK TIME: 30 MINS | VEG | GLUTEN FREE |

BULGUR CEREAL RISOTTO

½ cup (90g) bulgur, rinsed
2 tbsps flaxseed
Pinch of salt
½ cup (125ml) water
1 cup (250ml) milk of choice
75g blue cheese
½ cup (60g) almonds, chopped
2 tbsps chopped parsley

STEPS

1. Place bulgur in a medium saucepan with the flaxseed, salt, water and milk and bring to a boil. Reduce to a simmer, cover and cook for 10 minutes.
2. Remove from the stove and let sit for a further 10 minutes until the water has evaporated.
3. Fluff the cooked bulgur with a fork.
4. Serve in breakfast bowls topped with blue cheese, almonds and chopped parsley.

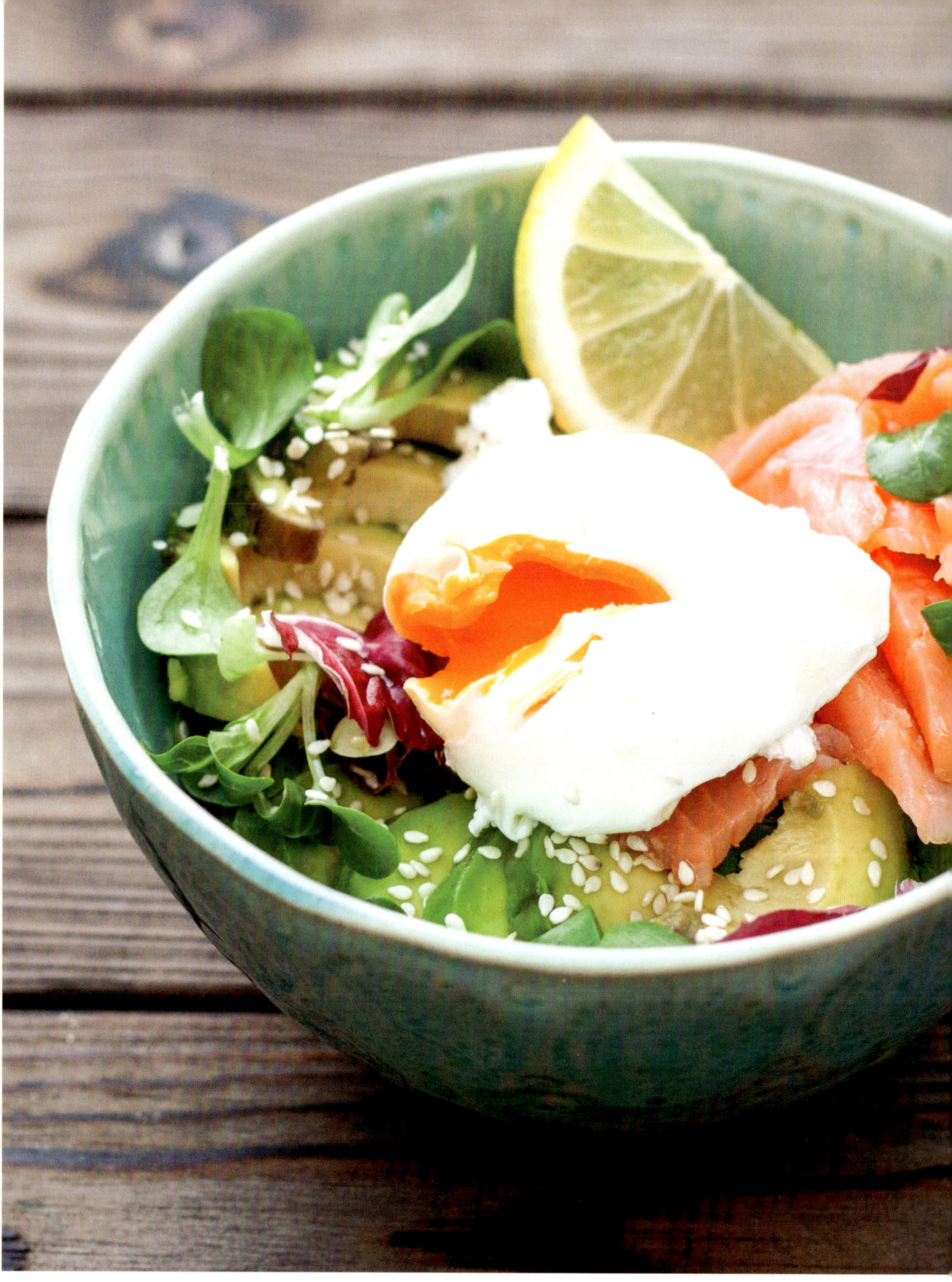

BREAKFAST BOWL

2 cups (80g) tightly packed mixed salad leaves

200g smoked salmon

1 small avocado

Dash of white vinegar

4 eggs

1 radish, thinly sliced

1 tbsp black sesame seeds

1 tbsp white sesame seeds

2 lemon wedges

STEPS

1. Split the salad leaves between two serving bowls. Place half the smoked salmon on top in each bowl. Slice the avocado and place half in each bowl.
2. To poach the eggs, add a small dash of vinegar to a pan of steadily simmering water – about 5cm deep. Crack each egg gently into a small shallow dish and use this to slide them into the water one at a time. Cook for 2½-3 minutes for a runny yolk and 3½-4 minutes for a set yolk.
3. Gently lift the eggs out with a slotted spoon and drain on a paper towel.
4. Place two eggs in each bowl to the side of the avocado.
5. Garnish with the sesame seeds and lemon wedges.

SERVES 2 | PREP + COOK TIME: 15 MINS | GLUTEN FREE | DAIRY FREE |

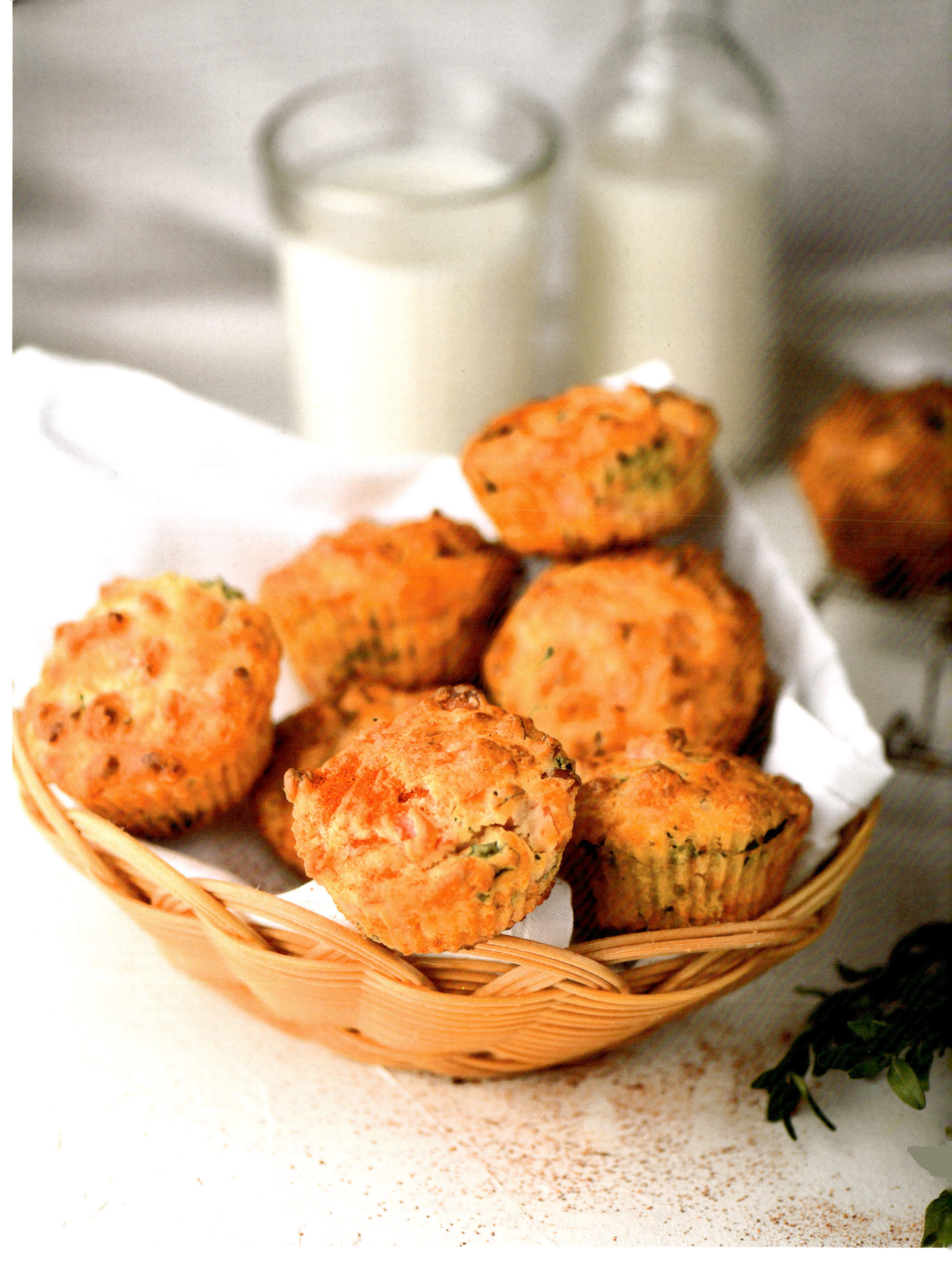

PAPRIKA CHEESE MUFFINS

2 cups (250g) plain flour
2 tsps baking powder
1 tsp paprika
2 spring onions, finely sliced
Salt and pepper, to taste
1 cup (125g) grated Cheddar cheese
¼ cup (25g) grated Parmesan cheese
1 cup (250ml) milk
60g unsalted butter, melted
1 large egg
1 tbsp chopped fresh parsley (optional)

STEPS

Preheat oven to 200°C.

1. In a large mixing bowl, whisk together the flour, baking powder, paprika, onions, salt and pepper.
2. Add the grated Cheddar cheese and grated Parmesan cheese to the dry ingredients.
3. In a separate bowl, whisk together the milk, melted butter, egg and chopped parsley.
4. Pour the wet ingredients into the dry ingredients and stir until just combined. Be careful not to over-mix; a few lumps are okay. Spoon the batter into a greased muffin tin, filling each cup about three-quarters full.
5. Bake in the preheated oven for about 18-20 minutes, or until the muffins are golden brown and a toothpick inserted into the centre comes out clean.

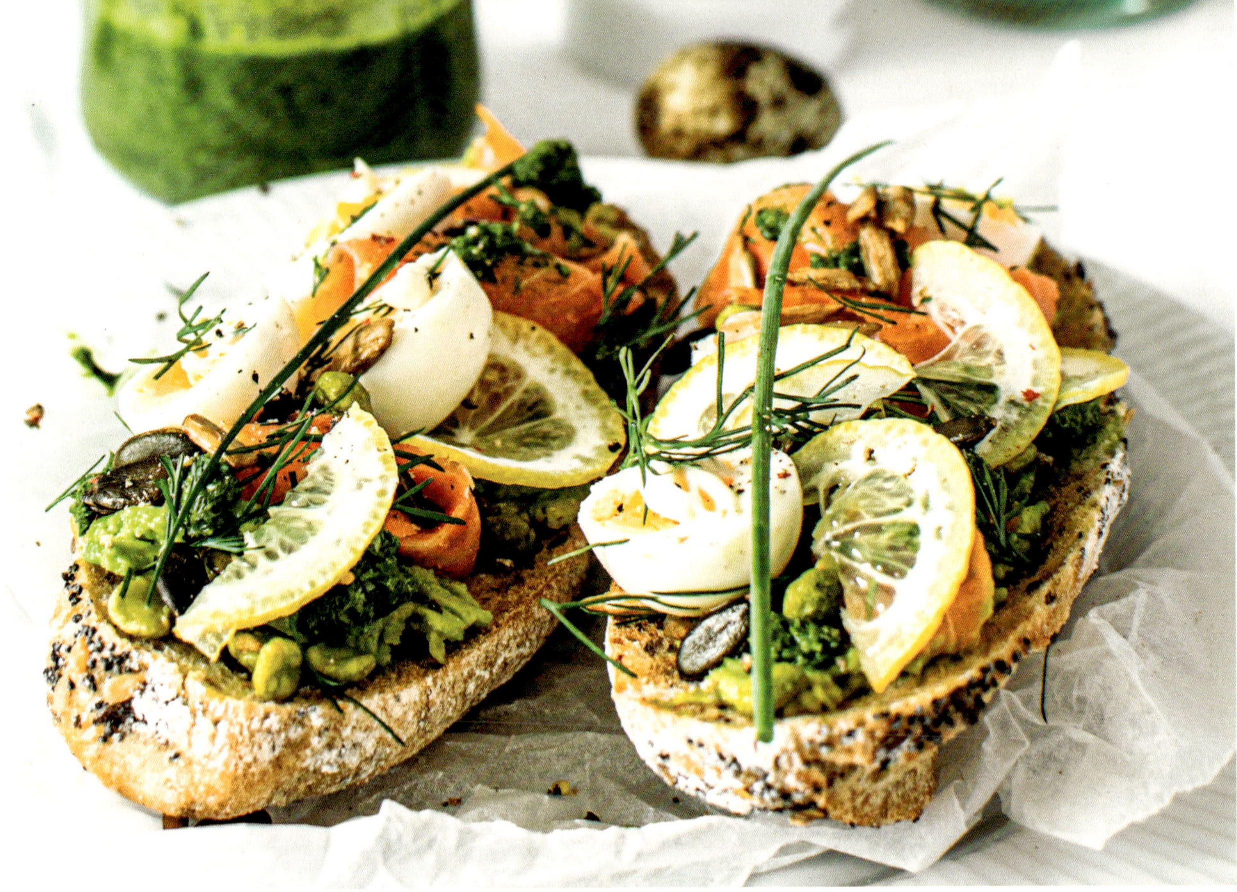

SALMON AVOCADO TOAST

1 large avocado

½ tsp lemon juice

½ tsp chopped dill + extra to garnish

Salt and pepper to taste

4 slices low-carb bread, toasted

400g smoked salmon slices

2 tbsps pesto (store-bought or see recipe page 69)

4 eggs, hard-boiled

Pepitas and lemon slices to serve (optional)

STEPS

1. In a small bowl mash together the avocado flesh with lemon juice and dill. Season with salt and pepper.
2. Divide the avocado mash between the four slices of toasted bread and spread it on each slice.
3. Top with the smoked salmon slices, dollops of pesto and halved boiled eggs.
4. Garnish with extra dill, pepitas and lemon slices.

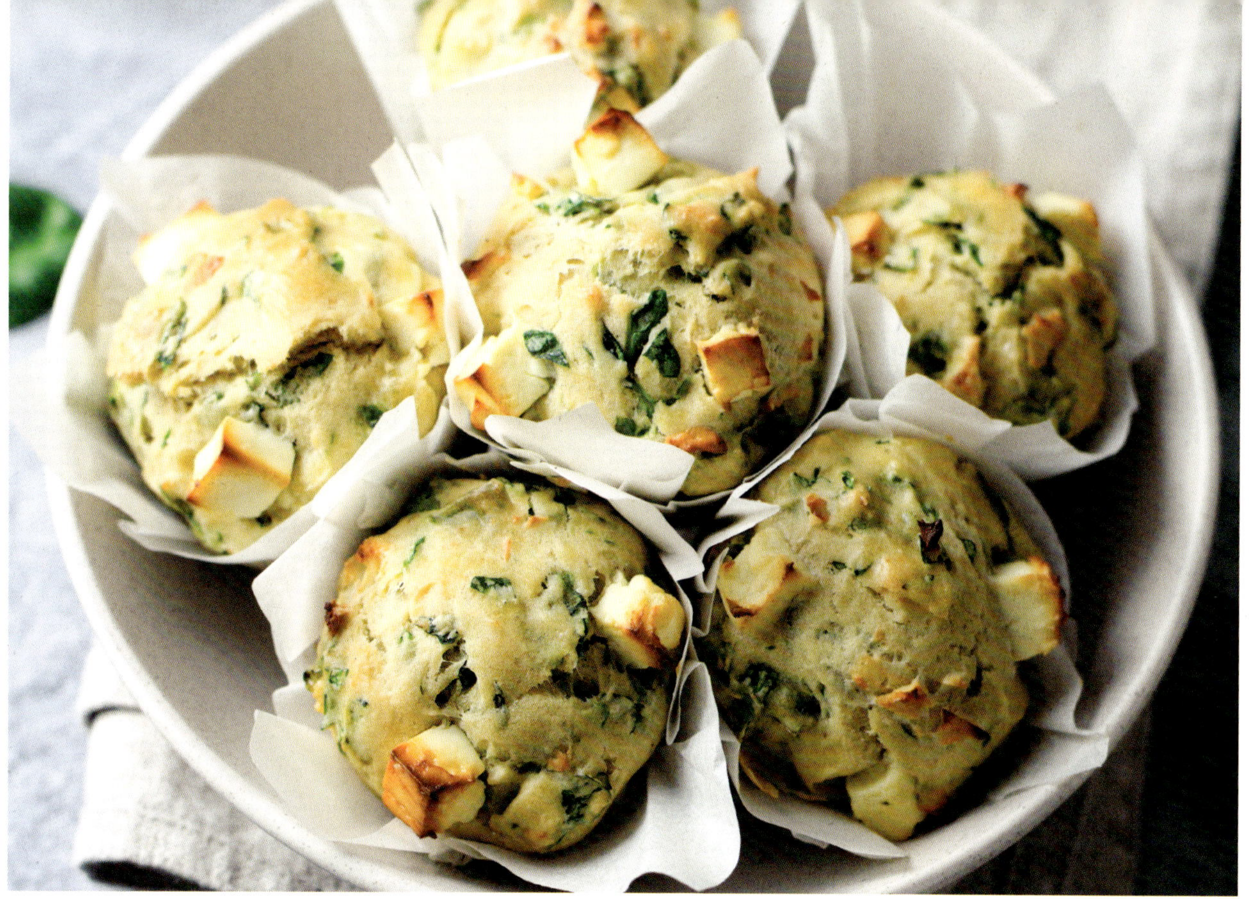

MAKES 8 | PREP + COOK TIME: 40 MINS | VEG | GLUTEN FREE |

SPINACH & FETA MUFFINS

4 eggs
60g butter, melted
¼ cup (60ml) water
Salt and pepper to taste
⅓ cup (30g) coconut flour
½ tsp baking powder
4 spring onions, chopped
1 zucchini, grated
½ cup (115g) cooked spinach
4 tbsps chopped fresh parsley
½ tsp ground nutmeg
¼ cup (25g) grated Parmesan cheese
150g feta cheese, diced

STEPS

Preheat oven to 200°C.

1. Combine eggs, butter, water, salt and pepper in a large bowl. Whisk thoroughly. Add coconut flour and baking powder and mix well.
2. Add in spring onions, zucchini, spinach, parsley and nutmeg. Mix thoroughly.
3. Stir through Parmesan and half the feta cheese. Add more water if the mixture is too stiff.
4. Spoon the mixture into a lined muffin tin, filling each cup two-thirds full. Top the muffins with the remaining feta cubes.
5. Bake for 20-25 minutes until firm and golden.

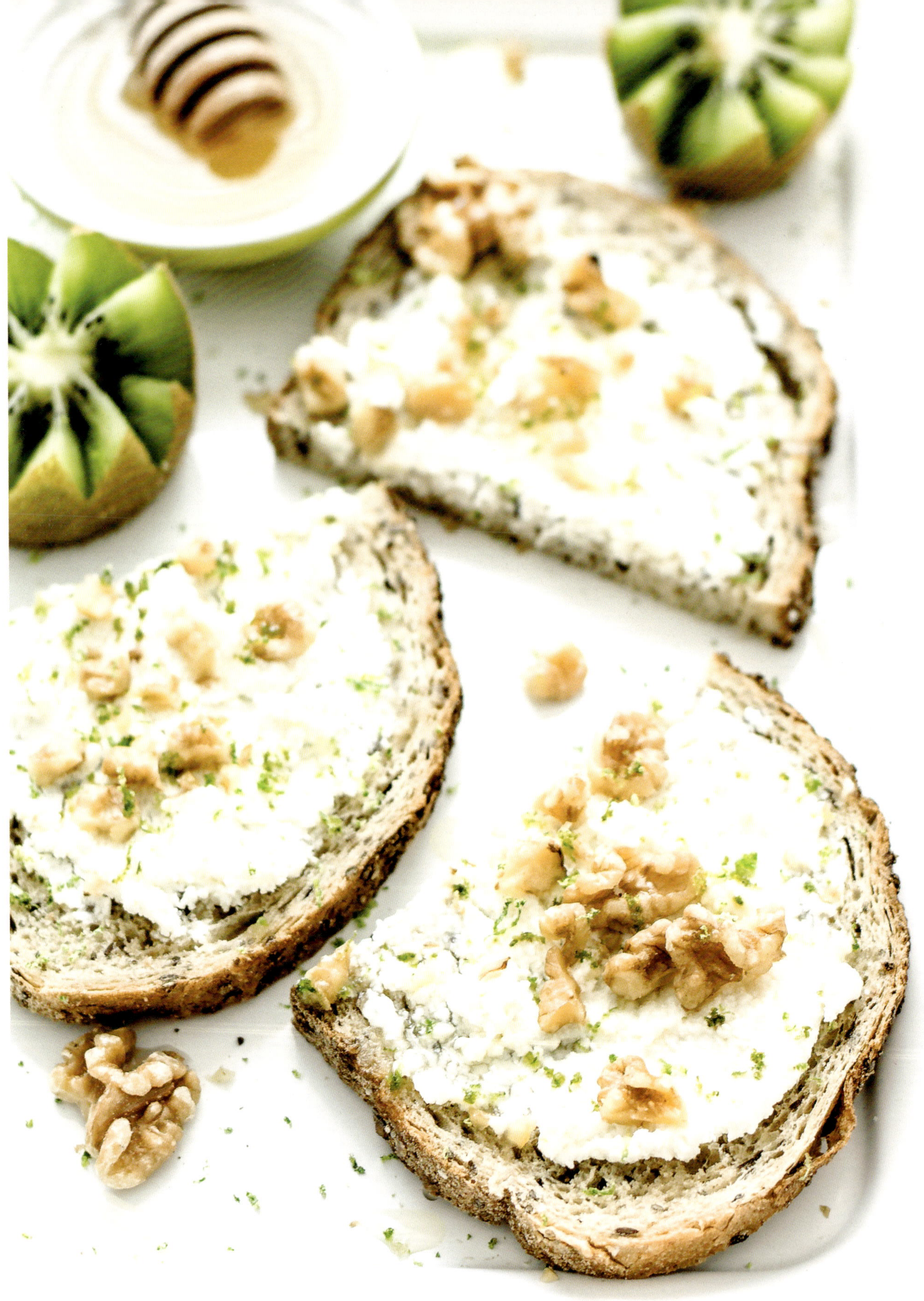

WHOLEGRAIN TOAST WITH HOMEMADE CREAM CHEESE

4 slices low-carb bread

2 tbsps walnuts, chopped

½ tsp grated lime zest

2 tsps honey

CREAM CHEESE
(MAKES APPROXIMATELY 1 CUP)

1 cup (260g) silken tofu

2 tbsps white chia seeds, finely ground

¼ cup (30g) raw cashews, roughly chopped

2 tsps agave syrup

2 tbsps water

Salt and pepper to taste

STEPS

1. Place all the ingredients for the cream cheese in a blender. Blend until thoroughly combined and smooth and creamy.
2. Place in the refrigerator for 2 hours to thicken to a cream cheese consistency.
3. When ready to eat remove from the refrigerator and season to taste with salt and pepper.
4. To assemble, toast the slices of bread. Spread 2 tablespoons of the cream cheese over each slice of toast. Top with chopped walnuts and lime zest.
5. Drizzle a teaspoon of honey over each to serve.

SERVES 2 | PREP: 20 MINS + CHILLING | VEG | DAIRY FREE |

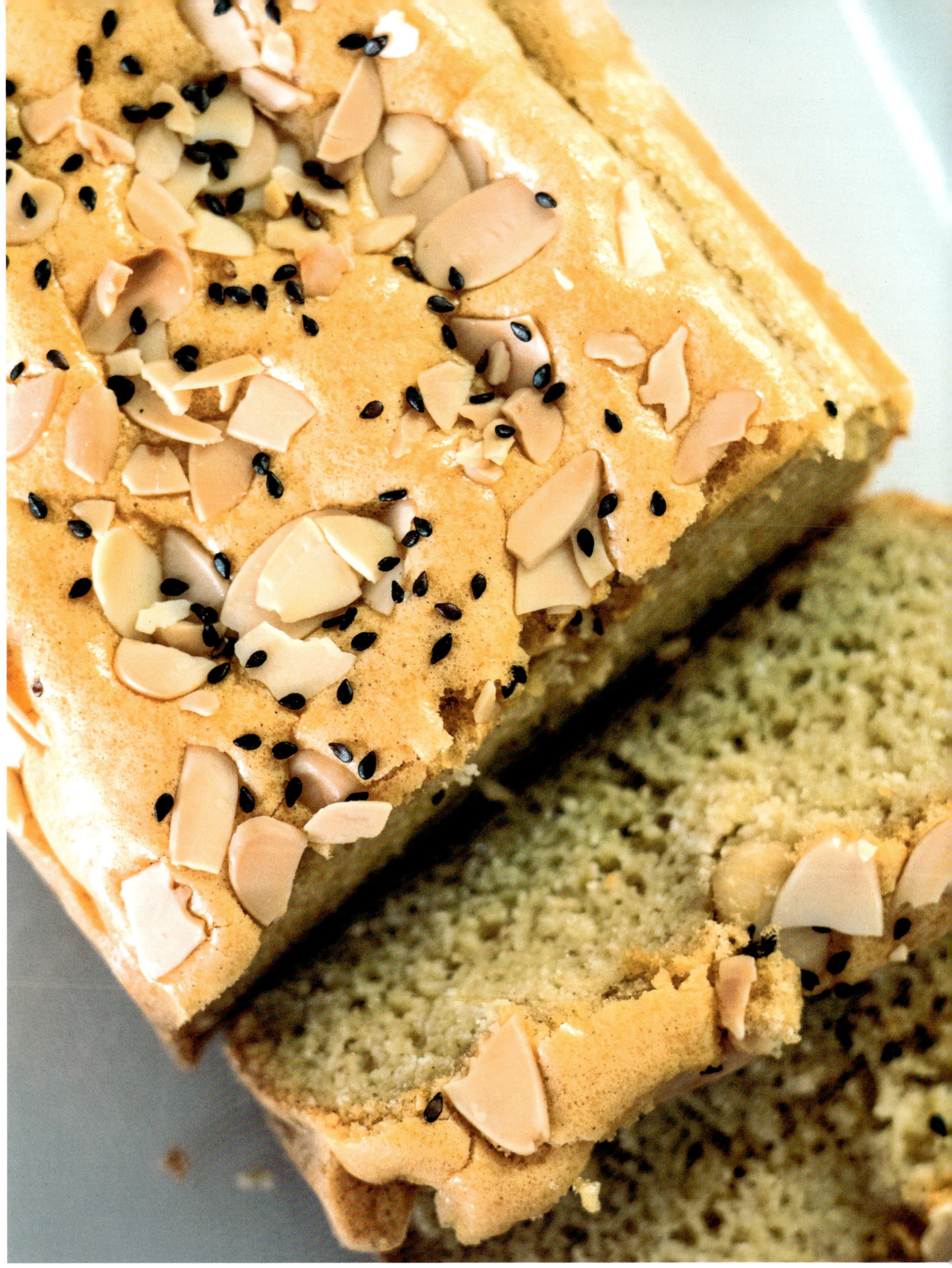

LOW-CARB BREAD

2 cups (200g) almond flour

¼ cup (25g) coconut flour

¼ cup (35g) ground flaxseed

¼ cup (20g) psyllium husk powder

1 tsp baking powder

½ tsp salt

4 large eggs

¼ cup (60ml) melted coconut oil or butter

½ cup (125ml) unsweetened almond milk

1 tbsp apple cider vinegar

1 tbsp black sesame seeds

¼ cup (30g) slivered almonds

STEPS

Preheat the oven to 180°C.

1. Grease a loaf tin and cover it with baking paper, making sure extra paper is hanging over the sides.
2. In a large bowl, combine the almond flour, coconut flour, ground flaxseed, psyllium husk powder, baking powder and salt.
3. In a separate bowl, whisk together the eggs, melted coconut oil or butter, almond milk and apple cider vinegar.
4. Pour the wet ingredients into the dry ingredients and stir until well combined. The mixture will be thick and sticky. Transfer the dough to the prepared loaf pan and smooth the top with a spatula. Sprinkle with sesame seeds and almonds.
5. Bake for 50-60 minutes, or until the loaf is golden brown and a toothpick inserted into the centre comes out clean. Remove from the oven and allow the bread to cool in the pan for a few minutes. Then transfer it to a wire rack to cool completely before slicing.

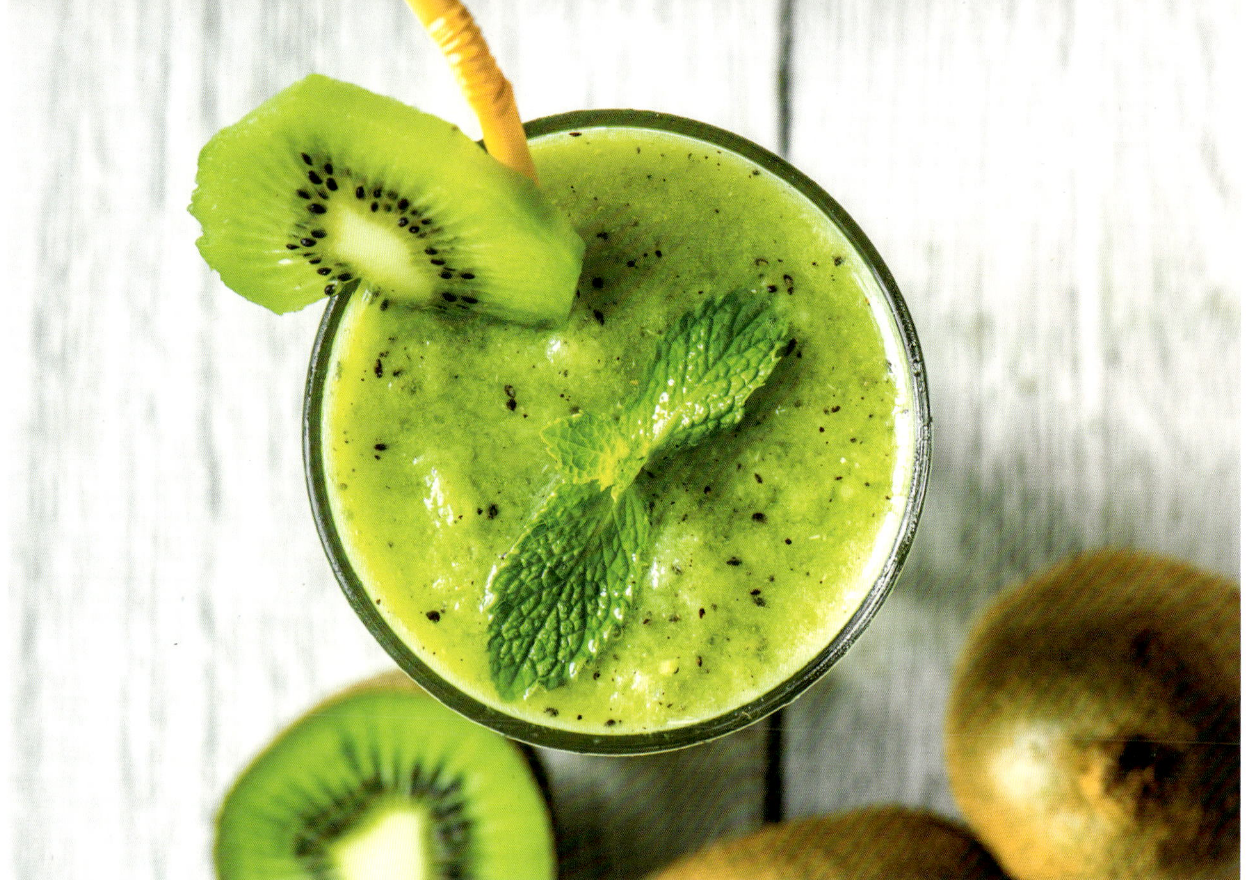

SERVES 2 | PREP + COOK TIME: 10 MINS | VEG | GLUTEN FREE | DAIRY FREE

ULTIMATE GREEN SMOOTHIE

1 banana, sliced

½ small Lebanese cucumber, roughly chopped

3 kiwi fruits, peeled and sliced, reserve some slices for garnish

1¼ cups (35g) spinach leaves, roughly chopped

1 green apple, cubed

1 cup (250ml) coconut water

1 cup (250ml) water

Mint leaves to serve (optional)

STEPS

1. Place the banana, cucumber, kiwi fruit, spinach, apple, coconut water and water in a blender and process until smooth.
2. Divide the smoothie between serving glasses and serve garnished with sliced kiwi fruit and mint leaves.

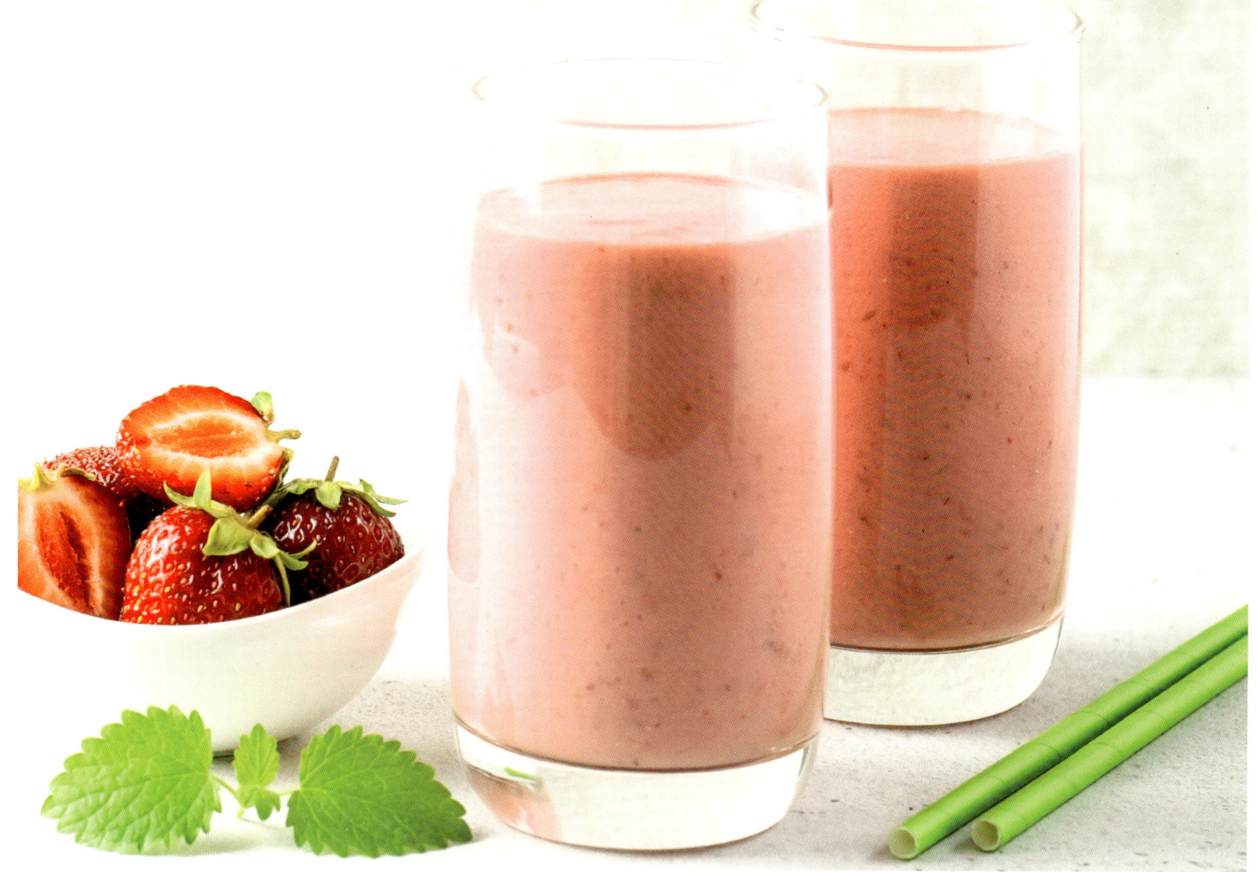

SERVES 2 | PREP + COOK TIME: 5 MINS | VEG | GLUTEN FREE | DAIRY FREE |

STRAWBERRY SMOOTHIE

2 frozen bananas

3 cups (600g) frozen strawberries

½ cup (125ml) macadamia milk or almond milk

STEPS

1. Add all the ingredients to your blender and blend until smooth.
2. Divide the smoothie between serving glasses.

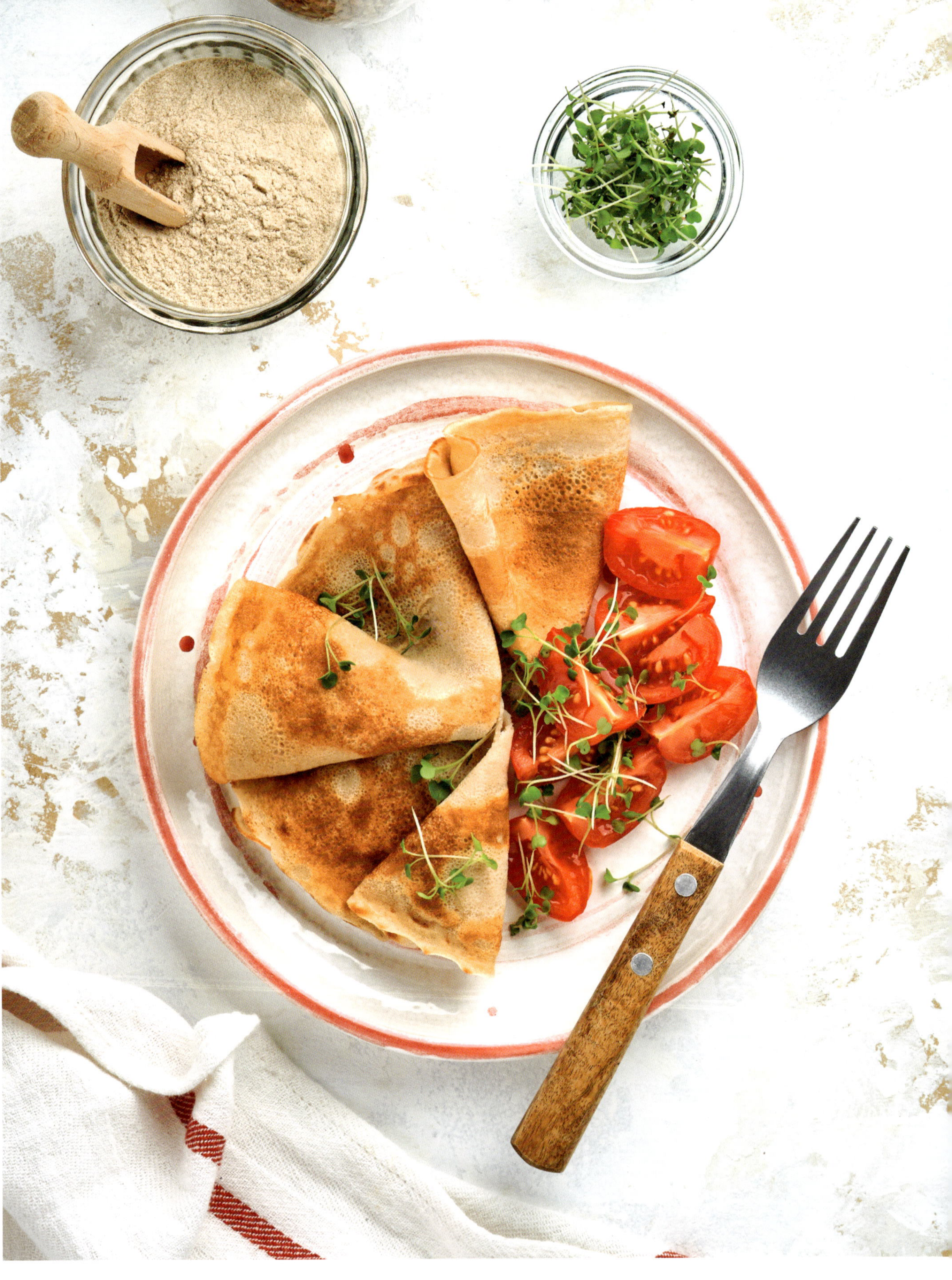

ALMOND FLOUR CREPES

CREPES

1 cup (100g) almond flour

1 tsp cornflour

4 eggs

1¼ cups (310ml) almond milk

½ tsp salt

Cooking spray or butter for frying

TO SERVE

4 Roma tomatoes, quartered

Micro herbs

STEPS

1. In a medium-sized bowl whisk the almond flour, cornflour, eggs, almond milk and salt together until a smooth batter forms. Let the batter sit for 5-10 minutes.
2. Heat a nonstick pan over a medium-high heat and add cooking spray or a little butter.
3. Use a ladle to spoon the batter into the pan, rotating the pan to help the batter spread out into a thin, even layer. Leave the batter to cook for 3-4 minutes before flipping.
4. Use a spatula to lift the edge of the crepe and flip, cook for another 1 minute than transfer crepe to a plate. Repeat with the remaining batter. Place greaseproof paper between the crepes on the plate to avoid them sticking together.
5. Serve crepes with fresh tomato and micro herbs (or your choice of toppings).

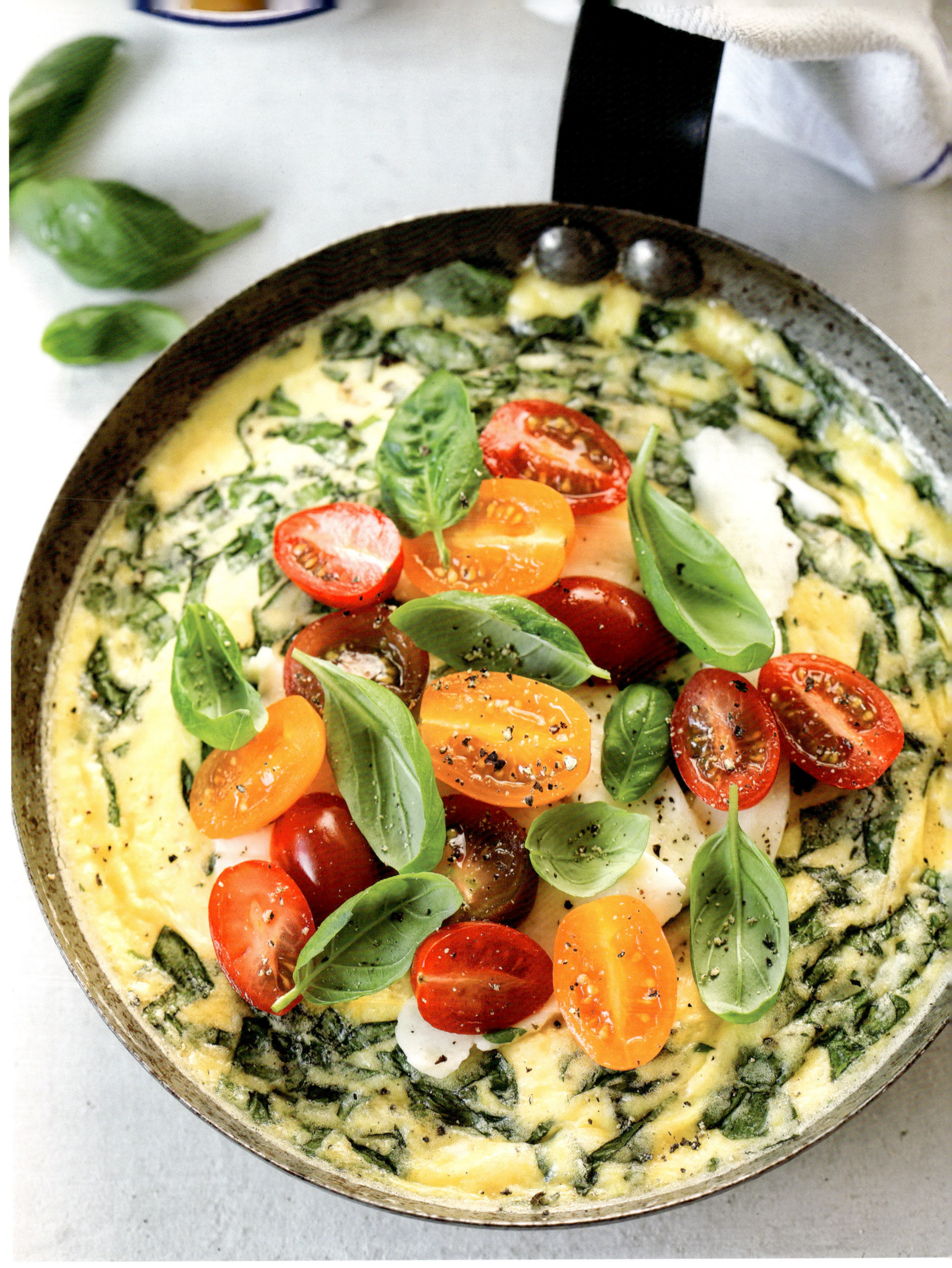

BASIL FRITTATA WITH HALLOUMI

SERVES 6 | PREP + COOK TIME: 25 MINS | VEG | GLUTEN FREE |

6 large eggs, roughly beaten

Salt and pepper to taste

1 cup (125g) grated tasty cheese

½ cup (125ml) thickened cream

2 cups (30g) fresh basil leaves, roughly chopped + ¼ cup (5g) whole leaves, to garnish

1 tbsp butter

250g mixed cherry tomatoes, halved

150g halloumi, cut into thin slices and halved

STEPS

Preheat oven to 180°C.

1. Season the eggs with salt and pepper and whisk through the grated cheese, cream and chopped basil.
2. Heat the butter in a medium, deep-sided ovenproof pan over medium heat. Pour the egg mixture into the pan and stir to combine. Place the pan in the oven and bake for 5 minutes. Remove from the oven, dot with half the tomatoes and the halloumi.
3. Return to the oven and bake for 7 minutes until the frittata is cooked through.
4. Serve garnished with remaining tomatoes and basil leaves.

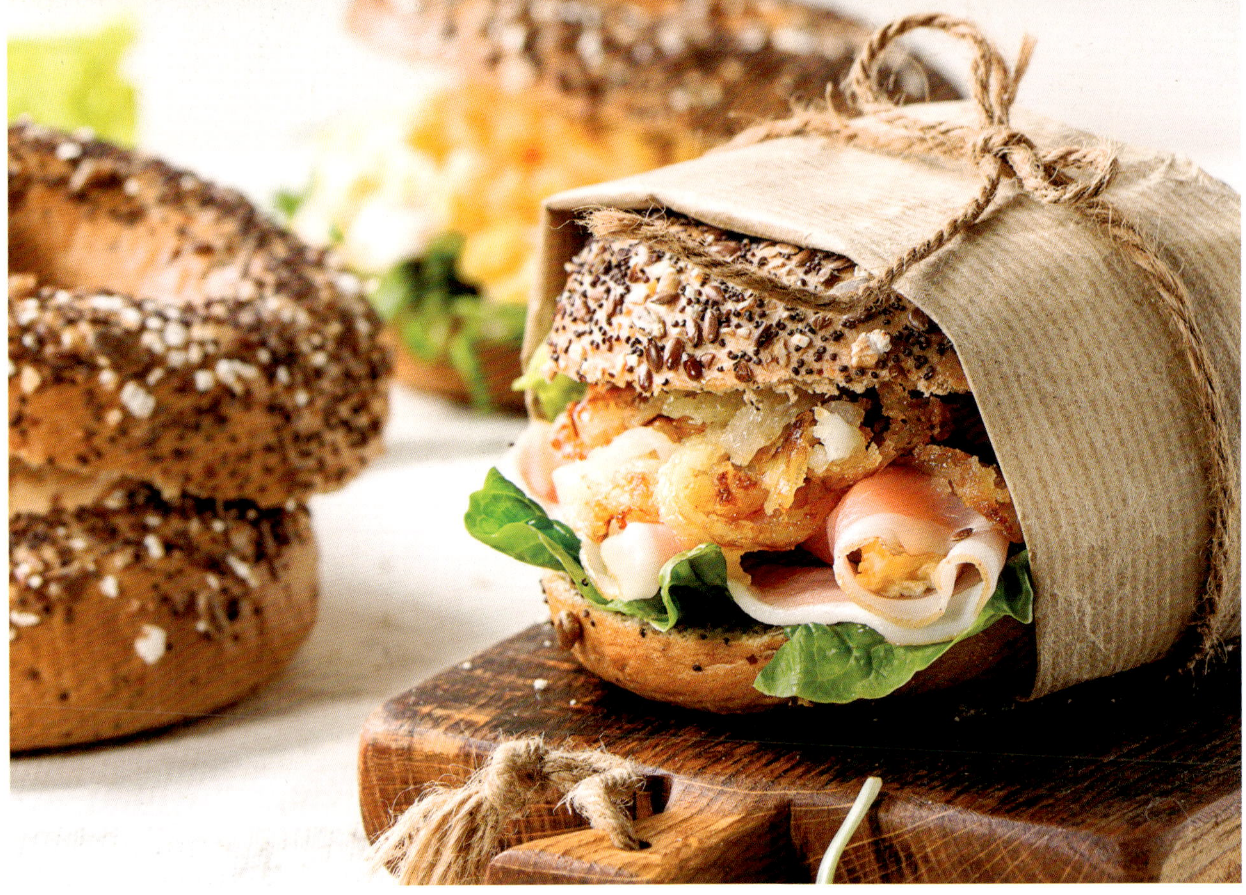

BREAKFAST BAGEL

1 tbsp rice flour

1 tbsp tapioca flour

Salt and pepper to taste

1 large onion, thickly sliced into rings

2 tbsps olive oil

2 low-carb bagels, halved

4 butter lettuce leaves

300g sliced prosciutto

½ cup (15g) watercress

STEPS

1. Stir together the flours, lightly season them and then toss with the onion rings so they are lightly coated.
2. Heat a small nonstick frying pan over medium heat. Heat the olive oil and then fry the onion slices for 8 minutes until they are softened but slightly crunchy on the outside.
3. Remove from the pan and drain on absorbent paper.
4. Lightly toast the bagel halves.
5. Layer each bagel with two lettuce leaves, half the prosciutto, half the onion and half the cress.

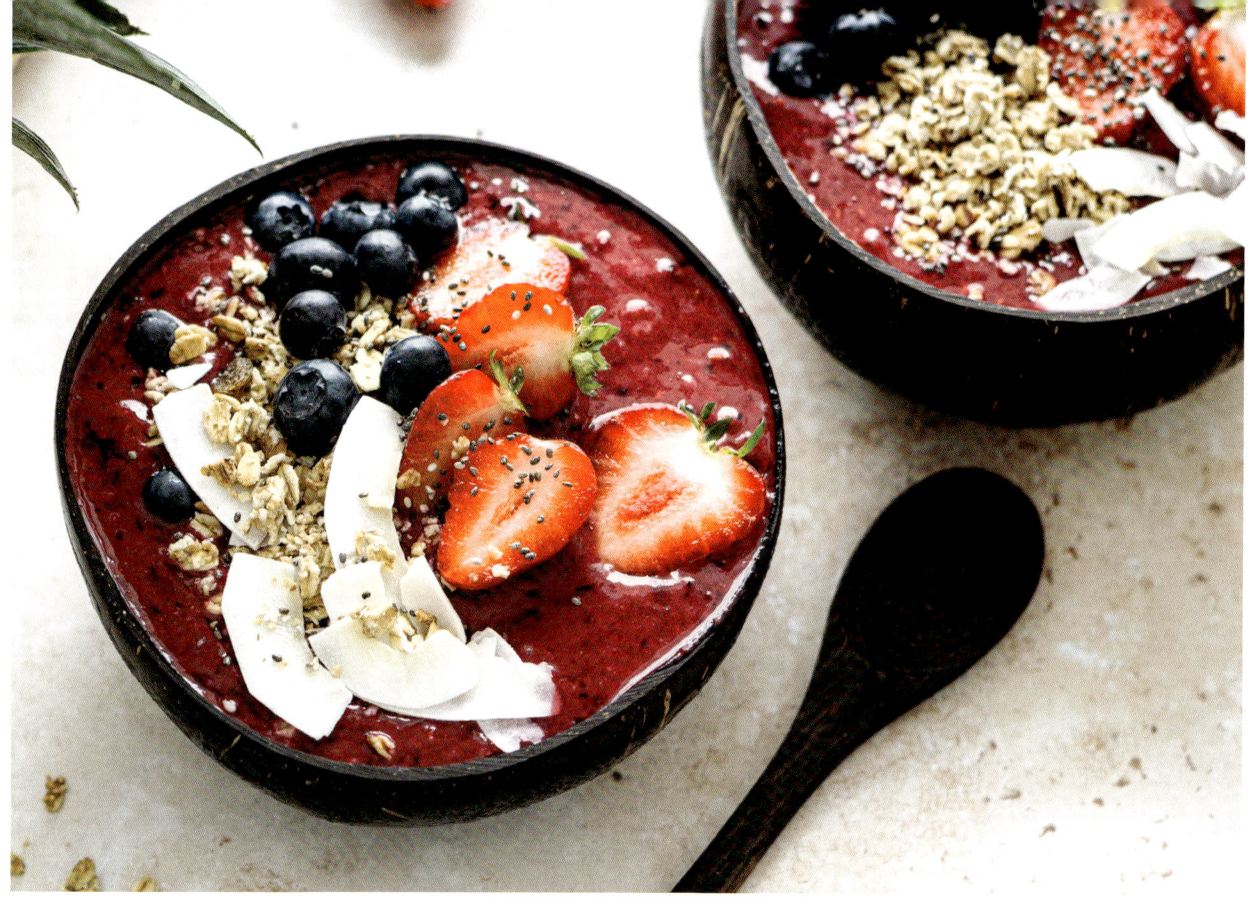

BERRY SMOOTHIE BOWLS

1 tsp psyllium husk powder

½ cup (60g) mixed berries

¼ cup (25g) chopped frozen cauliflower pieces

¼ cup (30g) raw almonds

2 cups (500ml) coconut milk

2 tsps shaved coconut

¼ cup (20g) store-bought muesli

STEPS

1. Place the psyllium, half of the berries, the cauliflower, almonds and coconut milk in a blender and puree until smooth. Let the smoothie sit for 5 minutes to thicken.
2. Pour into serving bowls and decorate with remaining berries.
3. Garnish with shaved coconut and a sprinkle of muesli.

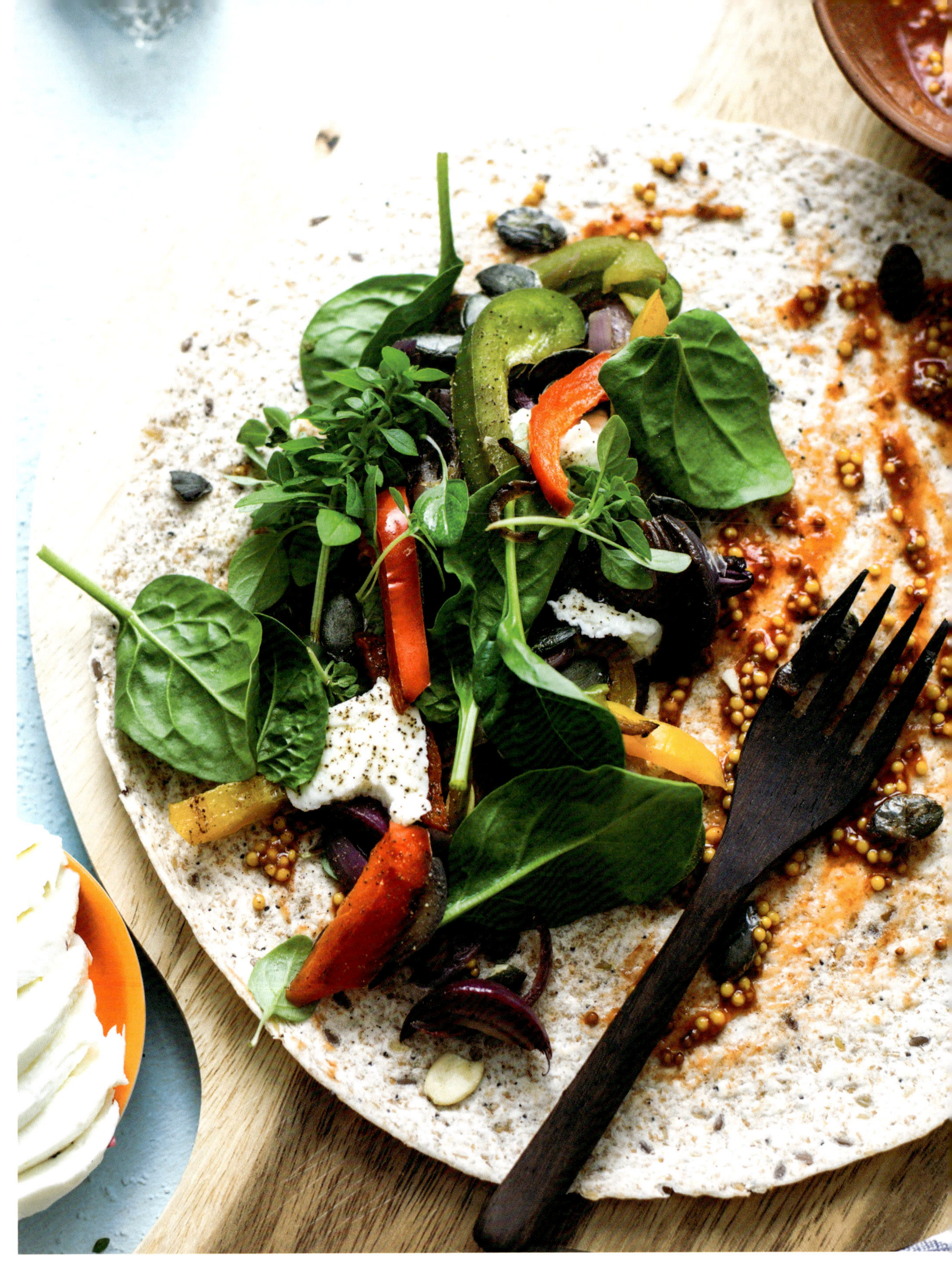

BREAKFAST BURRITO

2 tsps olive oil

1 red onion, sliced into wedges

2 cloves garlic, crushed

1 tsp ground cumin

1 tsp ground coriander

3 multicoloured capsicums, cut into strips

2 tbsps seeded mustard

3 tbsps Sriracha

4 large low-carb wholegrain tortillas

2 cups (60g) baby spinach

150g feta, crumbled

2 tbsps pepitas

Salt and pepper to taste

STEPS

1. Heat the olive oil in a small nonstick frying pan over medium heat. Add red onion wedges and garlic and saute until translucent.
2. Add the spices and fry off until fragrant then add capsicums and fry for a further 2 minutes, then set veg mix aside.
3. In a small bowl mix together seeded mustard and Sriracha sauce and set aside.
4. To assemble the burritos, spread a tablespoon of sauce on each tortilla then divide the veg mixture between the tortillas.
5. Add the baby spinach and crumbled feta to each tortilla and serve with a sprinkle of pepitas and salt and pepper to taste.

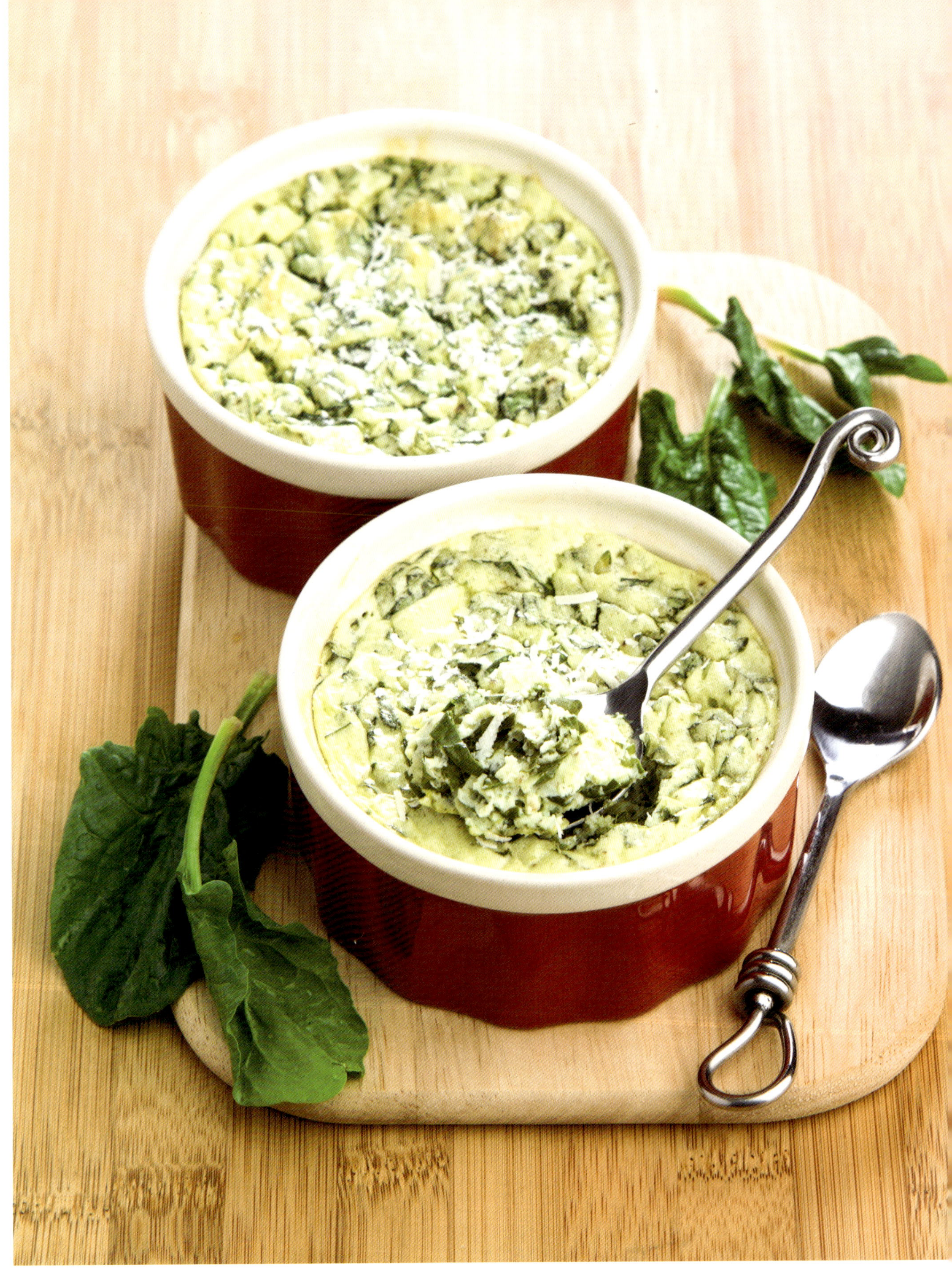

SIMPLE SPINACH SOUFFLE

30g butter

2 tbsps plain flour

¾ cup (185ml) milk

2 cups (60g) baby spinach, chopped

¾ cup (75g) finely grated Parmesan cheese

Salt and pepper to taste

4 eggs, separated

STEPS

Preheat oven to 200°C.

1. In a saucepan, melt the butter over medium heat. Add the flour and whisk continuously for about 1-2 minutes to form a roux. Gradually pour in the milk, whisking constantly until the mixture thickens and comes to a simmer. Add the chopped spinach and cook until wilted.

2. Remove the saucepan from the heat and add the grated cheese. Stir until the cheese is melted and the mixture is smooth. Season with salt and pepper to taste.

3. In a separate bowl, beat the egg yolks. Gradually whisk the beaten egg yolks into the cheese mixture.

4. In another clean bowl, beat the egg whites with a hand mixer until foamy. Gently fold about a third of the beaten egg whites into the cheese mixture to lighten it. Then, carefully fold in the remaining egg whites until well incorporated. Pour the mixture into greased ramekins, filling them about three-quarters full.

5. Place the ramekins in the preheated oven and bake for 20-25 minutes or until the souffle is puffed, golden brown, and set in the centre. Serve immediately while the souffle is still puffed and airy.

NOTE: Souffles are delicate and tend to deflate quickly, so it's best to serve them immediately after baking.

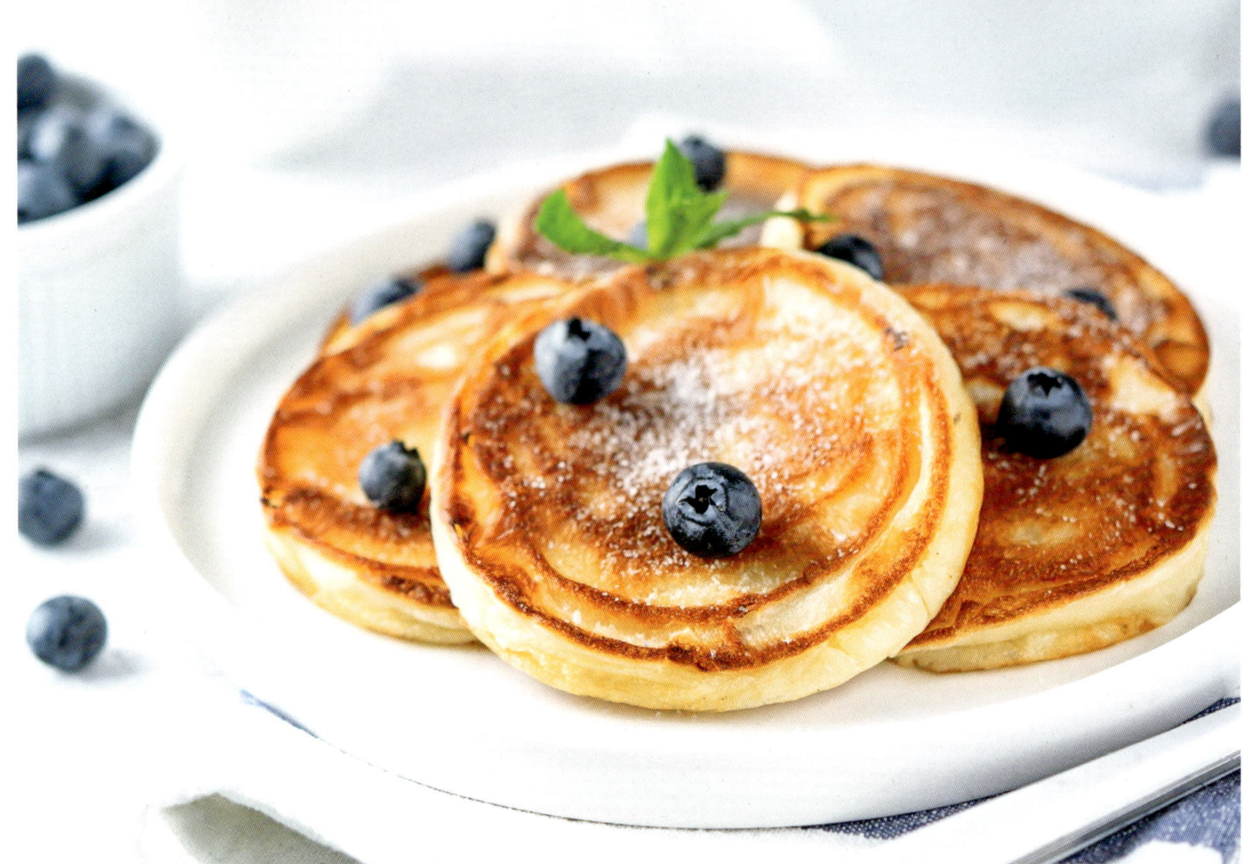

RICOTTA PANCAKES

1 cup (250g) ricotta cheese

4 large eggs

¼ cup (25g) almond flour

1 tsp baking powder

½ tsp vanilla extract

Sweetener of your choice (e.g. stevia or erythritol) to taste (optional)

Butter or coconut oil for greasing the pan

Toppings of your choice (e.g. fresh berries or chopped nuts)

STEPS

1. In a medium mixing bowl, whisk together the ricotta cheese and eggs until well combined.
2. Add the almond flour, baking powder, vanilla extract and sweetener (if using). Then mix until you have a smooth batter.
3. Heat a nonstick pan over a medium heat and melt a tablespoon of butter or coconut oil, then spoon the batter onto the pan to form pancakes. Cook for 2-3 minutes on one side until bubbles start to form on the surface, then flip the pancakes and cook for an additional 1-2 minutes.
4. Remove the pancakes from the pan and repeat the process with the remaining batter.
5. Serve the pancakes with your favourite toppings such as fresh berries or chopped nuts.

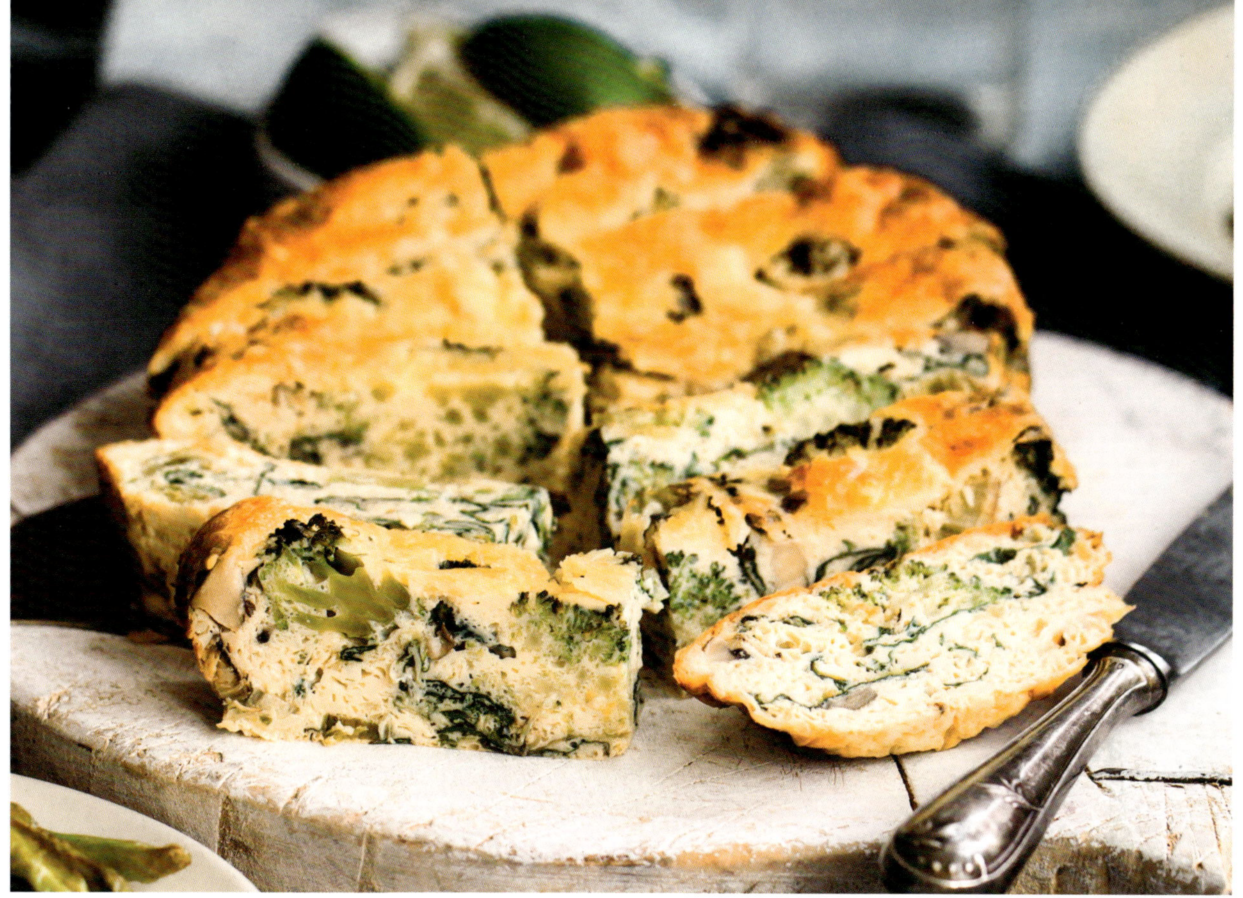

SERVES 5 | PREP + COOK TIME: 40 MINS | VEG | GLUTEN FREE |

SPINACH, BROCCOLI & CHEESE FRITTATA

8 large eggs, room temperature, lightly beaten

⅓ cup (80ml) cream

Salt and pepper to taste

2 tbsps water

2½ cups (415g) lightly steamed broccoli, roughly chopped

3 cups (90g) baby spinach leaves, roughly chopped

1¼ cups (155g) grated Cheddar cheese

2 tbsps olive oil

2 medium cloves garlic, crushed

STEPS

Preheat oven to 220°C.

1. Whisk the eggs with the cream, a pinch each of salt and pepper and the water in a large mixing bowl. Stir through the broccoli and spinach and 1 cup of the cheese.
2. Heat the oil a large, deep-sided ovenproof frying pan over medium heat. Fry the garlic for 1 minute.
3. Add the garlic to the egg mixture and stir through. Wipe the pan down, lightly oil and pour in the frittata mixture. Sprinkle with remaining cheese.
4. Bake for 15 minutes until just set in the middle. Remove from oven and allow it to cool for 5 minutes before serving.

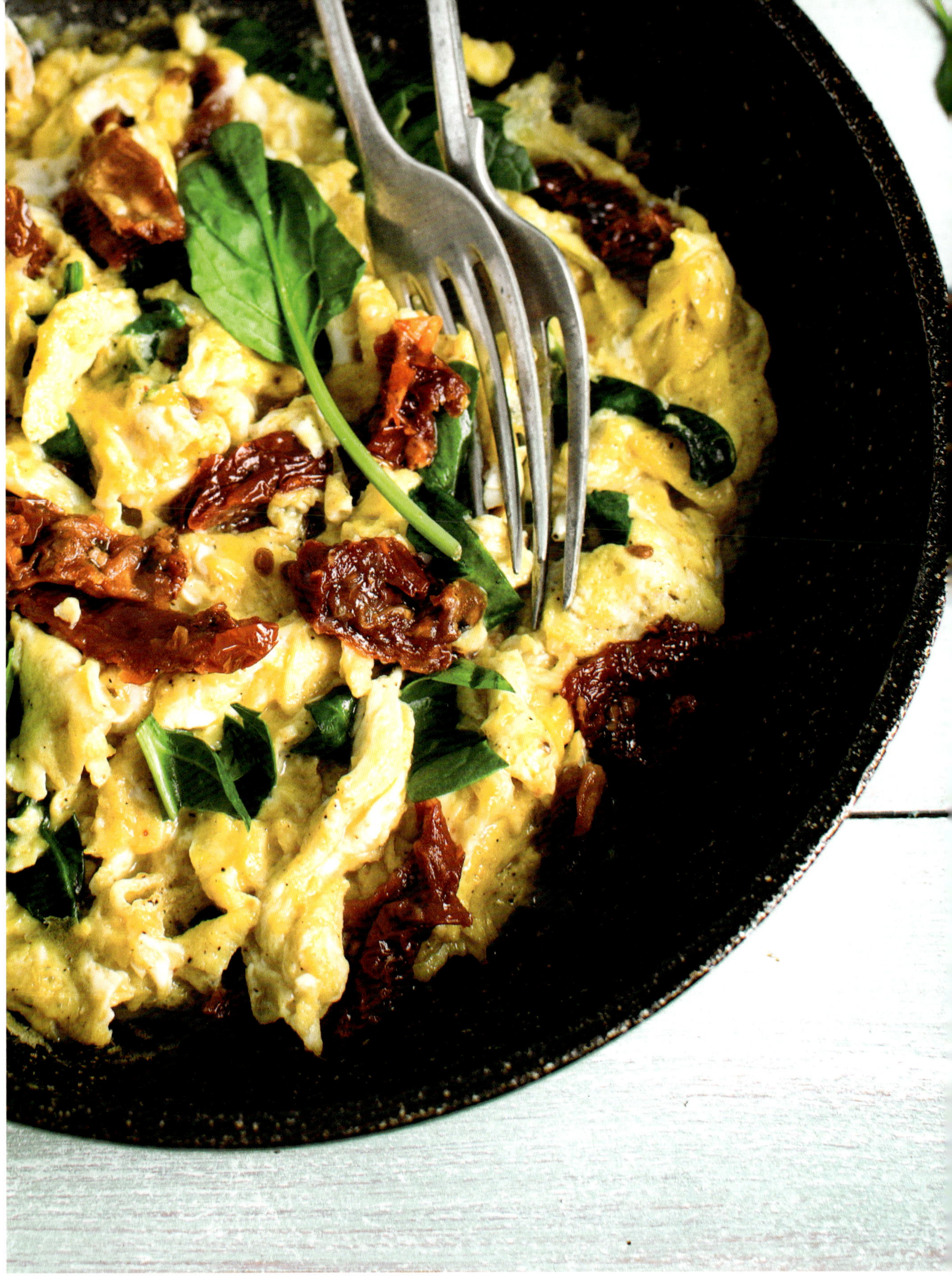

SUN-DRIED TOMATO SCRAMBLED EGGS

4 large eggs

½ cup (110g) cottage cheese

1 tbsp butter or ghee

2 cups (60g) baby spinach

½ cup (30g) semi-dried tomatoes, roughly chopped

Salt and pepper to taste

STEPS

1. Thoroughly whisk the eggs and cottage cheese in a bowl for at least 1 minute.

2. Heat butter in a medium nonstick frying pan over medium heat. Add spinach and semi-dried tomatoes and saute until spinach is wilted.

3. Pour the beaten egg mixture into the pan and cook for 1 minute. Then use a spatula to scramble the eggs until they are just set, around 2-3 minutes.

4. Season with salt and pepper and garnish with some extra semi-dried tomatoes. Serve immediately.

SERVES 2 | PREP + COOK TIME: 10 MINS | VEG | GLUTEN FREE |

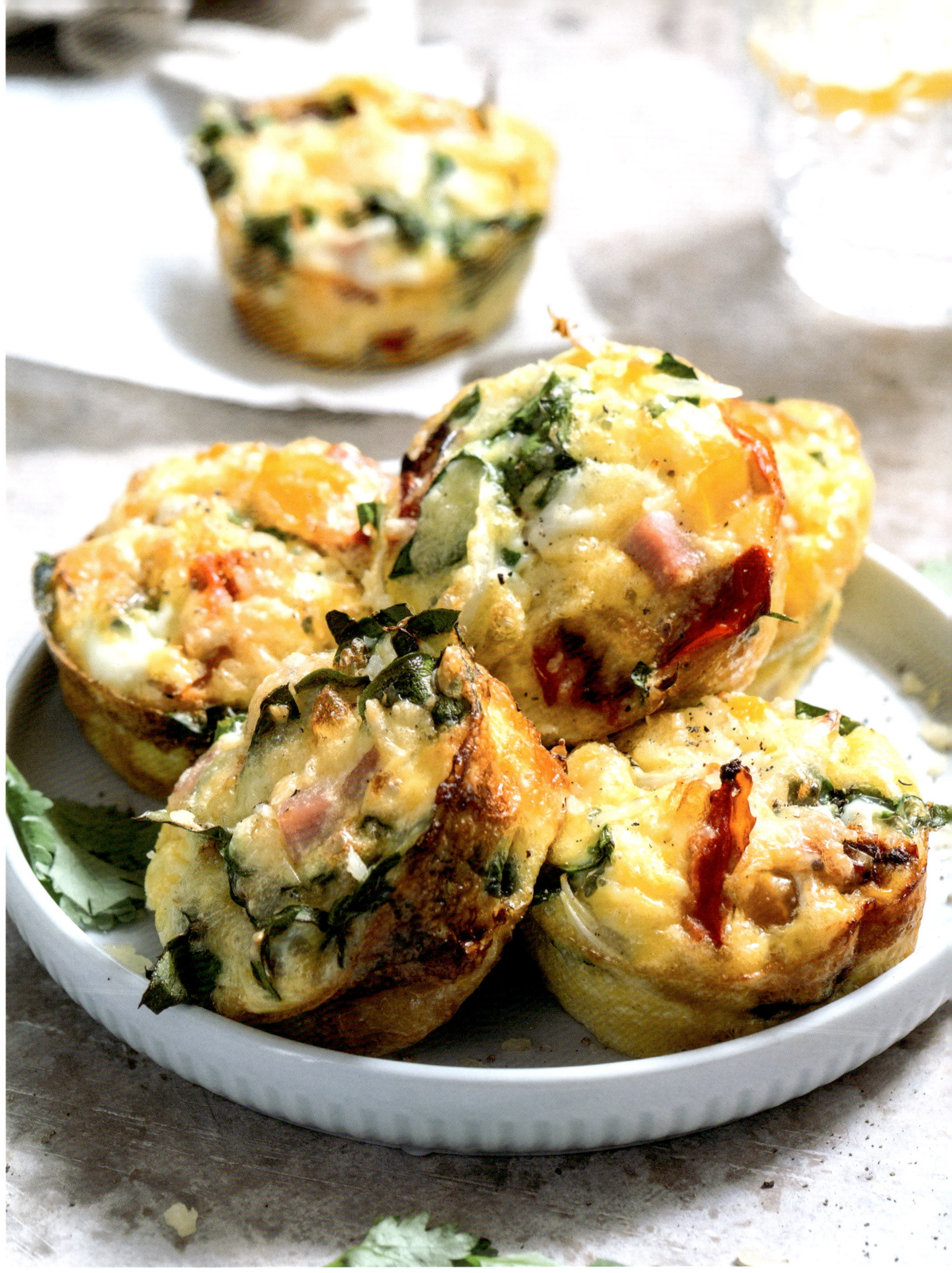

EGG & BACON MUFFINS

8 eggs

¼ cup (60ml) cream

⅓ cup (80g) crumbled feta cheese

⅛ tsp garlic powder

⅛ tsp onion powder

½ tsp chilli flakes

3 spring onions, chopped

1 cup (30g) baby spinach leaves, chopped

Salt and pepper to taste

STEPS

Preheat the oven to 180°C.

1. In a large bowl beat the eggs with the cream until frothy.
2. Place the feta, garlic powder, onion powder, chilli flakes, spring onions, spinach, salt and pepper to the bowl with the beaten eggs. Fold until all the ingredients are well incorporated.
3. Grease a muffin tin and half-fill the holes with the mixture.
4. Bake for 20 minutes or until eggs are fully set.
5. Serve immediately or store in the fridge for up to 5 days.

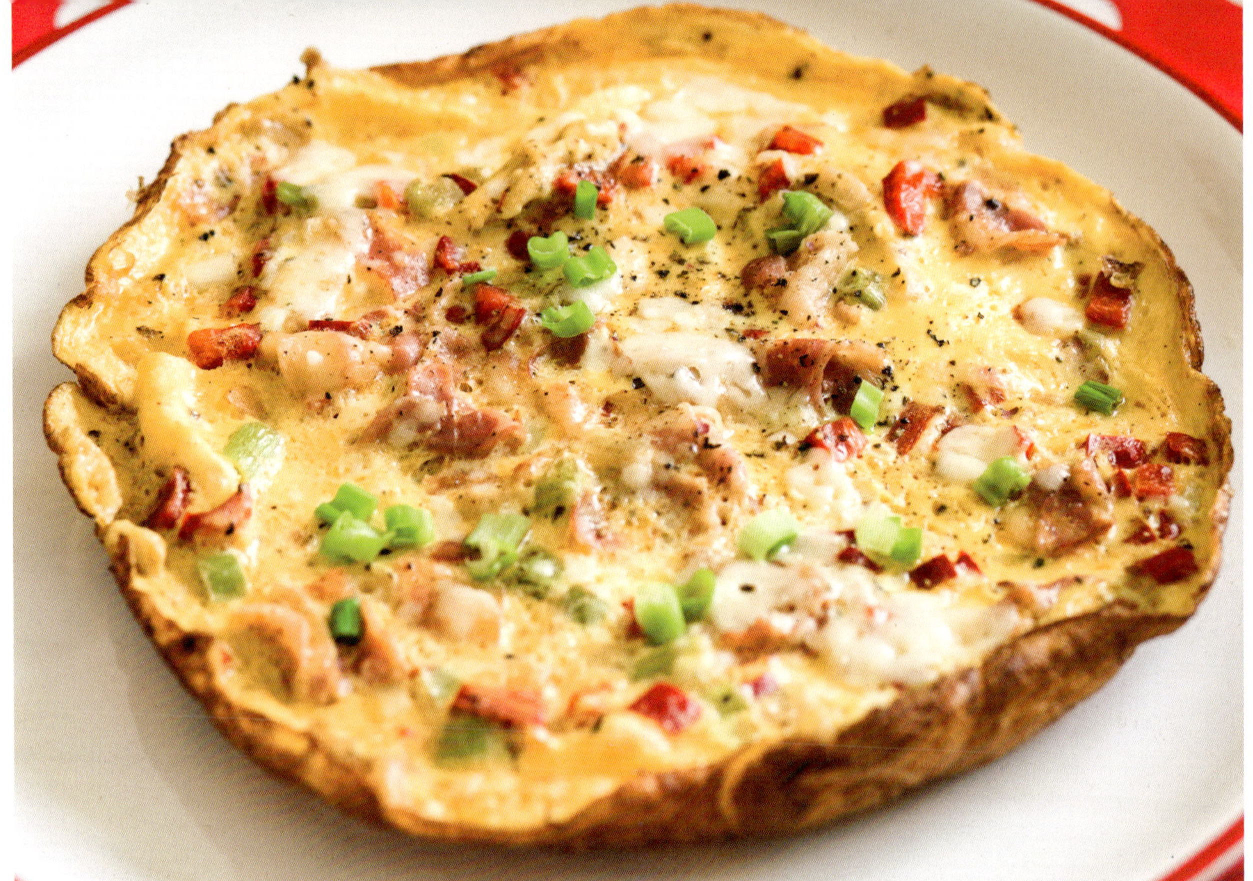

SERVES 2 | PREP + COOK TIME: 55 MINS | GLUTEN FREE

DEEP DISH OMELETTE

6 large eggs

½ cup (125ml) milk

½ tsp salt

¼ tsp pepper

1 cup (135g) cooked ham or cooked bacon, diced

1 cup (125g) grated Cheddar cheese (or any cheese of your choice)

½ cup (85g) diced capsicum

½ cup (75g) diced onion

½ cup (40g) sliced mushrooms

¼ cup (10g) chopped fresh herbs (such as parsley, chives or basil)

Spring onions, sliced, to garnish

STEPS

Preheat oven to 190°C.

1. In a large mixing bowl, whisk together the eggs, milk, salt and pepper until well combined. Add the diced ham or bacon, grated cheese, capsicum, onions, mushrooms and fresh herbs to the egg mixture. Stir to combine.
2. Pour the mixture into a greased shallow baking dish, spreading it evenly.
3. Bake in the preheated oven for 35-40 minutes or until the omelette is set in the centre and lightly golden on top.
4. Remove from the oven and let it cool for a few minutes. Serve warm, sprinkled with spring onions.

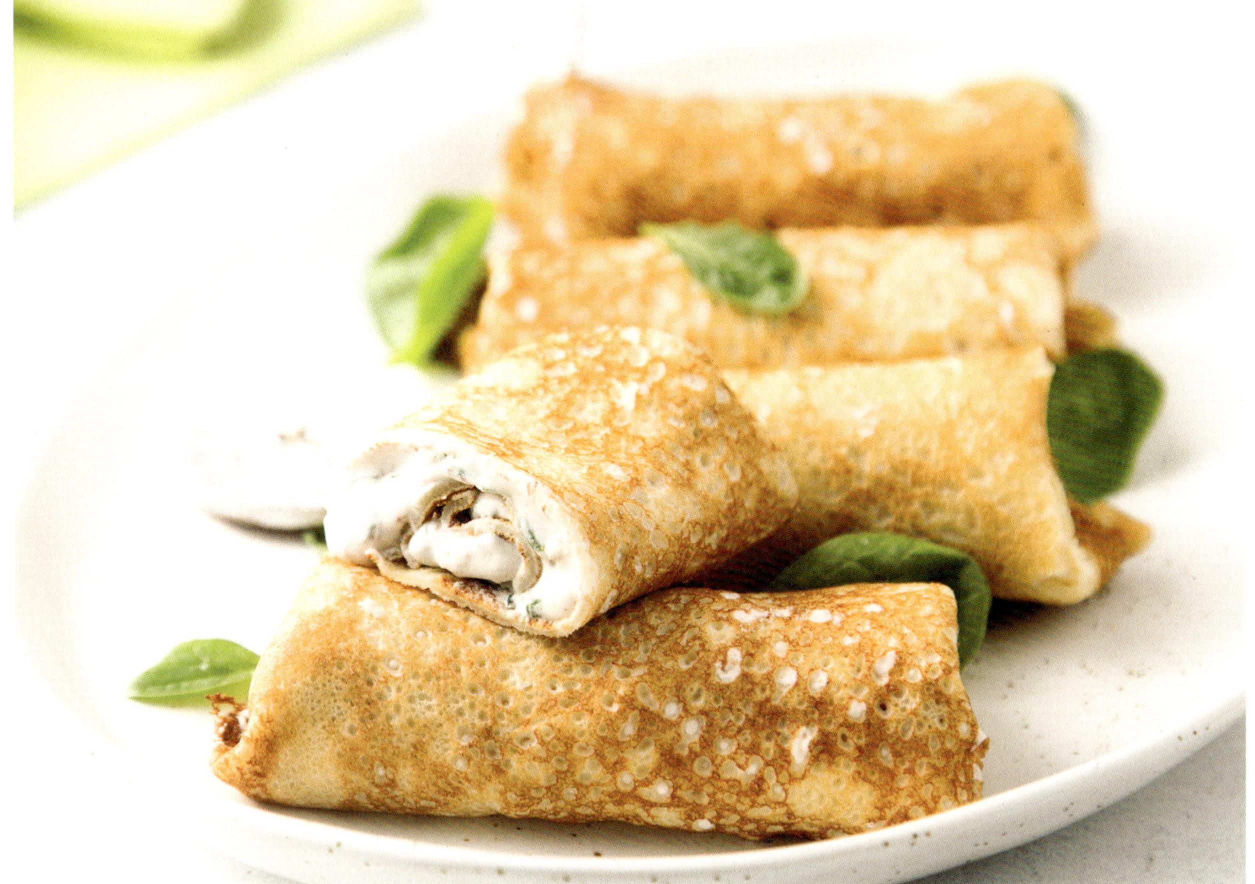

SAVOURY CREPE WITH CREAM CHEESE

CREPES

2 large eggs

2 tbsps almond flour

1 tbsp coconut flour

¼ cup (60ml) unsweetened almond milk

¼ tsp salt

¼ tsp garlic powder (optional)

Cooking spray or butter for frying

CREAM CHEESE FILLING

100g cream cheese, softened

1 tbsp chopped fresh herbs (such as parsley, dill or chives)

Salt and pepper to taste

STEPS

1. In a medium-sized bowl, whisk eggs, flours, milk, salt and garlic powder until combined. Let the batter sit for a few minutes to thicken.
2. Heat a nonstick frying pan over medium heat and add cooking spray or butter. Pour about ¼ cup of batter into the pan and tilt to spread the batter into a thin, round shape. Cook for 1-2 minutes on one side, then flip and cook for an additional 1-2 minutes on the other side. Set aside on a plate.
3. Remove from the pan and repeat the process with the remaining batter.
4. In a small bowl, mix together cream cheese, fresh herbs, salt and pepper until well combined.
5. Spread a thin layer of the cream cheese mixture onto each crepe, then tuck the ends in and roll up firmly to enclose the filling. Serve immediately.

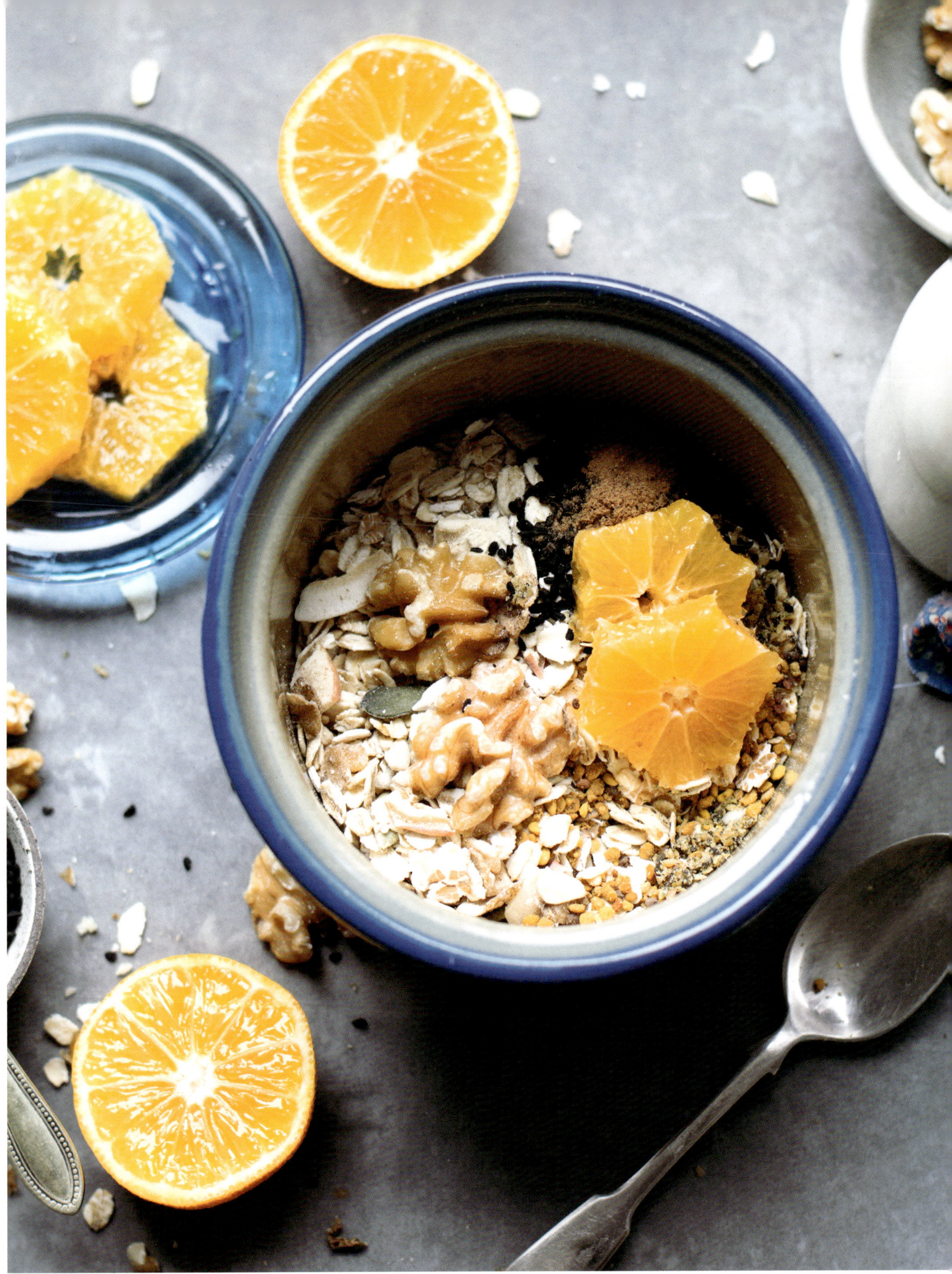

HOMEMADE MUESLI

1 cup (125g) flaked almonds

1 cup (90g) coconut flakes

1 cup (125g) pecans, chopped

1 cup (125g) walnuts, chopped

1 cup (90g) rolled oats

½ cup (60g) sunflower seeds

1 tbsp brown sugar

1 tsp cinnamon

½ tsp nutmeg

TO SERVE (OPTIONAL)

Almond milk

Mixed seeds

Fresh fruit, sliced

STEPS

Preheat oven to 180°C.

1. Mix all ingredients together in a large bowl.
2. Spread evenly over a lined baking tray.
3. Bake in the oven for 8 minutes then remove and allow to cool.
4. Serve with almond milk and a sprinkle of seed mix and finish with slices of fresh fruit.

NOTE: Will keep in an airtight container for 2 weeks.

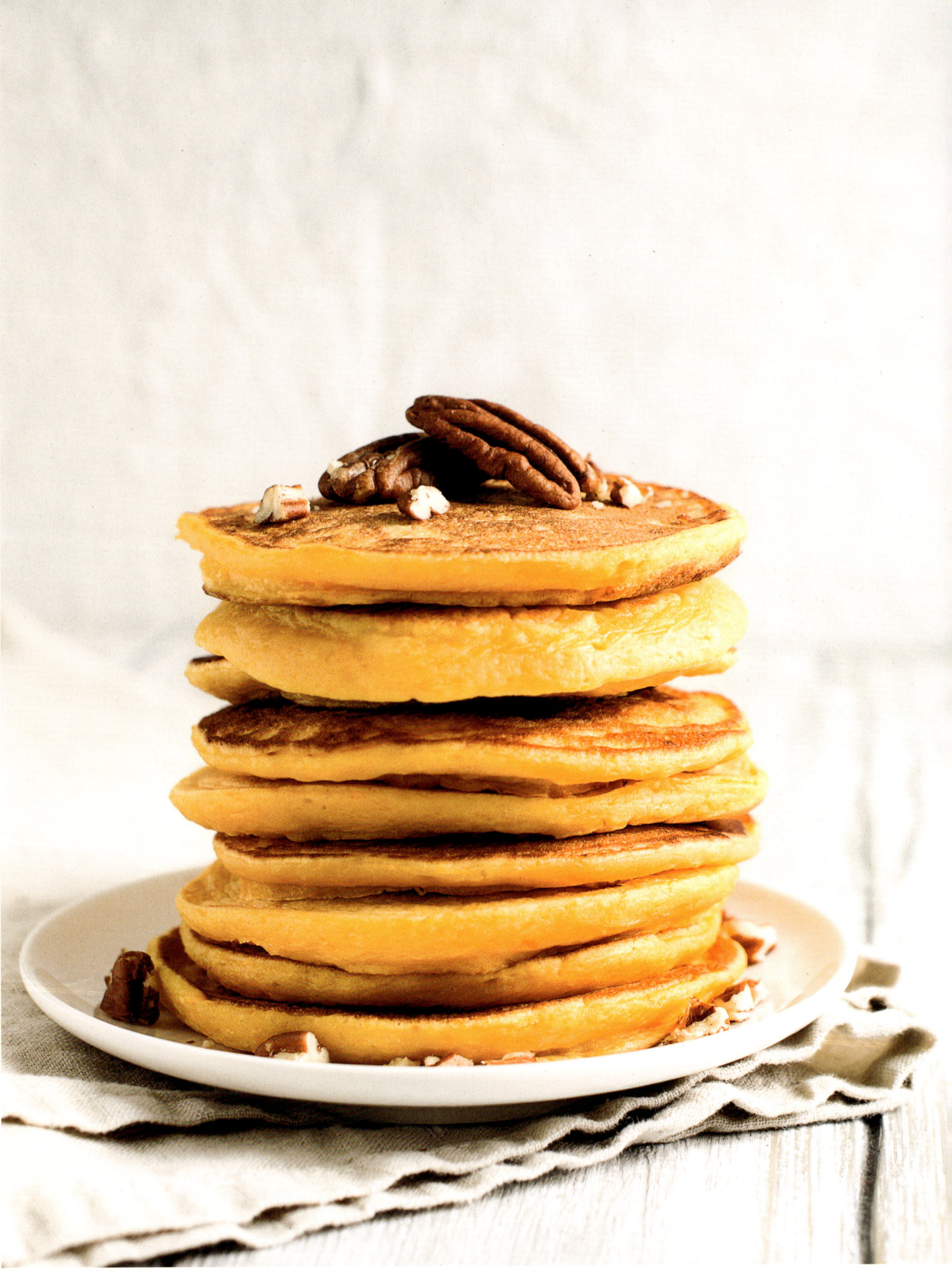

PROTEIN-POWERED PUMPKIN PANCAKES

6 large eggs, room temperature

½ cup (110g) mashed cooked pumpkin

⅓ cup (65g) Baker's Secret (brown sugar replacement)

60g butter, melted

1 tsp vanilla extract

½ cup (50g) coconut flour

⅓ cup (30g) unflavoured whey protein powder

2 tsps cinnamon

¼ tsp ground cloves

¼ tsp ground nutmeg

¼ tsp ground ginger

1 tsp baking powder

¼ tsp salt

2 tbsps almond milk

Oil for frying

Chopped pecans to serve (optional)

STEPS

1. In a large bowl, whisk together the eggs, pumpkin and brown sugar replacement. Add the butter and vanilla extract and stir until smooth. Add the coconut flour, protein powder, spices, baking powder and salt, and whisk well to combine. Add almond milk and whisk to incorporate.
2. Lightly oil a large frying pan and heat over medium heat. Scoop about two heaped tablespoons of batter onto the pan and spread into a 10cm circle.
3. Cook for 2-3 minutes until the bottom is golden brown and the top is set around the edges. Flip carefully and continue to cook until the second side is golden brown. Repeat with the remaining batter.
4. Scatter with chopped pecans or your choice of toppings to serve.

NOTE: Brown sugar replacement is available to purchase at major supermarkets under various brand names such as Truvia or Whole Earth Baker's Secret.

SERVES 4 | PREP + COOK TIME: 30 MINS | VEG | GLUTEN FREE |

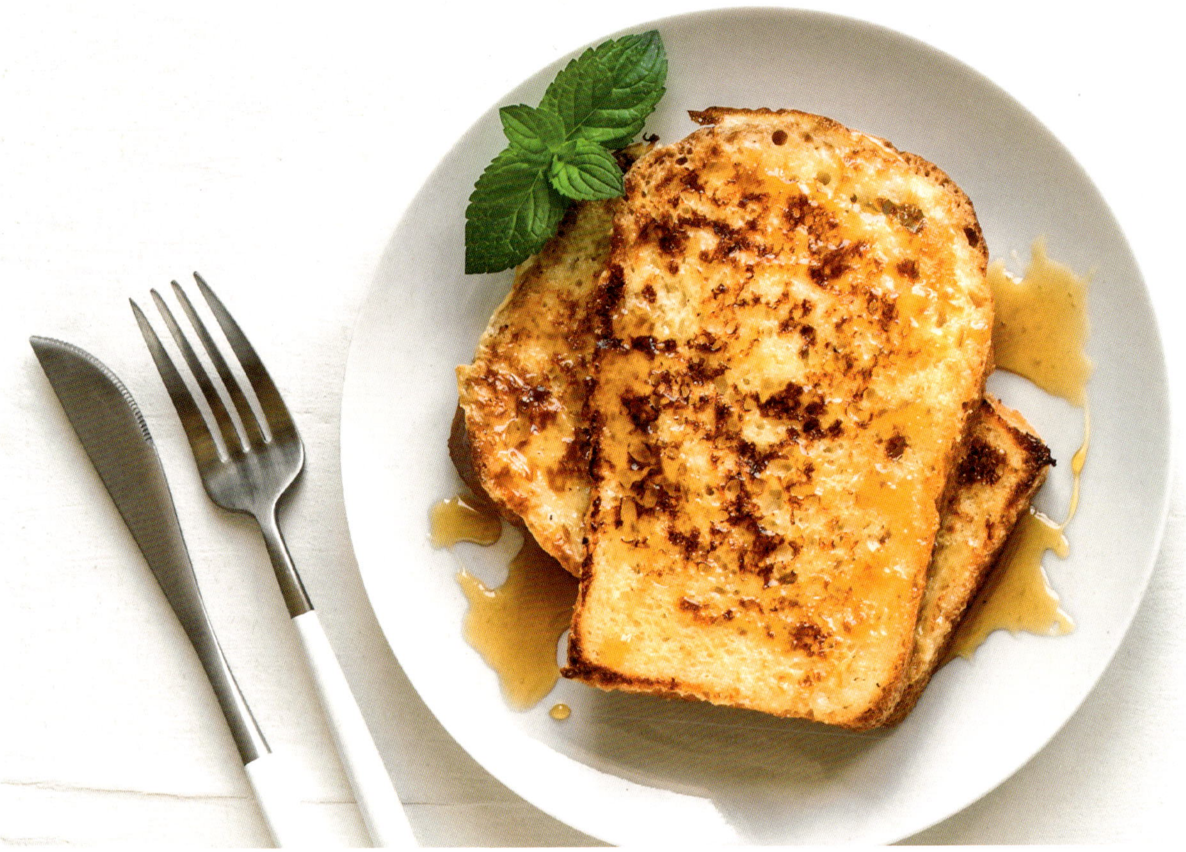

SERVES 2 | PREP + COOK TIME: 15 MINS | VEG

SUNDAY FRENCH TOAST

4 eggs

⅓ cup (80ml) milk (non-dairy or dairy)

1 tsp ground cinnamon

Olive oil spray for frying

4 slices low-carb bread

Maple syrup (if using) or Bakers Classic Syrup

STEPS

1. Lightly beat the eggs with the milk and cinnamon.
2. Spray a nonstick frying pan with olive oil and heat over medium heat.
3. Soak each piece of bread thoroughly in the egg mixture.
4. Fry the egg-soaked bread slices for 1 minute on each side or until browned.
5. Serve warm with maple syrup.

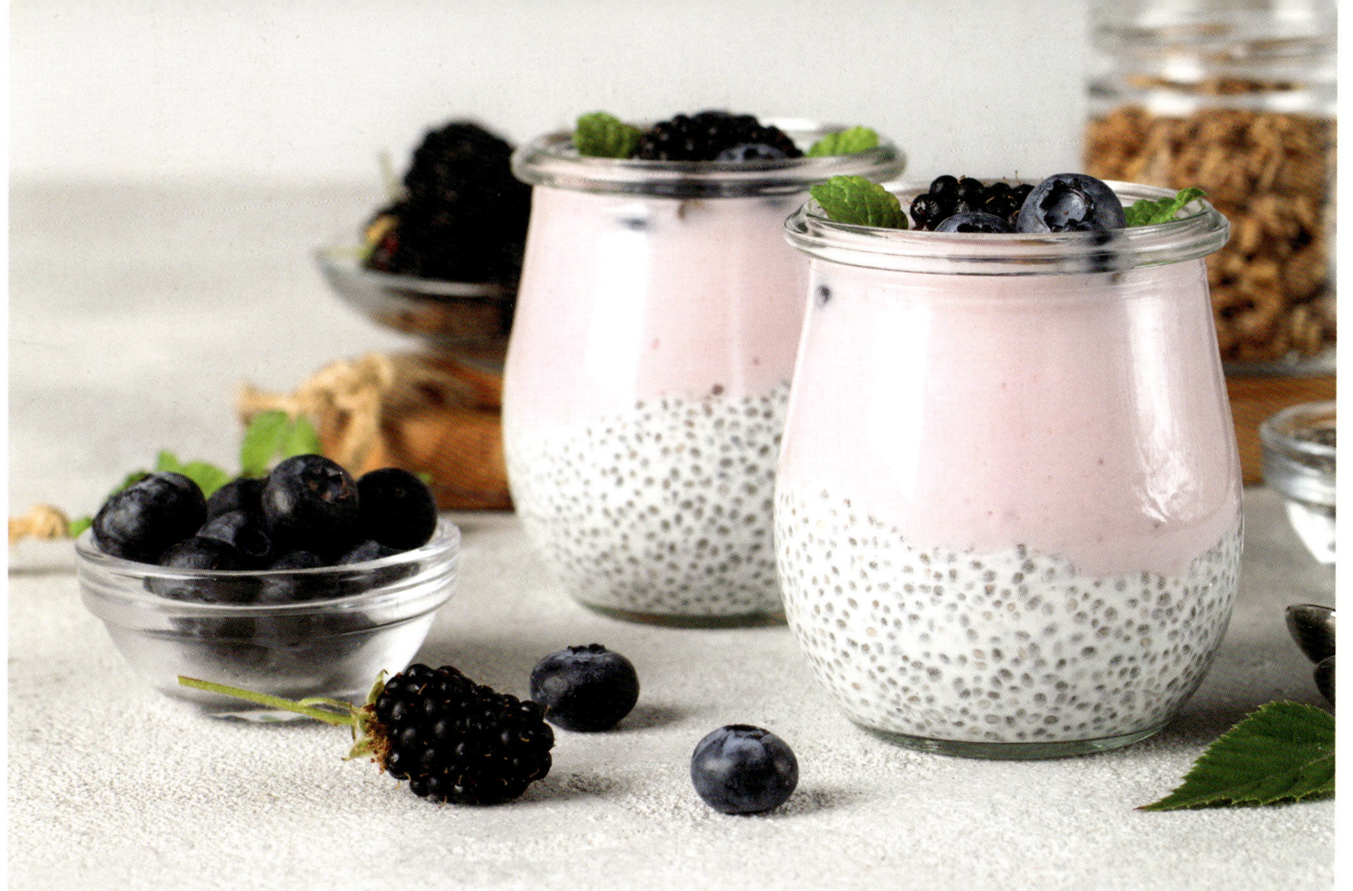

SERVES 2 | PREP + COOK TIME: 10 MINS + CHILLING | VEG | GLUTEN FREE |

BLUEBERRY CREAM CHIA POTS

4 tbsps chia seeds

1 cup (250ml) almond milk

2 tbsps agave syrup

½ tsp cinnamon

1 cup (75g) fresh blueberries

½ cup (125ml) Greek yoghurt

STEPS

1. Combine the chia seeds, almond milk, agave syrup and cinnamon in a bowl. Cover and place in the refrigerator overnight.
2. Using a fork, mash half the fresh blueberries in a small bowl. Add the yoghurt and mix well to combine.
3. Divide the chia pudding mix between two serving glasses.
4. Dollop half the blueberry yoghurt over each.
5. Top with fresh blueberries.

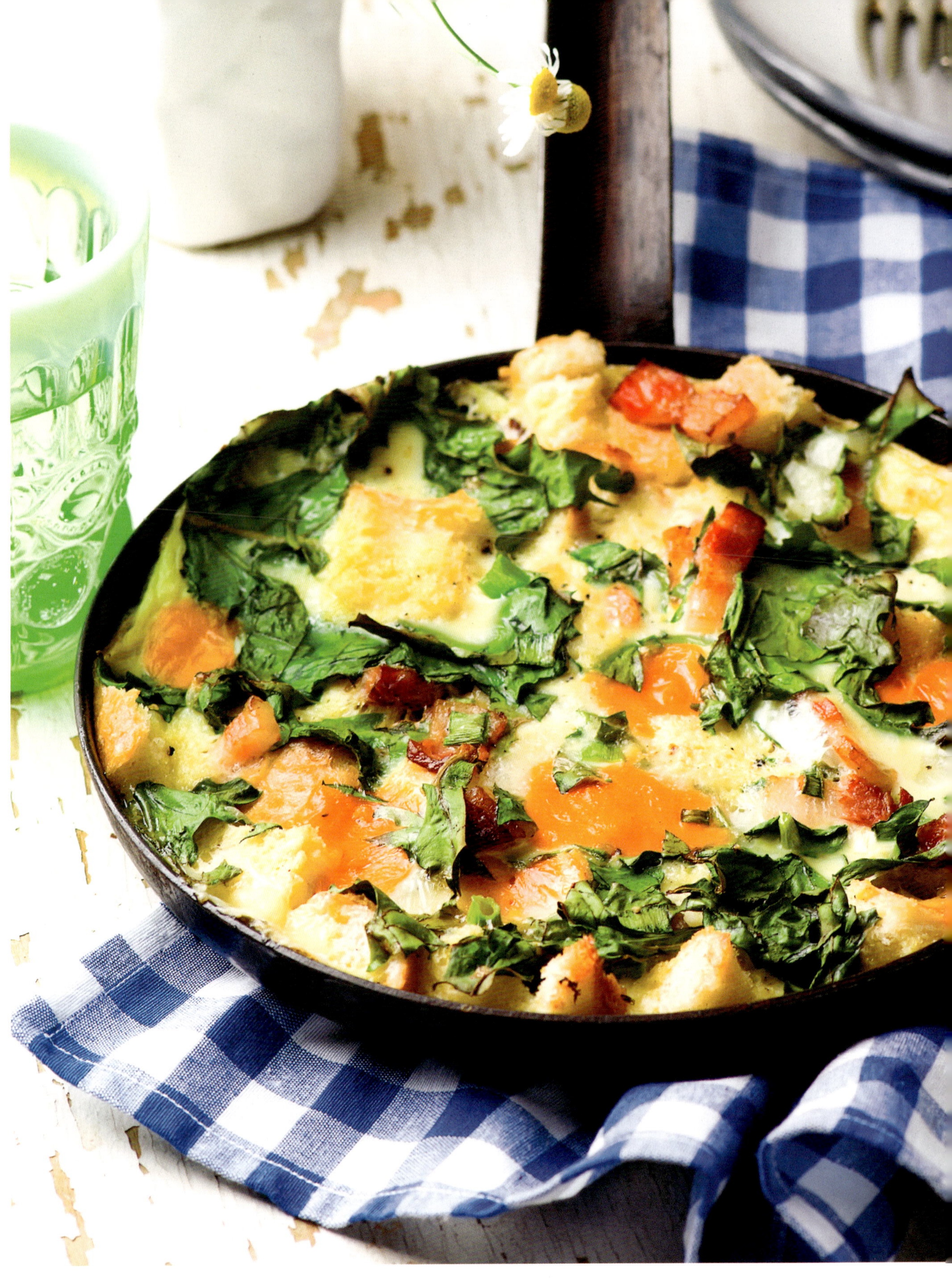

BREAKFAST STRATA WITH BACON, EGGS & GREENS

6 rashers bacon, chopped

1 small onion, finely chopped

2 cloves garlic, minced

4 cups (120g) low-carb bread cubes (store-bought or see recipe page 23)

2 cups (120g) chopped mixed greens (such as spinach, kale or Swiss chard)

6 large eggs

1½ cups (375ml) milk

1 cup (125g) grated cheese (such as Cheddar or Gruyere)

Salt and pepper to taste

STEPS

Preheat oven to 190°C.

1. In a large ovenproof pan, cook the chopped bacon over medium heat until crispy. Remove the bacon from the pan and set it aside.
2. In the same pan, add the chopped onion and minced garlic and saute them until they become fragrant and translucent.
3. Add the bread cubes to the skillet and toss them in the onion and garlic mixture. Cook for a few minutes until the bread cubes are lightly toasted. Add the chopped mixed greens to the skillet and cook until they wilt down. Add the bacon back to the pan and mix well.
4. In a separate bowl, whisk together the eggs and milk, salt and pepper. Pour the egg and milk mixture over the bread, greens and bacon in the pan. Gently press down the ingredients with a spatula to ensure they are evenly distributed.
5. Sprinkle the shredded cheese over the top of the mixture and transfer pan to the preheated oven and bake for about 25-30 minutes, or until the strata is set and the top is golden brown.

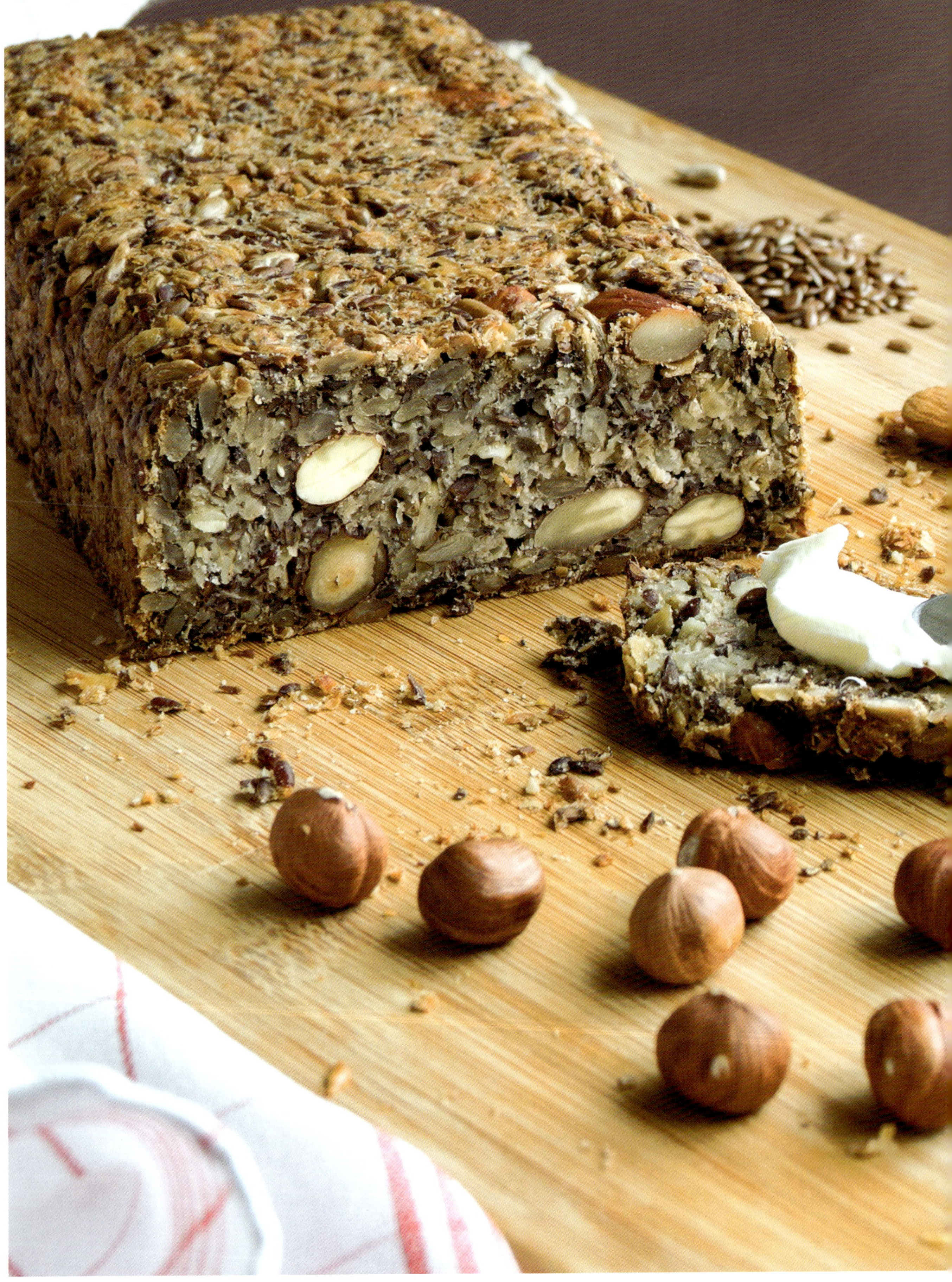

NUT & SEED LOAF

1 cup (100g) almond flour
½ cup (70g) ground flaxseed
½ cup (60g) sunflower seeds
½ cup (65g) pepitas
¼ cup (40g) chia seeds
¼ cup (40g) sesame seeds
1 tsp baking powder
½ tsp salt
4 large eggs
¼ cup (60ml) melted coconut oil or olive oil

STEPS

Preheat oven to 160°C.

1. In a large mixing bowl, combine the almond flour, ground flaxseed, sunflower seeds, pepitas, chia seeds, sesame seeds, baking powder and salt.
2. In a separate bowl, whisk together the eggs and melted coconut oil or olive oil. Pour the wet ingredients into the dry ingredients and mix until well combined. The mixture will be thick and sticky.
3. Transfer the mixture into a greased and lined loaf pan and smooth the top with a spatula.
4. Bake for about 40-45 minutes, or until the loaf is golden brown and a toothpick inserted into the centre comes out clean.
5. Remove from the oven and let it cool in the pan for a few minutes. Then transfer it to a wire rack to cool completely before slicing.

NOTE: Try different combinations of nuts and seeds, but be sure not to miss out the ground flaxseed as this works as a binding agent.

MAKES 1 LOAF | PREP + COOK TIME: 1 HOUR 5 MINS | VEG | GLUTEN FREE | DAIRY FREE |

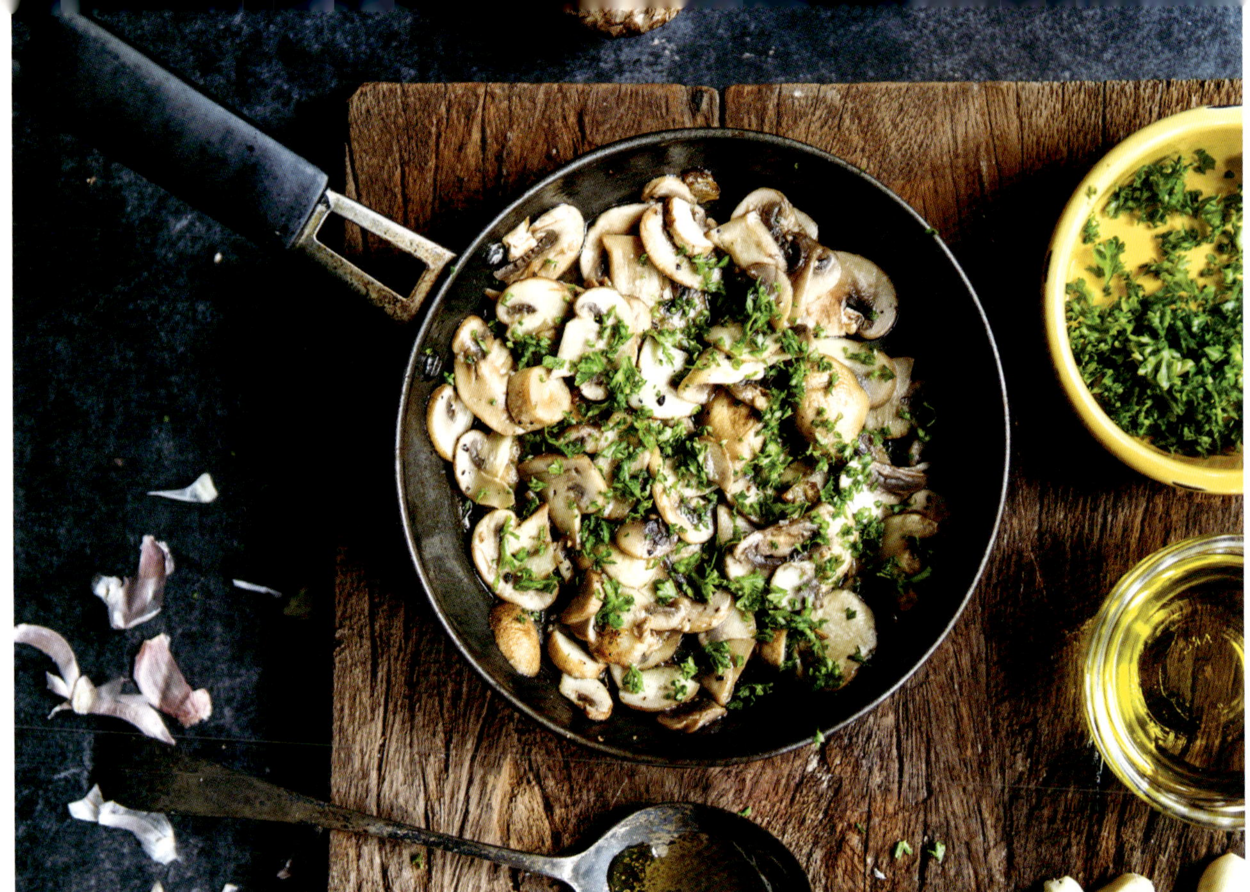

GARLIC MUSHROOMS WITH SOUR CREAM

2 tbsps olive oil

500g mushrooms, sliced

4 cloves garlic, minced

2 tbsps sour cream

Salt and pepper to taste

Parsley to serve (optional)

STEPS

1. Heat olive oil in a large frying pan over medium heat. Add mushrooms and cook, stirring regularly, for 7-8 minutes until the mushrooms release their liquid and become golden brown and tender.
2. Add the garlic and cook for another minute until fragrant.
3. Stir in the sour cream.
4. Season to taste with salt and pepper and garnish with chopped parsley.

NOTE: Thyme also works well in this dish. If preferred, add in place of parsley when you add the garlic.

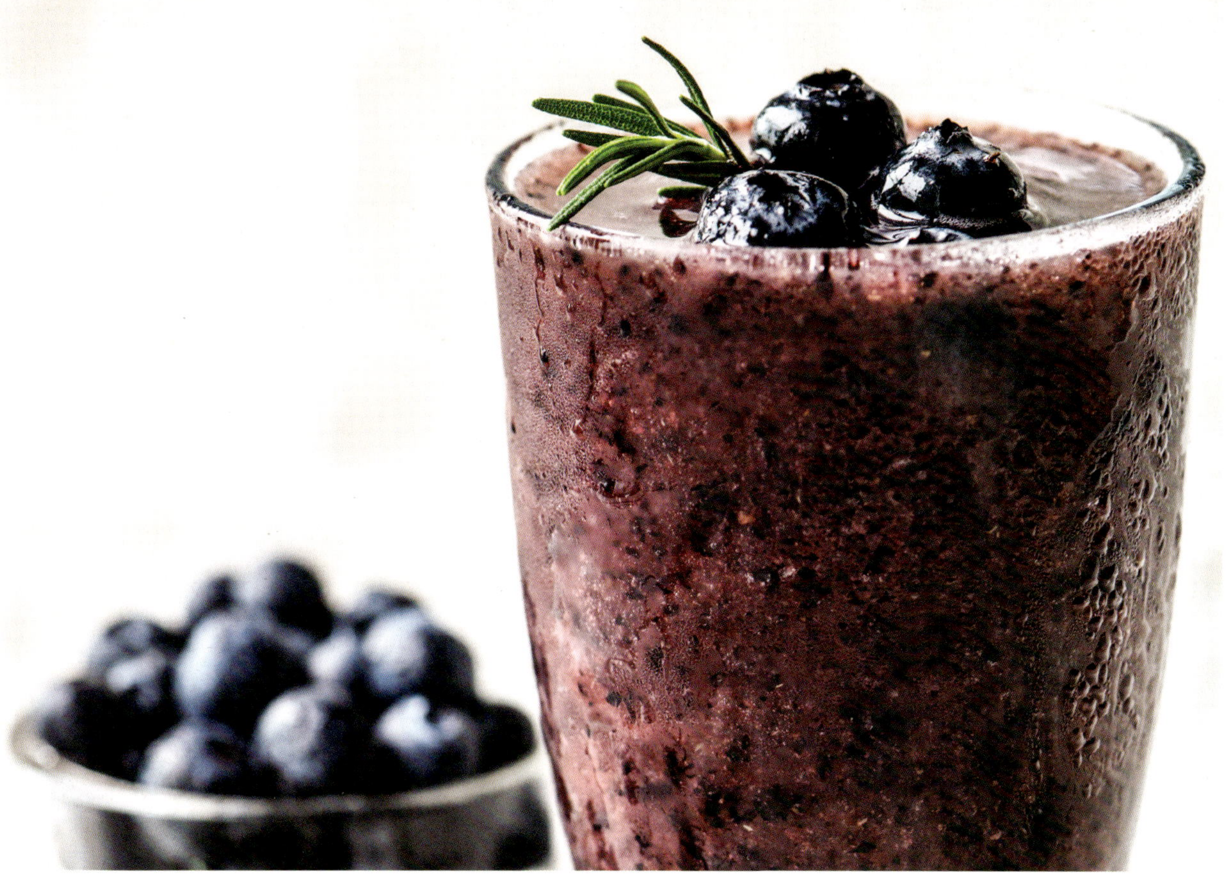

SERVES 2 | PREP + COOK TIME: 5 MINS | VEG | GLUTE FREE | DAIRY FREE |

BLUEBERRY SMOOTHIE

½ cup (60g) frozen blackberries
½ cup (60g) frozen blueberries
2 cups (500ml) coconut water
1 tsp chia seeds

STEPS

1. Place all ingredients into a high-speed blender. Blend on high for 30 seconds until well combined.
2. Pour into bottles or glasses to serve.

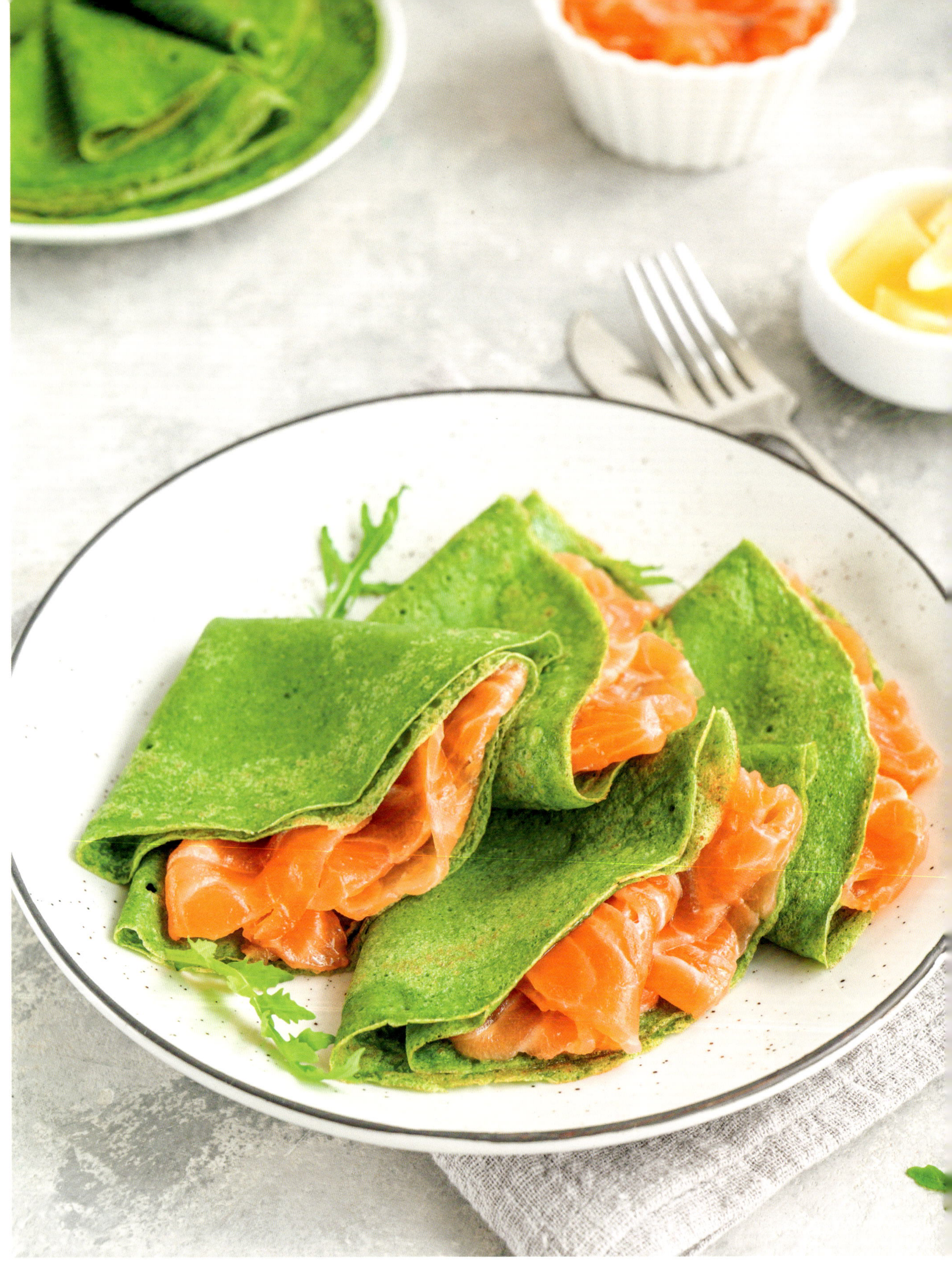

SPINACH CREPES

SERVES 2 | PREP + COOK TIME: 30 MINS | GLUTEN FREE |

CREPES

4 eggs

30g frozen spinach, thawed and squeezed

¼ cup (25g) coconut flour

1½ tbsps arrowroot flour

½ cup (125ml) almond milk

Pinch of salt

½ tsp olive oil

TO SERVE

110g cream cheese

200g smoked salmon slices

Rocket leaves

STEPS

1. To make the crepes, place the eggs, spinach, coconut flour, arrowroot, almond milk and salt into a blender and blend until smooth. Add more almond milk if necessary to achieve a pourable consistency.

2. Heat a medium frying pan over a medium heat. Brush with olive oil. Pour ¼ cup batter into the pan and swirl to cover base. Cook until the top of the crepe is no longer wet and the bottom has turned light brown.

3. Run a spatula around the edge of the pan to loosen then flip and cook for 1 minute or until cooked through. Transfer to a plate and cover with foil to keep warm. Repeat with remaining batter.

4. Fill each crepe with a spread of cream cheese and sliced smoked salmon. Then fold into quarters, and serve with rocket leaves.

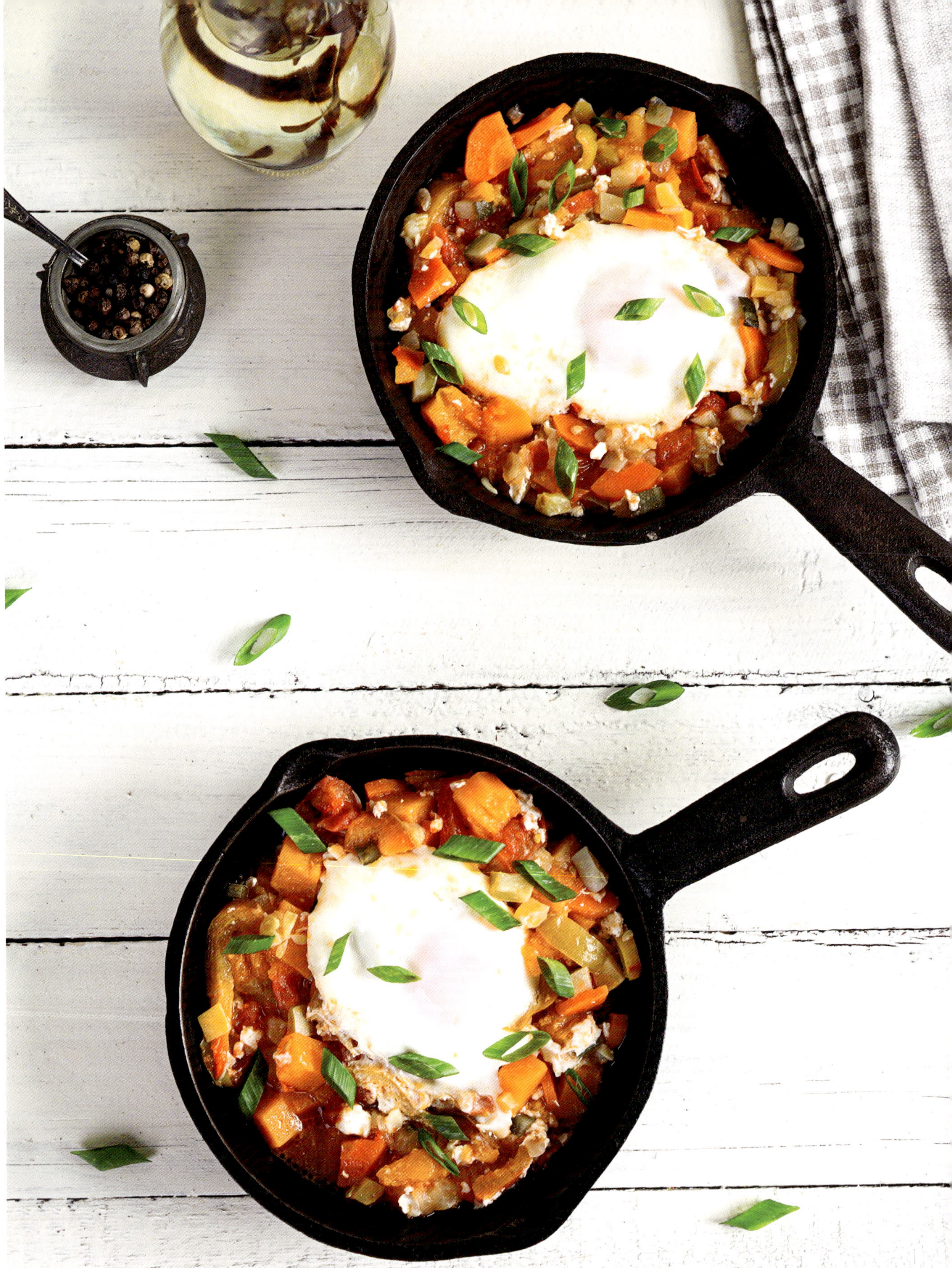

VEGGIE SHAKSHUKA

- 1 tbsp olive oil
- 1 small red onion, chopped
- 1 small red capsicum, chopped
- 1 carrot, quartered and sliced
- 2 tbsps pickled jalapeno chilli, finely chopped
- 2 cloves garlic, crushed
- 1 tsp ground cumin
- 1 tsp ground oregano
- 1 tsp sweet paprika
- 1 x 400g can chopped tomatoes
- 1 x 400g can kidney beans
- 4 eggs
- Spring onions, chopped, to garnish

STEPS

Preheat oven to 180°C.

1. Heat the olive oil in a medium, heavy, ovenproof frying pan over medium heat. Fry the onion, capsicum, carrot, chilli and garlic for 5 minutes, or until the onion is softened.
2. Stir through the cumin, oregano and paprika. Add the tomatoes and kidney beans and bring to a boil.
3. Reduce heat to a low simmer and cook for 15 minutes or until vegetables have softened.
4. Remove from the heat then make four hollows in the mixture and gently crack the eggs into them, being careful not to break the yolks. Transfer the frying pan to the oven and bake for 10 minutes, or until the eggs are cooked to your liking.
5. Let sit for 5 minutes once out of the oven then garnish with sliced spring onions.

SERVES 2 | PREP + COOK TIME: 35 MINS | VEG | GLUTEN FREE | DAIRY FREE |

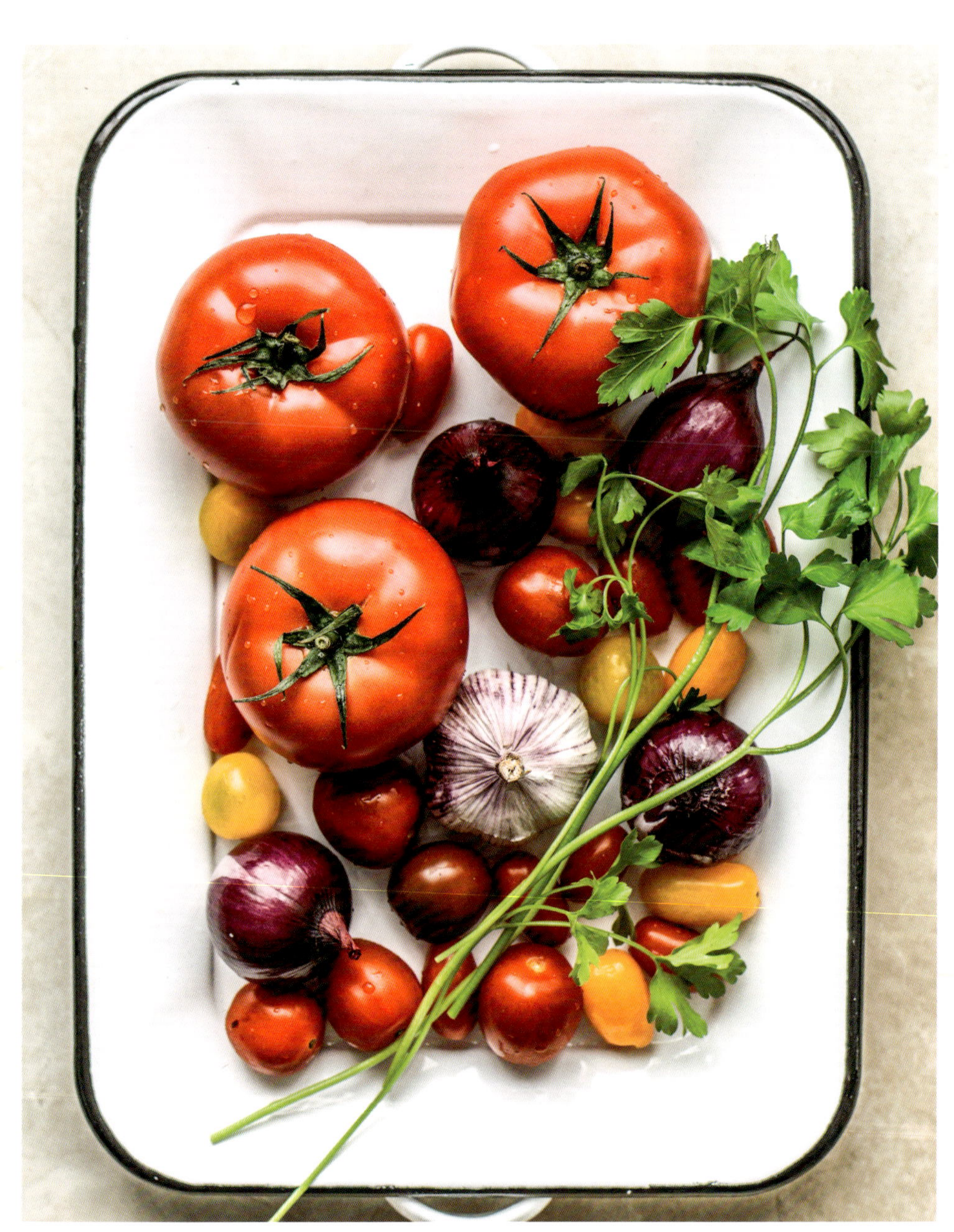

TASTY LUNCHES

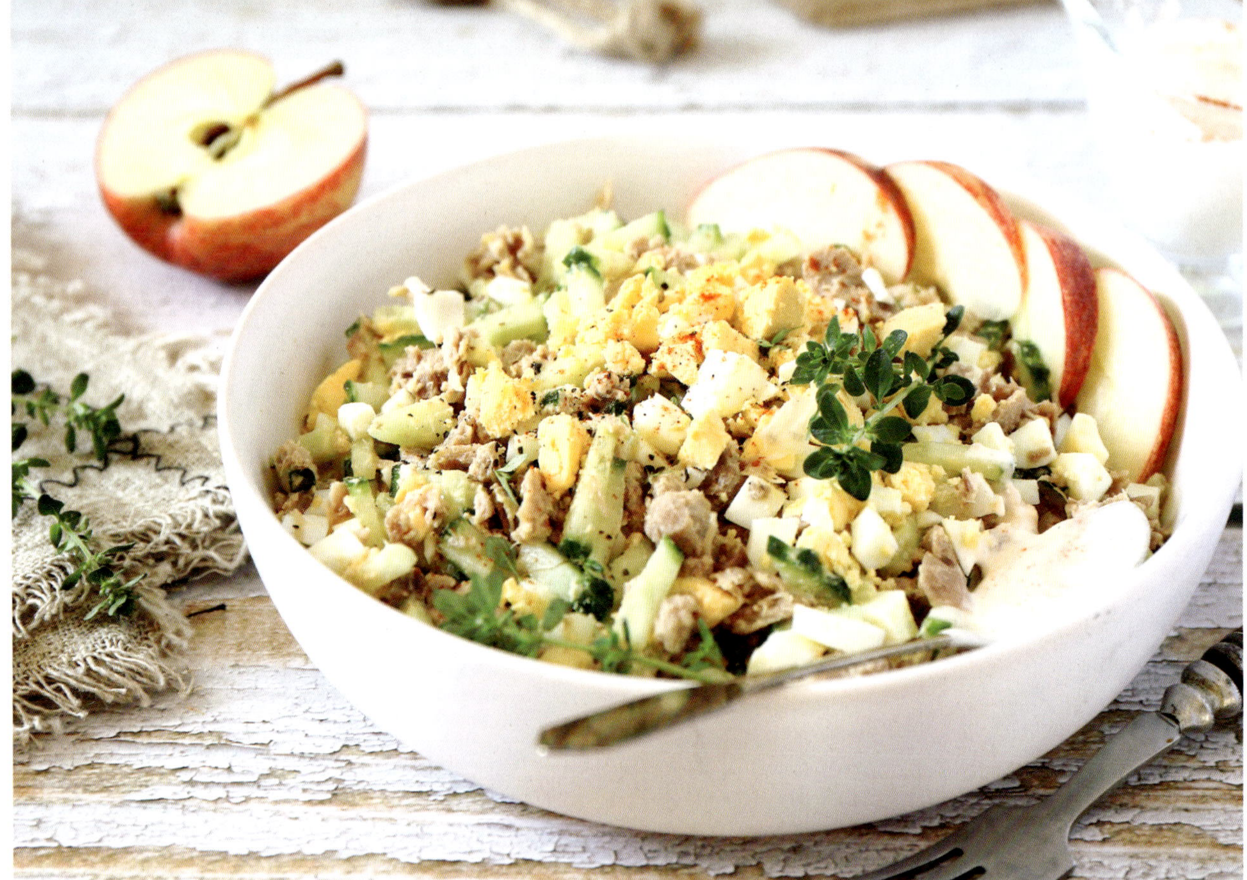

EGG & TUNA CHOPPED SALAD

1 x 425g can tuna, drained

2 eggs, hard-boiled, peeled and chopped

1 large apple, cored and thinly sliced, reserve 8 slices for garnish

½ small cucumber, diced

½ small red onion, diced

¼ cup (10g) chopped fresh parsley

¼ cup (60g) mayonnaise

1 tbsp Dijon mustard

1 tbsp lemon juice

Salt and pepper to taste

Lettuce or salad greens

Fresh herbs to serve

STEPS

1. In a large mixing bowl, combine the drained tuna, chopped hard-boiled eggs, apple, cucumber, red onion and fresh parsley.
2. In a separate small bowl, whisk together the mayonnaise, Dijon mustard, lemon juice, salt and pepper until well combined.
3. Pour the dressing over the tuna mixture and gently toss to coat all the ingredients evenly.
4. To serve, place a bed of lettuce or salad greens in individual bowls. Spoon the tuna, egg and apple mixture over the greens.
5. Garnish the salad with sliced apple and fresh parsley or mixed herbs.

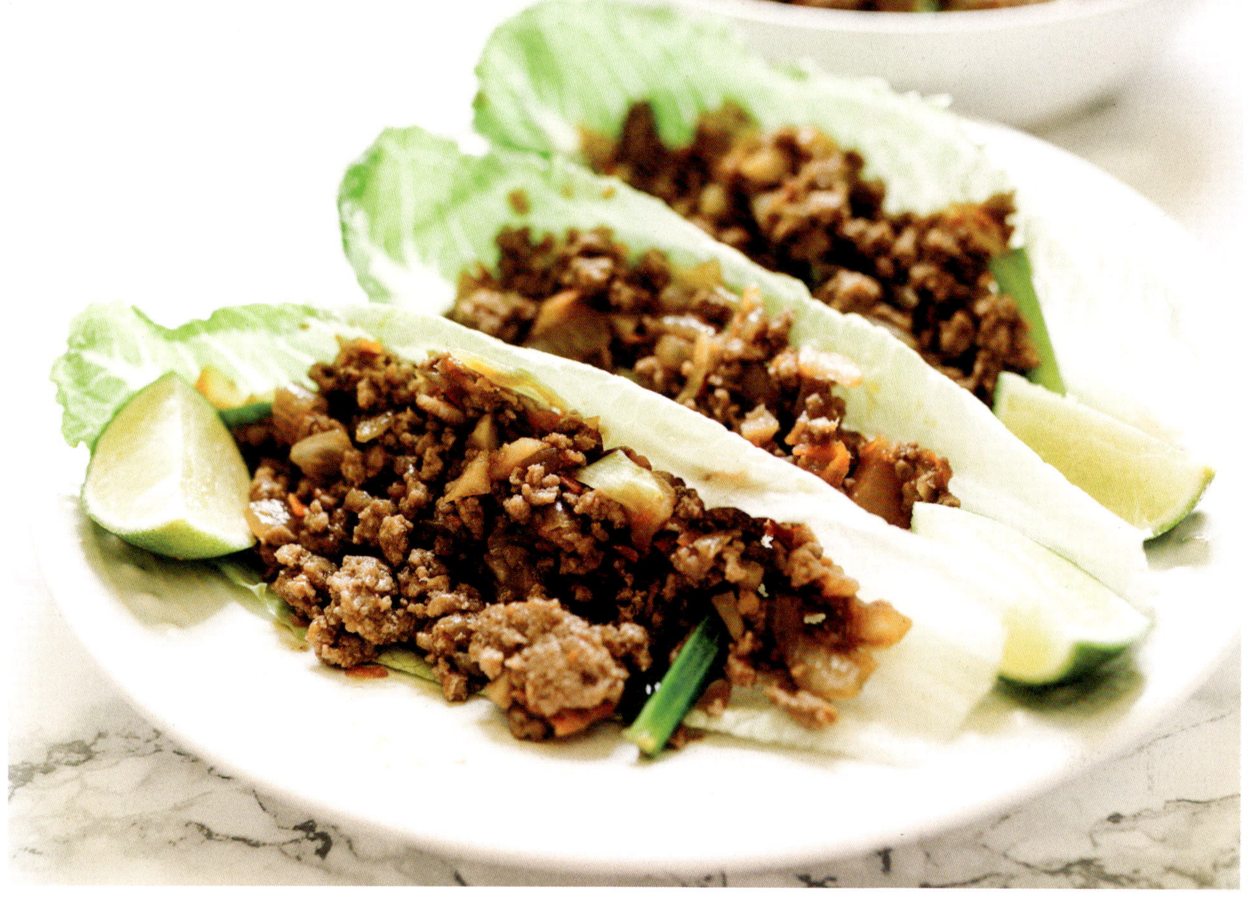

ASIAN BEEF LETTUCE WRAPS

2 tbsps coconut oil

500g beef mince

1 carrot, grated

2 tbsps tamari

3 small spring onions, finely sliced

2 tsps rice wine vinegar

Salt and pepper to taste

8 large cos lettuce leaves

1 small red chilli, finely chopped (optional)

STEPS

1. Heat the oil in a large frying pan over medium-high heat. Fry the mince for 6 minutes until browned. Add the carrot and tamari and cook for another 5 minutes.
2. Add half the spring onions and vinegar then fry a further 4 minutes. Season to taste.
3. Serve ⅓ cup portions of the mince on the lettuce leaves, garnished with the remaining spring onions and chilli (if using).

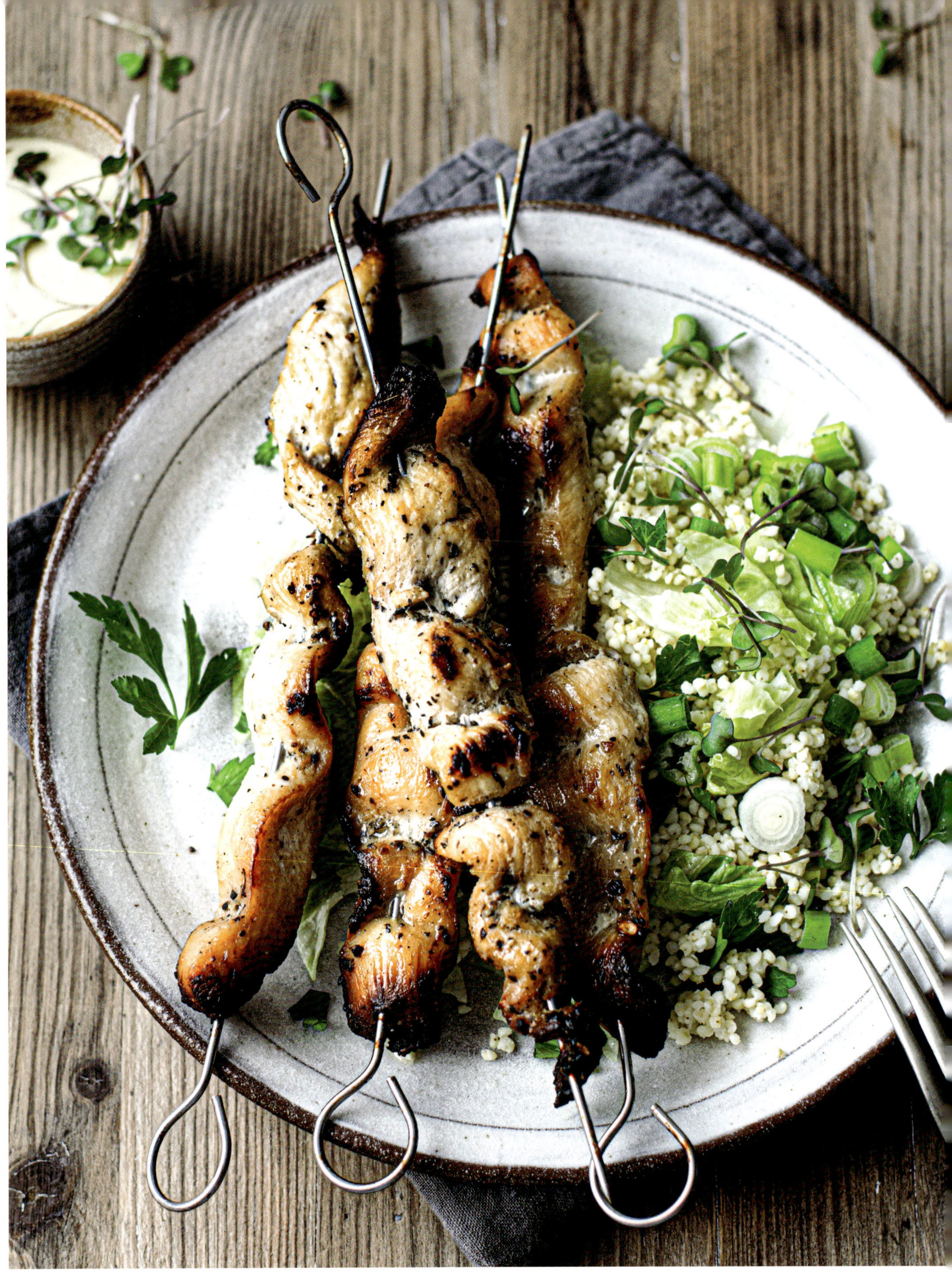

YOGHURT-MARINATED CHICKEN SKEWERS

CHICKEN

1 clove garlic, crushed

1 tbsp lemon juice

¼ tsp dried oregano

½ tsp ground cumin

1 cup (250ml) Greek yoghurt

1 tbsp olive oil

2 x 150g chicken breasts, cut into 2cm cubes

SALAD

2 cups (90g) packed salad leaves, chopped

2 spring onions, finely sliced

1 cup (185g) cooked millet

2 tbsps chopped parsley

1 tbsp lemon juice

2 tbsps olive oil

Salt and pepper to taste

STEPS

1. Mix the garlic, lemon juice, dried oregano, cumin, yoghurt and olive oil together in a small bowl. Add the chicken cubes to the bowl and mix until pieces are well coated.

2. Thread the chicken pieces evenly onto metal or soaked wooden skewers, place on a tray and refrigerate until you are ready to cook them.

3. To make the salad, combine salad leaves, spring onions, cooked millet and parsley in a bowl, then add lemon juice, 1 tablespoon of olive oil and salt and pepper. Mix to combine.

4. Heat remaining oil in a large frying pan on a medium to high heat and cook the chicken skewers in batches until cooked through and slightly charred.

5. Divide the salad onto serving plates and arrange chicken skewers on top.

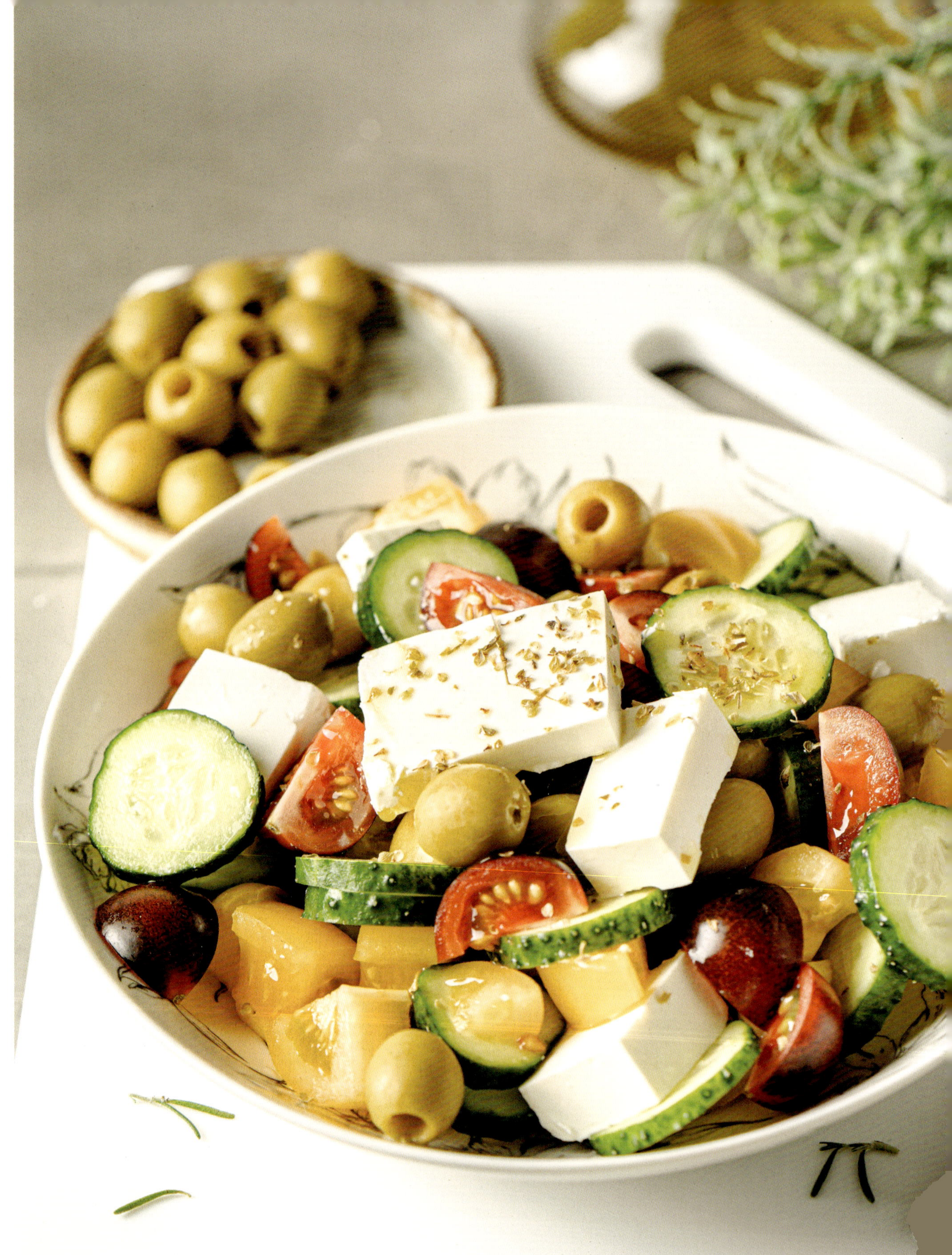

FETA & OLIVE SALAD

SERVES 4 | PREP + COOK TIME: 20 MINS | VEG | GLUTEN FREE |

1 cup (225g) cherry tomatoes, halved
½ small cucumber, sliced
¼ cup (35g) pitted green olives
60g Danish feta cheese, cubed
2 tbsps olive oil
1 tsp lemon juice
1 tbsp red wine vinegar
1 clove garlic, crushed
½ tsp dried oregano + extra to serve
Salt and pepper to taste

STEPS

1. In a large bowl, add cherry tomatoes, sliced cucumber, olives and feta cheese.
2. To make the dressing, whisk together the olive oil, lemon juice, red wine vinegar, garlic, dried oregano and salt and pepper to in a small bowl, mix well to combine.
3. Pour the dressing over the salad and toss well to coat all the ingredients.
4. Serve immediately with a little cracked pepper and dried oregano to garnish.

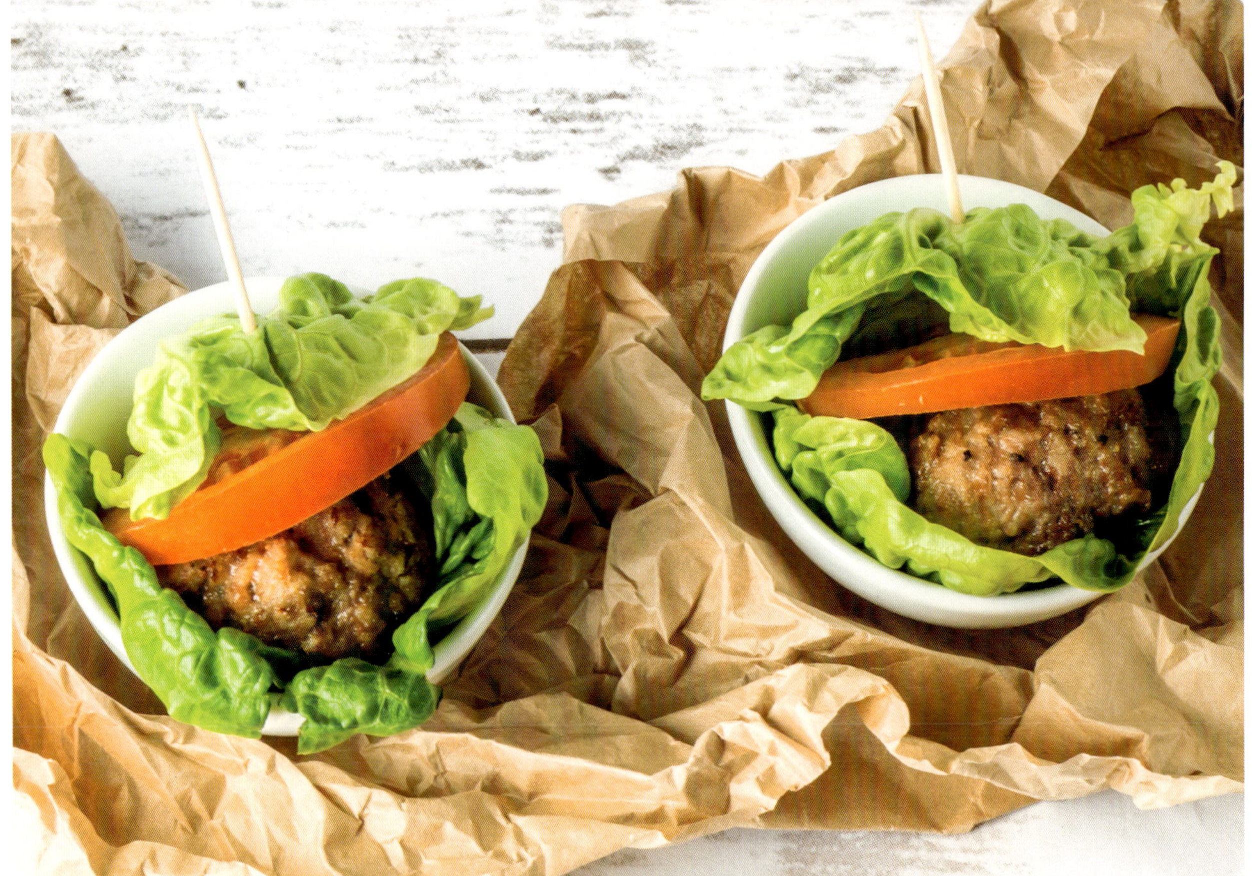

MINI TURKEY BURGERS

500g turkey mince

½ cup (125g) crumbled feta cheese

1 red onion, finely chopped

1 tbsp chopped parsley

1 tbsp chopped mint

1 tbsp milk

1 egg

½ tsp salt

⅛ tsp pepper

1 tbsp olive oil

10 oak lettuce leaves

1 medium tomato, sliced

2 tbsps store-bought mayonnaise

STEPS

1. In a large bowl combine turkey, feta, onion, parsley, mint, milk, egg, salt and pepper. Using your hands, mix until thoroughly combined.
2. Evenly divide the mixture and shape into eight balls. Press each ball flat with hands to form eight small patties.
3. Heat oil in a large frying pan over medium heat.
4. Cook each patty for 3-4 minutes on each side, until golden brown and turkey is cooked through.
5. Serve in lettuce cups with sliced tomato and a dollop of mayonnaise.

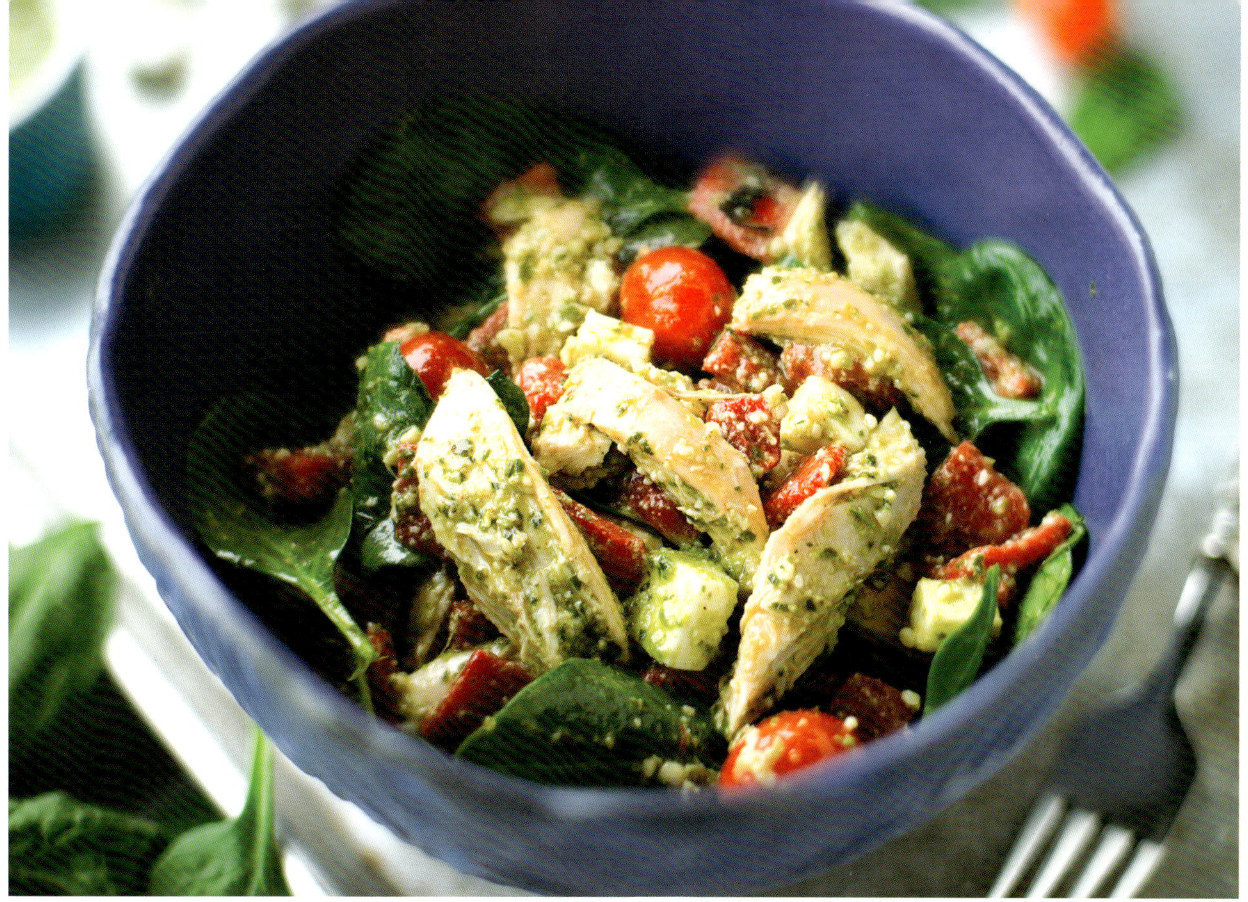

CHICKEN PESTO SALAD

PESTO

2½ cups (80g) fresh basil leaves

½ cup (70g) pine nuts

¾ cup (75g) grated Parmesan cheese

Salt and pepper to taste

⅓ cup (80ml) olive oil

SALAD

600g cooked chicken breasts, cut into small strips

250g cherry tomatoes, halved

¾ cup (40g) semi-dried tomatoes, halved

500g baby spinach leaves

300g feta, cubed

STEPS

1. Place basil leaves and pine nuts in a food processor with Parmesan and salt and pepper to taste. With the motor running, add oil gradually, until the pesto forms a smooth paste.
2. In a large serving bowl toss together the chicken, tomatoes, semi-dried tomatoes, spinach leaves and feta along with the pesto.

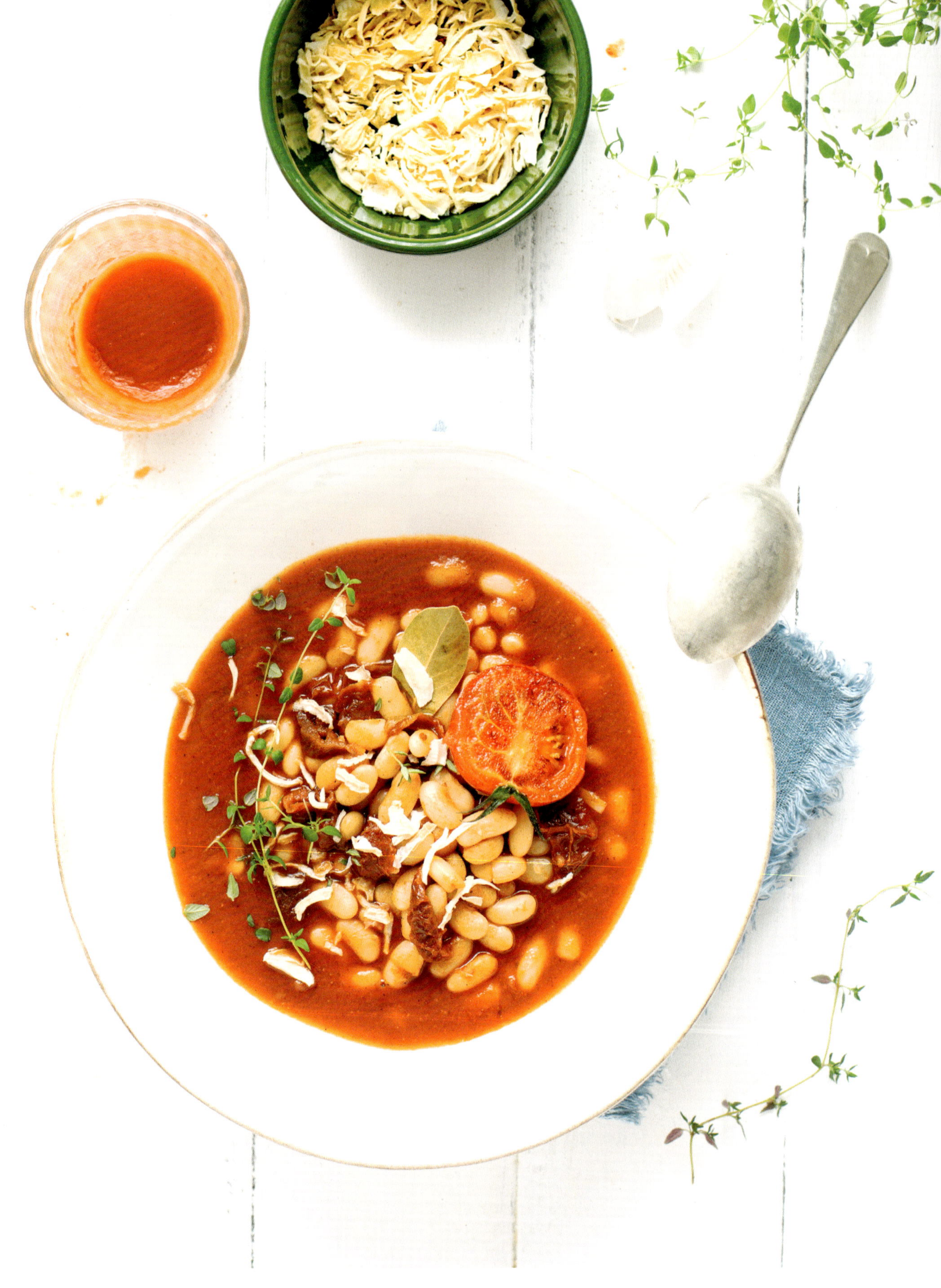

TOMATO & WHITE BEAN SOUP

1 tbsp olive oil

1 medium brown onion, finely chopped

2 cloves garlic, crushed

1 tsp Italian dried mixed herbs

3 large tomatoes, roughly chopped

1 x 400g can crushed tomatoes

1 tbsp tomato paste

3 cups (750ml) vegetable stock

1 tsp Worcestershire sauce

1 x 400g can white beans, rinsed and drained

½ cup (30g) sun-dried tomatoes, roughly chopped

Salt and pepper to taste

STEPS

1. In a large saucepan, heat olive oil over medium-high heat.
2. Add onion, garlic and herbs and cook for about 2-3 minutes until onions are translucent and garlic is fragrant.
3. Add in fresh and tinned tomatoes, tomato paste, vegetable stock and Worcestershire sauce. Bring to a boil and then reduce heat and simmer for 5 minutes, stirring occasionally.
4. Stir in beans and sun-dried tomatoes and continue to simmer gently until all the flavours are combined.
5. Divide into bowls and season with salt and pepper. Add sprigs of thyme to garnish.

NOTE: Beans do contain some carbs, so do not exceed the amount stated in the recipe. A 400g can of white beans contains 15g of carbs. This recipe contains 100g per person but feel free to leave them out altogether if you wish.

SERVES 4 | PREP + COOK TIME: 30 MINS | VEG | GLUTEN FREE | DAIRY FREE |

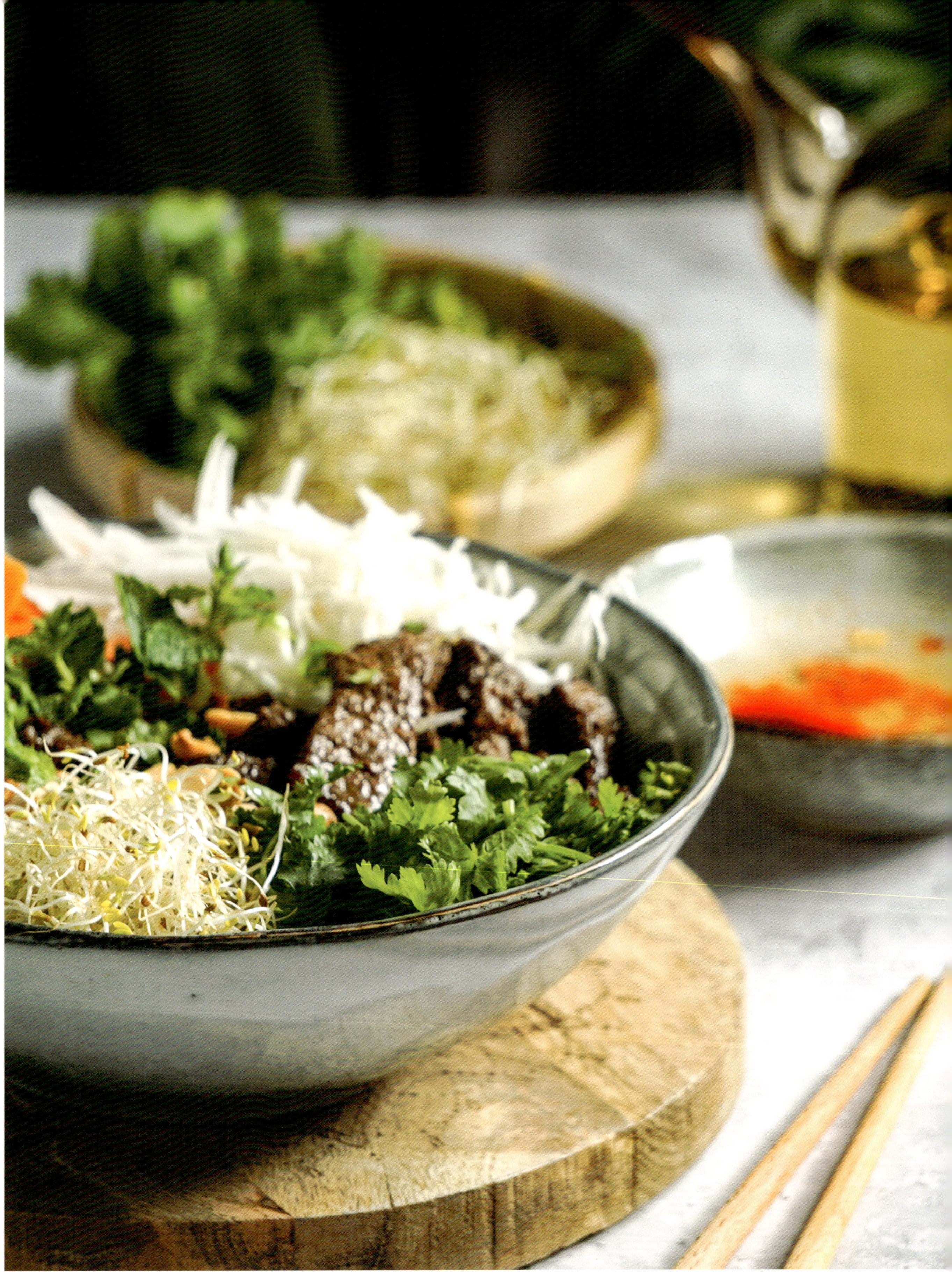

VIETNAMESE BEEF SALAD

BEEF

2 tbsps soy sauce

2 tbsps fish sauce

2 tbsps oyster sauce

2 cloves garlic, minced

1 tbsp white sugar

1 tbsp vegetable oil

450g beef sirloin, thinly sliced

DRESSING

½ tbsp fish sauce

½ tbsp brown sugar

½ tbsp rice wine vinegar

1½ tbsps fresh lime juice

1 clove garlic, crushed

1 tbsp fresh ginger, grated

1 tsp chilli paste (optional)

SALAD

250g rice vermicelli noodles, cooked according to package instructions

1 cup (35g) alfalfa sprouts

Fresh herbs, finely chopped (such as mint and coriander)

1 cucumber, sliced

1 carrot, sliced

Crushed peanuts to garnish

Lime wedges to serve

STEPS

1. In a bowl, combine the soy sauce, fish sauce, oyster sauce, minced garlic, sugar and vegetable oil. Add the sliced beef and marinate for at least 30 minutes.

2. Heat a frying pan over medium-high heat. Cook the marinated beef for about 2-3 minutes on each side, or until cooked to your liking. Remove from heat and set aside.

3. For the dressing, in a small bowl, whisk together the fish sauce, sugar, rice wine vinegar, lime juice, garlic, ginger and chilli paste (if using). Set aside for serving.

4. Assemble the bowls by placing a portion of cooked rice vermicelli noodles in each bowl. Top with the cooked beef, alfalfa sprouts, fresh herbs, sliced cucumber and sliced carrot.

5. Drizzle the dressing over the ingredients in each bowl and sprinkle with crushed peanuts. Serve bun bo nam bo with lime wedges on the side.

SERVES 2 | PREP + COOK TIME: 20 MINS + MARINATING | DAIRY FREE |

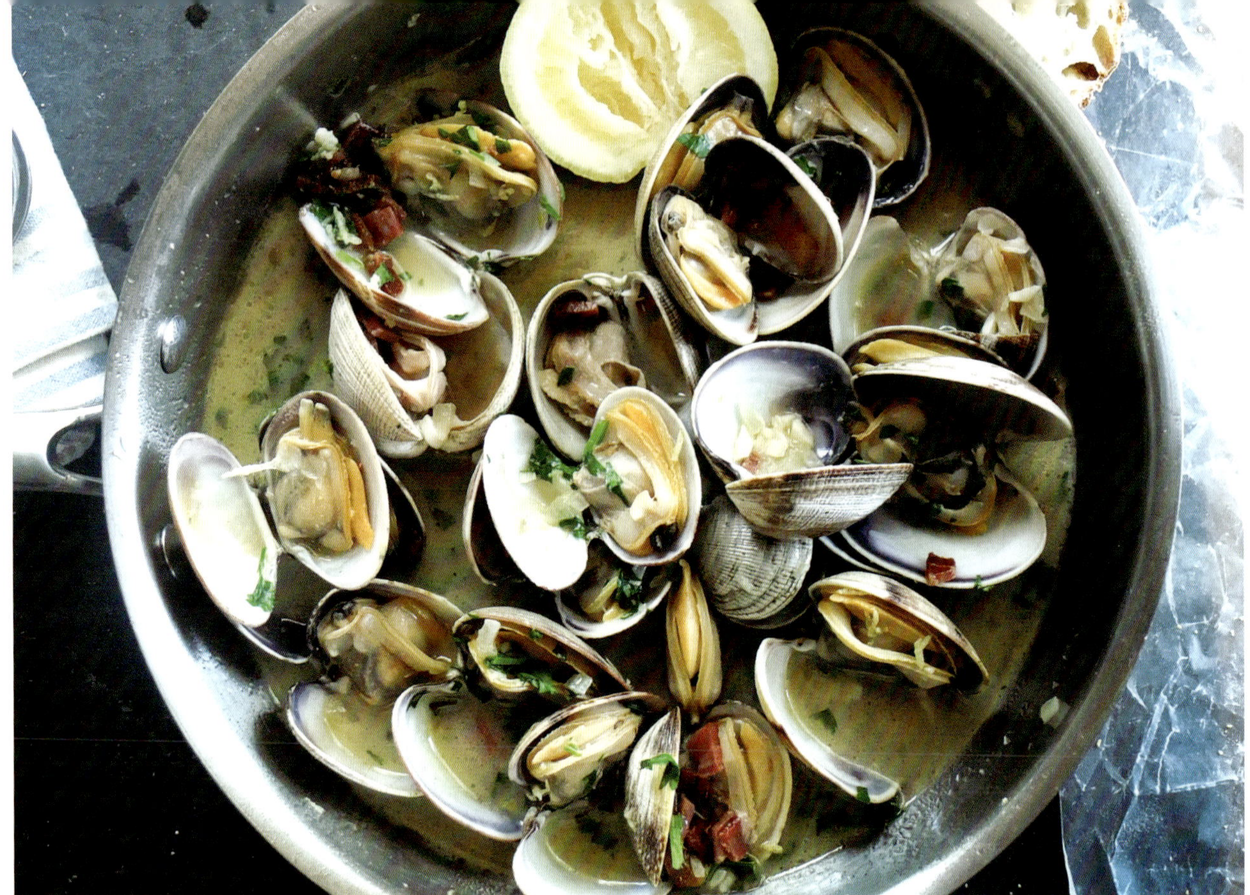

PIPIS WITH WHITE WINE & HERBS

2 tbsps olive oil

2 tbsps butter

1 small onion, finely chopped

2 cloves garlic, crushed

200g bacon, finely chopped

¼ cup (60ml) dry white wine

750g fresh pipis, rinsed thoroughly

3 tbsps parsley, finely chopped

½ cup (125ml) thickened cream

Salt and pepper to taste

Lemon wedges to serve

STEPS

1. In a large, heavy-based saucepan heat olive oil and butter on low-medium heat. Add onion, garlic and bacon and saute until the onion is translucent and garlic is fragrant.
2. Add wine and bring to a simmer and then reduce liquid slightly.
3. Add pipis, stir and cover with a lid; cook for 2 minutes or until pipis start to open.
4. Remove lid and add half the parsley and all of the cream; stir into the pipis and continue to cook until all pipi shells have opened.
5. Transfer the pipis to serving dishes and check the remaining liquid and season to taste. Pour it over the pipis and scatter the rest of the parsley on top. Serve with lemon wedges.

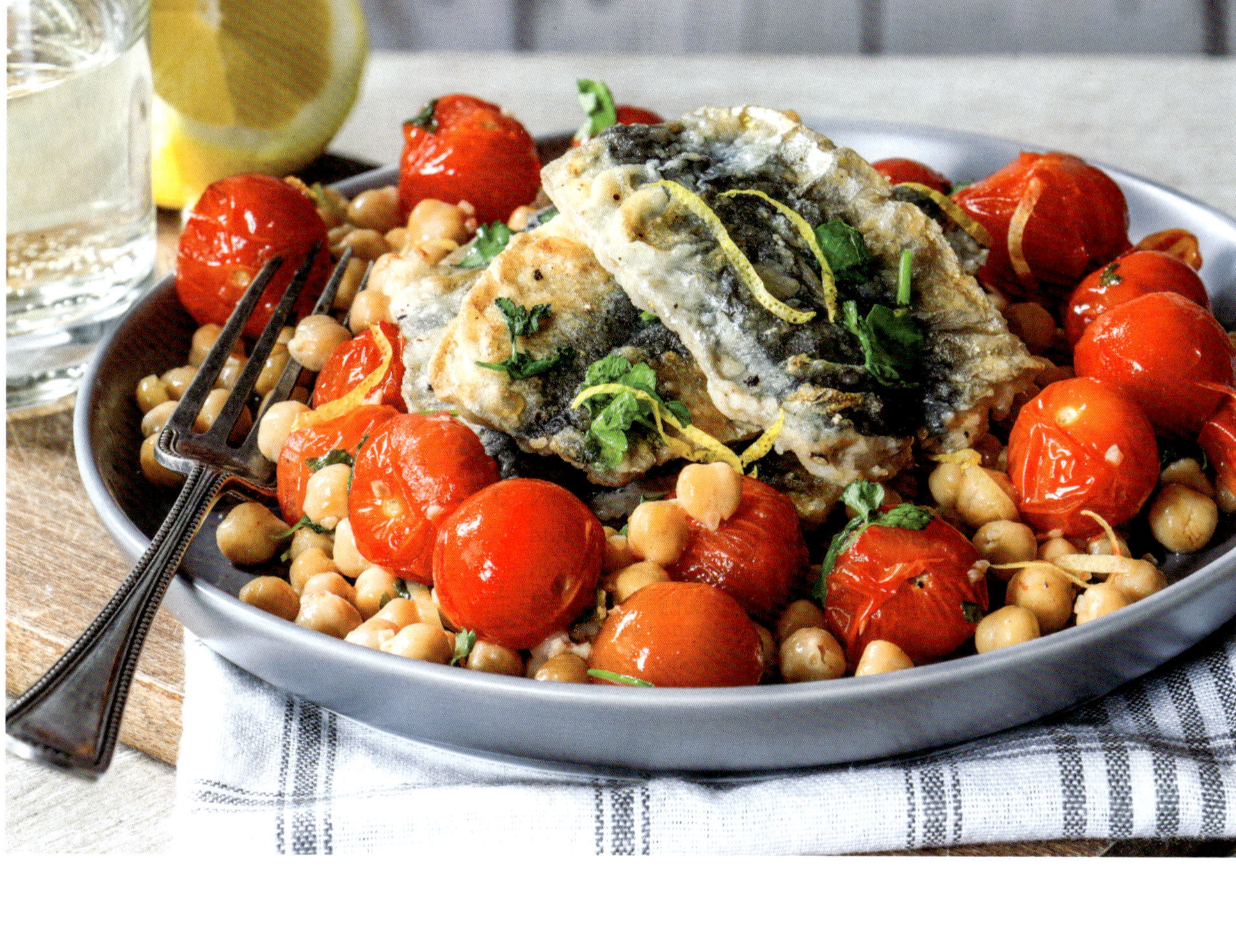

LEMON SARDINES WITH CHICKPEAS

SARDINES

3 cloves garlic, finely minced

¼ cup (60ml) olive oil

1 lemon, juiced

2 tbsps parsley, chopped

½ tsp pepper

8-10 fresh sardines

CHICKPEA SALAD

250g cherry tomatoes, roasted (or serve fresh to save time)

1 x 400g can chickpeas

2 cloves garlic, crushed

1 tbsp fresh thyme leaves

¼ cup (60ml) olive oil

Salt and pepper to taste

Parsley, finely chopped to serve

STEPS

Preheat grill to medium.

1. In a small bowl whisk garlic, oil, lemon juice, parsley and pepper together.
2. Layer sardines flat in a shallow baking dish. Pour over lemon juice mixture. Cover and allow to marinate for 30 minutes.
3. Grill sardines on a medium-high heat for 2-3 minutes or until cooked through, flipping over halfway. Remove from the grill and set aside for serving.
4. To make the salad, place tomatoes, chickpeas, garlic, thyme, olive oil and salt and pepper in a medium bowl. Toss well, making sure chickpeas and cherry tomatoes are well coated.
5. Divide salad among bowls and place fish fillets on top. Serve warm, garnished with fresh parsley.

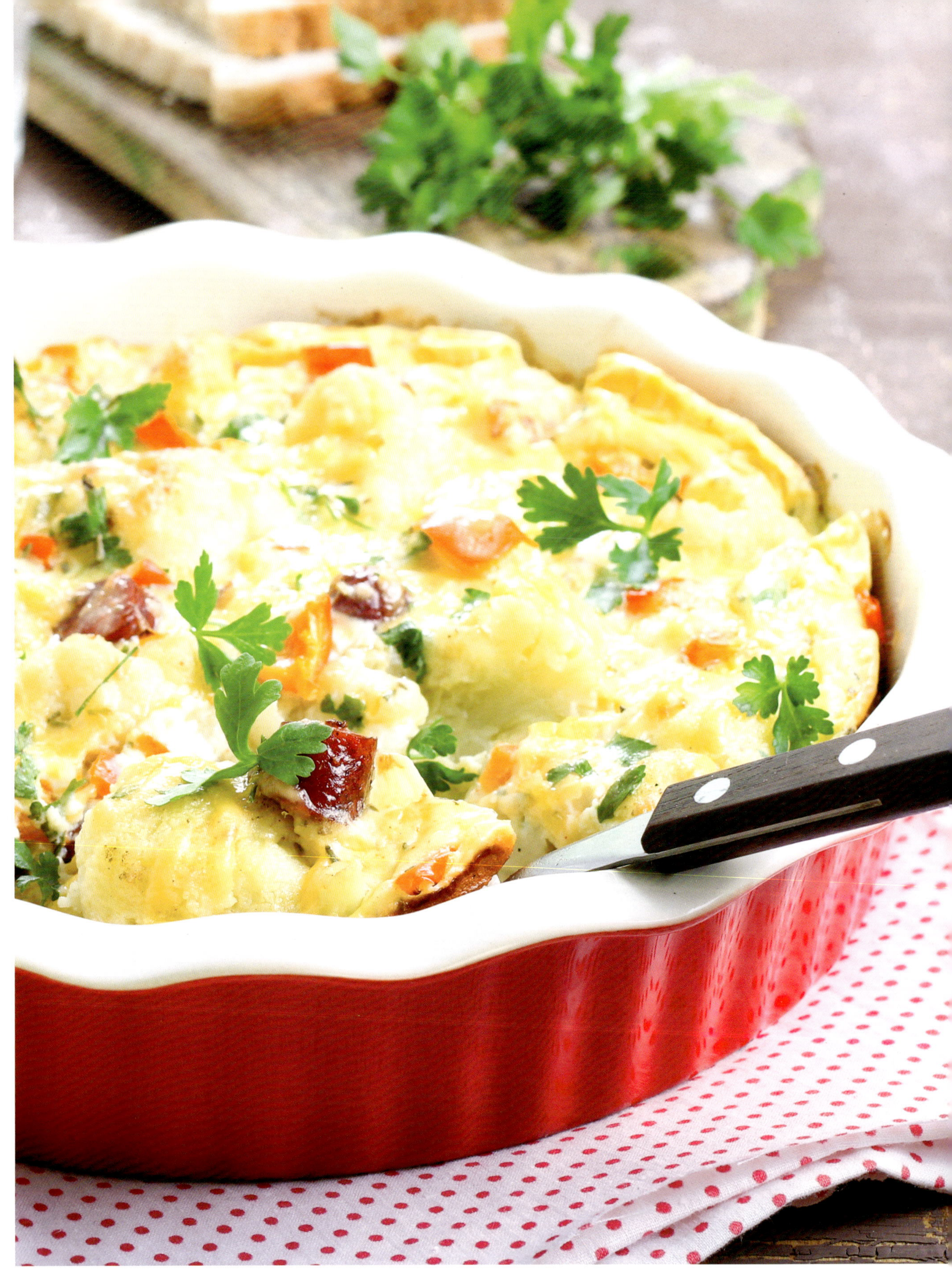

CAULIFLOWER CHORIZO BAKE

SERVES 6 | PREP + COOK TIME: 1 HOUR | GLUTEN FREE |

2 tbsps olive oil

450g chorizo sausage, diced

1 small onion, thinly sliced

3 cloves garlic, crushed

1 tsp paprika

½ tsp dried thyme

Salt and pepper to taste

1 medium head cauliflower, cut into florets and blanched

1 cup (125g) grated Cheddar cheese

½ cup (125ml) cream

Fresh parsley, chopped, to garnish

STEPS

Preheat oven to 180°C.

1. Heat oil in a pan over medium heat, add the chorizo and cook until browned. Remove from the pan and set aside.
2. In the same pan, add onion and garlic. Cook until onion is softened. Return the sausage to the pan and add paprika, dried thyme, salt and pepper. Stir to combine.
3. In a baking dish, layer half of the cauliflower. Top with half of the sausage mixture and sprinkle with half of the cheese. Repeat the layers with the remaining cauliflower, sausage and cheese.
4. Drizzle the cream over the top of the cauliflower and sausage layers and bake in the oven for about 20-25 minutes, or until the cheese is melted and bubbly. Garnish with fresh parsley.

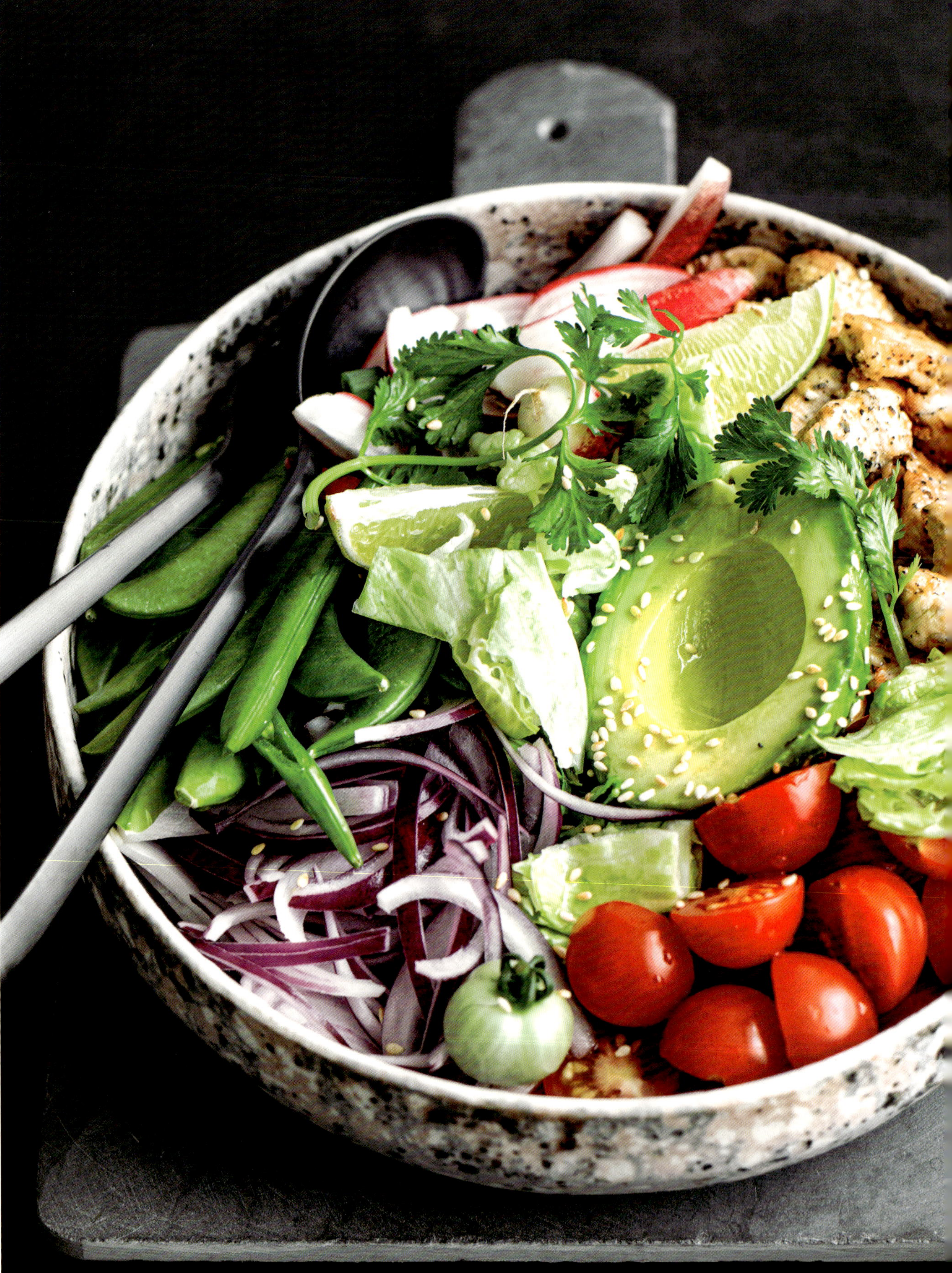

CHICKEN SALAD BOWL WITH MEDITERRANEAN DRESSING

2 x 150g chicken breasts

Salt and pepper to taste

1 tsp olive oil

2 cups (70g) salad leaves, chopped

1 cup (220g) sugar snap peas

½ red onion, sliced

½ cup (110g) cherry tomatoes, halved

3 radishes, halved and thinly sliced

1 avocado, halved

1 tsp white sesame seeds to serve

DRESSING

2 cloves garlic, crushed

½ tsp dried oregano

1 tbsp red wine vinegar

1 tbsp lemon juice

1 tbsp water

¼ cup (60ml) olive oil

STEPS

Preheat oven to 200°C.

1. Coat chicken breast evenly with salt, pepper and olive oil and place onto a prepared oven tray.
2. Bake chicken for 20 minutes or until cooked through. Remove from oven and set aside to rest. Once cooled, slice the chicken into 2cm lengths.
3. To make the dressing, add garlic, oregano, vinegar, lemon juice, water and olive oil to a jar and shake until the dressing is combined and slightly thickened.
4. To assemble the salad, divide salad leaves, sugar snap peas, onion, cherry tomatoes, radishes and avocado into the bowls.
5. Add sliced chicken and pour dressing over the salad; sprinkle with sesame seeds and salt and pepper to taste.

SERVES 2 | PREP + COOK TIME: 45 MINS | GLUTEN FREE | DAIRY FREE |

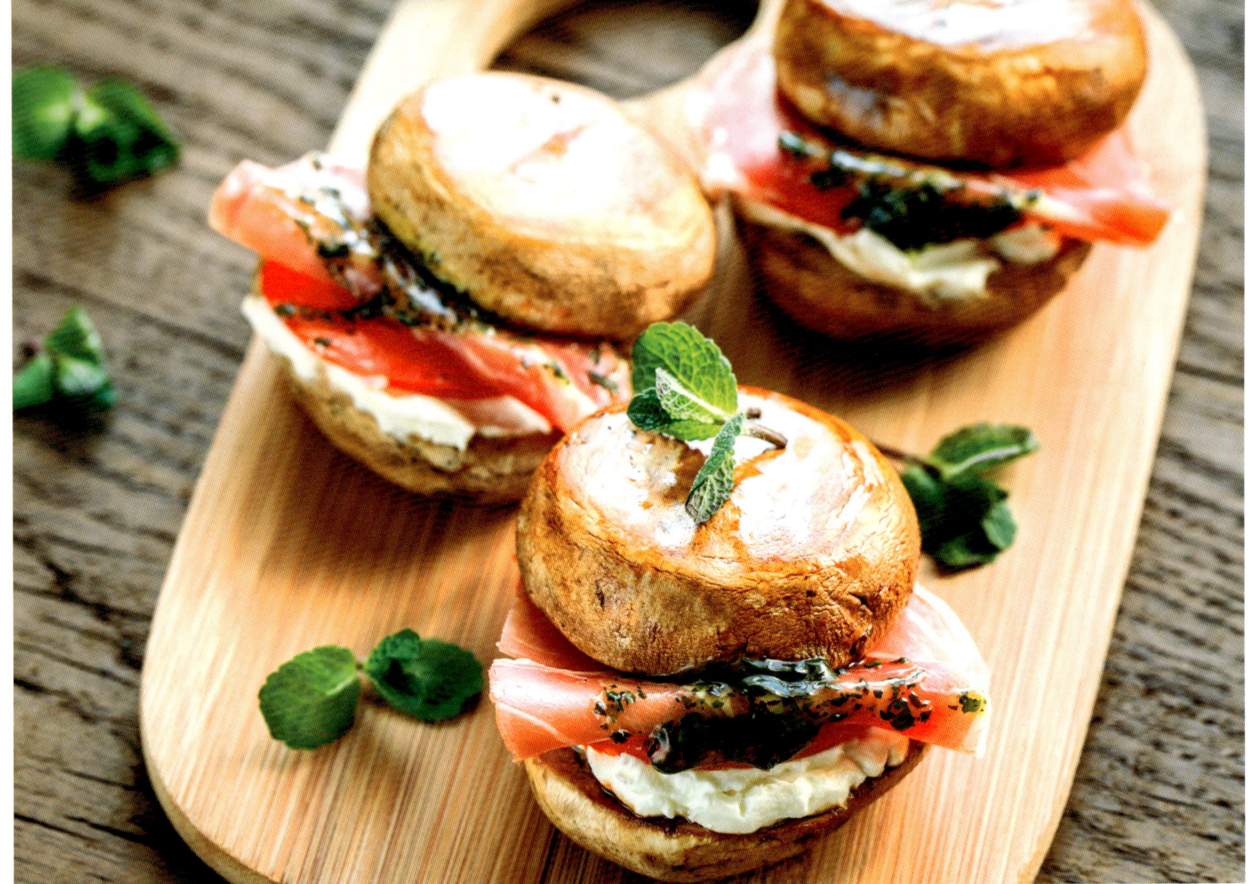

HAM & MINT SAUCE MUSHROOM BURGERS

⅔ cup (160ml) apple cider vinegar

Pinch of stevia powder

3 tbsps finely chopped fresh mint

Salt and pepper to taste

2 tbsps tamari

2 tbsps olive oil

8 large portobello mushrooms, cleaned and stalks removed

115g cream cheese

500g prosciutto

STEPS

1. Place the vinegar and stevia in a small saucepan over medium-high heat and bring to a simmer for 8 minutes. Remove from the heat, stir in the mint and a pinch of salt. Set aside to cool.
2. Mix together the tamari and olive oil as well as a couple of grinds of salt and pepper and lightly brush the mushrooms with the mix.
3. Heat a grill pan or barbecue to medium-high heat. Grill the mushrooms for 3 minutes on each side until just cooked.
4. Top half the mushrooms with a quarter of the cream cheese, a quarter of the ham and some of the mint sauce. Top with the remaining mushrooms to form burgers.

SERVES 2 | PREP + COOK TIME: 20 MINS | GLUTEN FREE | DAIRY FREE |

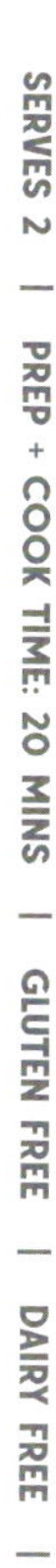

PISTACHIO SEARED TUNA

2 tsps olive oil

1 tbsp finely chopped pistachios

½ tbsp pepper

½ tsp lemon zest

½ tsp red wine vinegar

1 tsp fresh rosemary, chopped

2 x 150g tuna steaks

Salad greens to serve

¼ cup (35g) green olives, pitted and sliced to serve

STEPS

1. Mix together in a small bowl the oil, pistachios, pepper, zest, vinegar and rosemary. Rub the mix into the tuna steaks.
2. Heat a nonstick frying pan to high heat.
3. Fry the steaks for 1½ minutes on each side to sear them.
4. Remove from pan and slice into 1cm-thick slices.
5. Serve with fresh salad greens and olives sprinkled over.

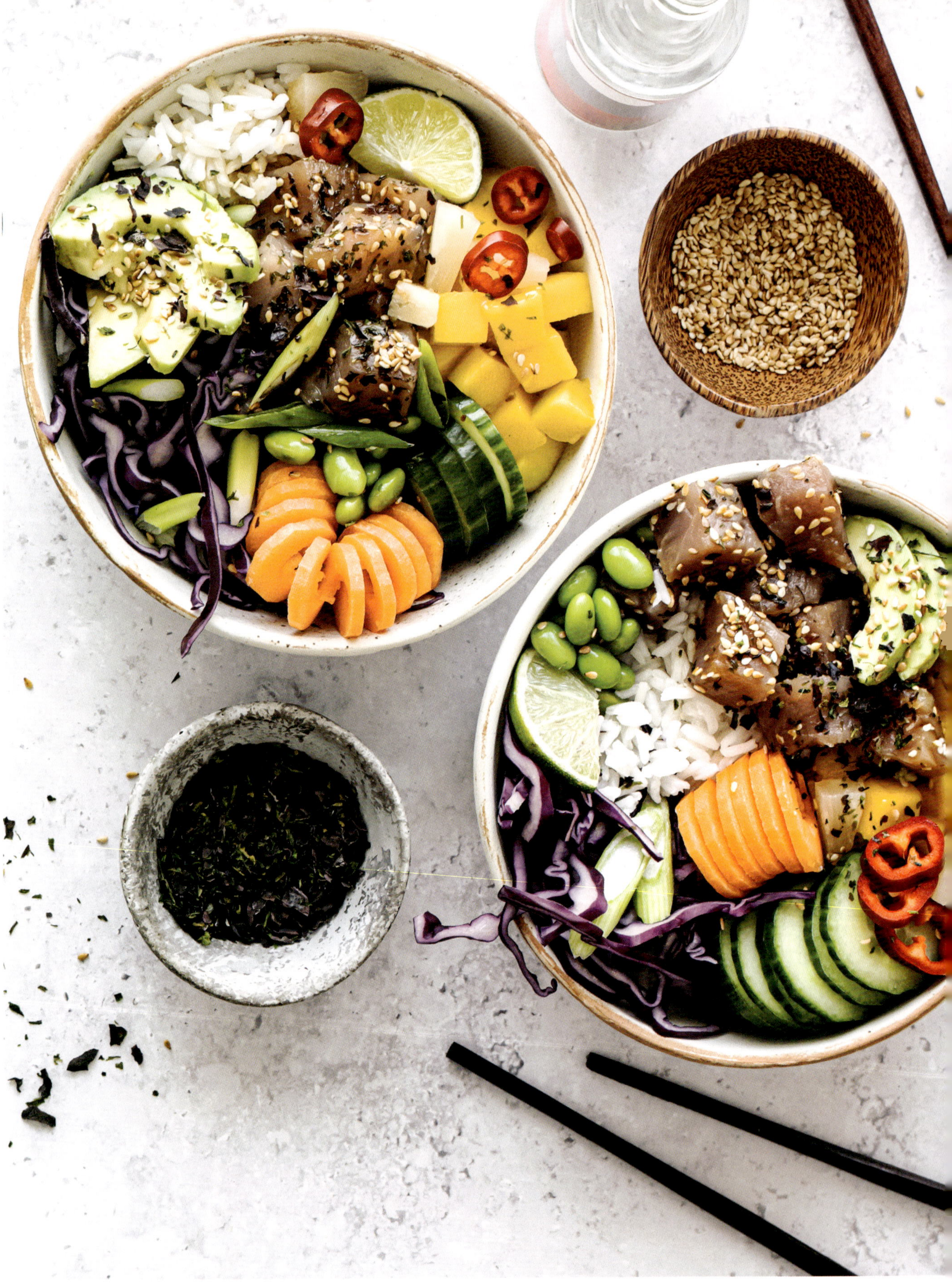

TUNA POKE BOWLS

2 tbsps soy sauce

1 tsp sesame oil

1 tbsp lime juice

1 tsp finely grated ginger

½ tsp Sriracha

1 tsp sesame seeds

400g of sashimi-grade tuna, cubed (see note)

SALAD

2 cups (310g) white or brown rice

1 large cucumber, sliced

½ mango, cubed

1 carrot, sliced

1 cup (100g) finely shredded red cabbage

1 avocado, sliced

½ cup (90g) edamame

3 large spring onions, sliced on an angle

TO GARNISH (OPTIONAL)

Sesame seeds

Seaweed flakes

Limes wedges

Fresh chilli slices

STEPS

1. In a large bowl mix together soy sauce, sesame oil, lime juice, ginger, Sriracha and sesame seeds. Add tuna and gently mix, being careful not break the tuna up. Set aside.
2. Cook rice according to packet instructions and set aside to cool.
3. Build your bowls by adding rice on the bottom then add your prepared vegetables and fruit on top, arranging them around the outside of the bowls and moving inward as you go.
4. Divide the marinated tuna mix between the bowls and top with extra sesame seeds, seaweed flakes, lime wedges and chilli, if desired.

NOTE: Check your local supermarket for vacuum-packed sashimi-grade fish, or ask your fishmonger.

SERVES 4 | PREP + COOK TIME: 15 MINS | DAIRY FREE |

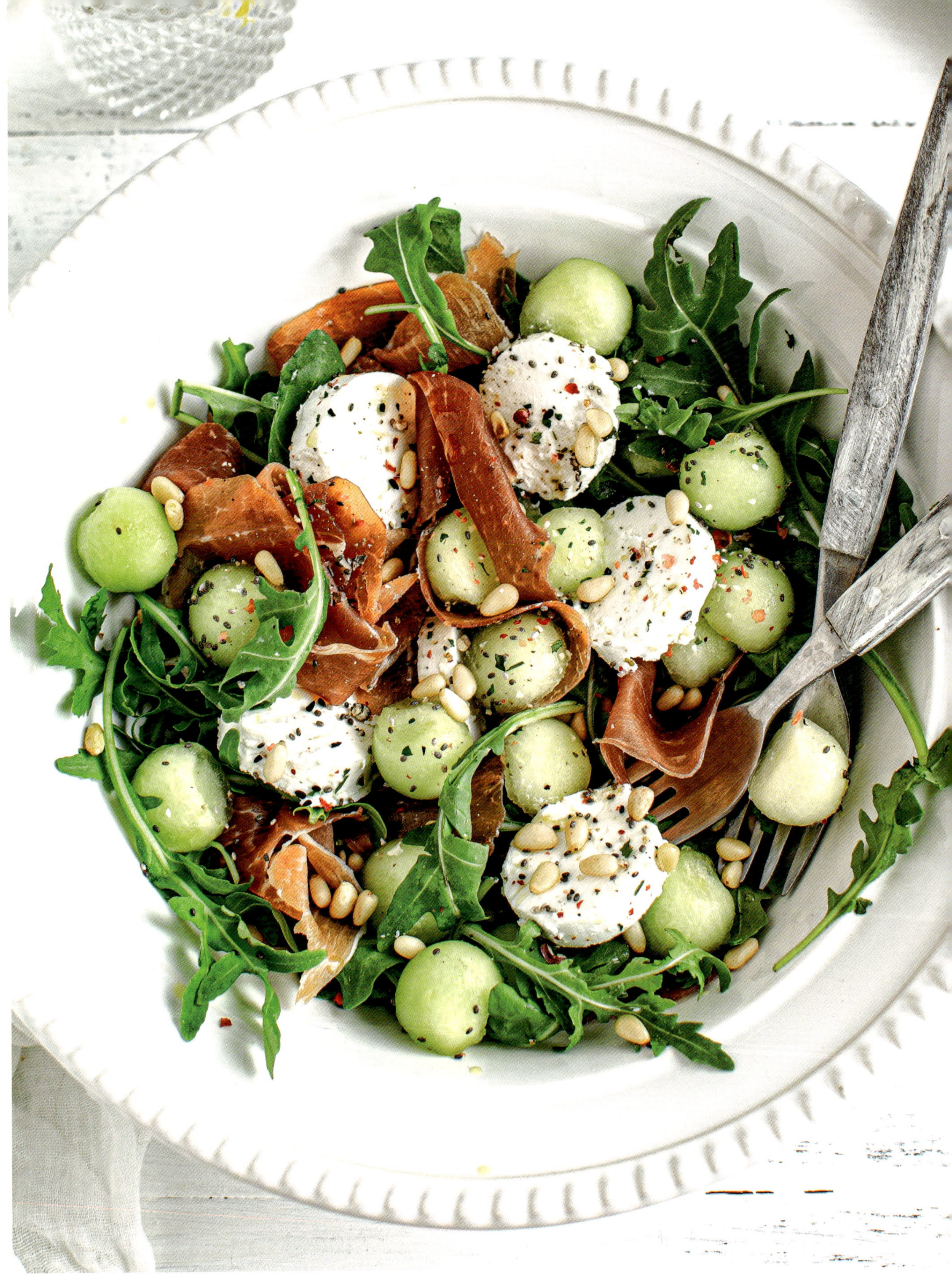

SUMMER SALAD BOWL WITH PARMA HAM

120g rocket leaves

1 honey dew melon, balled or sliced

200g buffalo mozzarella, sliced

6-8 slices of Parma ham, torn

¼ cup (35g) pine nuts, toasted

Salt and pepper to taste

DRESSING

1 tsp mixed Italian dried herbs

3 tbsps olive oil

1 tbsp balsamic vinegar

1 tsp Dijon mustard

STEPS

1. In a large bowl add rocket leaves, melon, sliced mozzarella and Parma ham and toss to combine.
2. For the dressing, in a small bowl add dried herbs, oil, balsamic vinegar and mustard; whisk thoroughly and set aside.
3. To assemble, drizzle the dressing on top of the salad and toss to make sure all the components are coated evenly.
4. Sprinkle with pine nuts and season with salt and pepper. Serve immediately.

SERVES 2 | PREP + COOK TIME: 20 MINS | GLUTEN FREE |

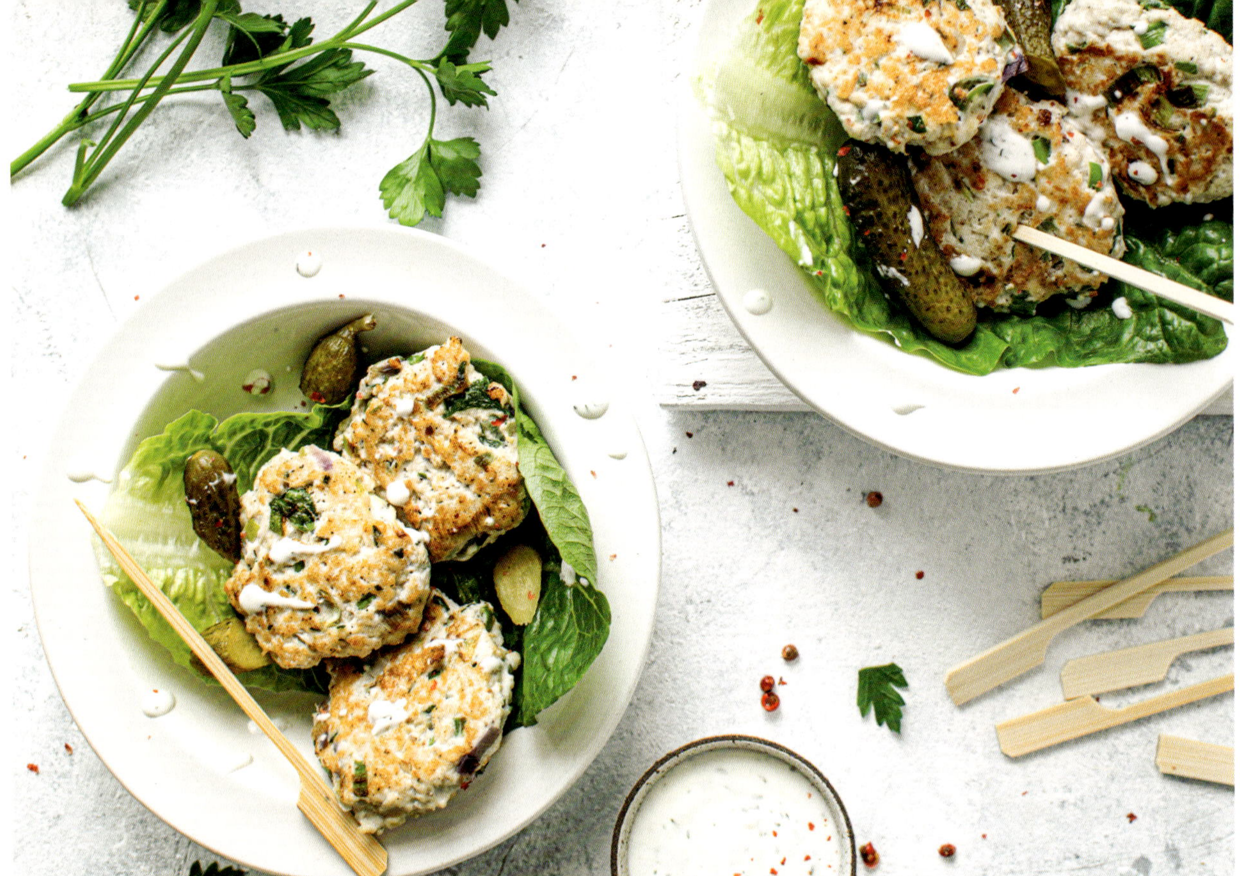

CHICKEN & CORIANDER PATTIES

3 tsps lemon juice

4 tbsps Greek yoghurt

2 tsps parsley, finely chopped

½ birdseye chilli, finely chopped (optional)

Salt and pepper to taste

300g chicken mince

1 small red onion, finely chopped

1 egg

1 clove garlic, crushed

½ tsp chilli powder

½ tsp ground cumin

2 tbsps coriander finely chopped

¼ tsp salt

2 tsps coconut oil

6 baby cos lettuce leaves

¼ cup (40g) sliced gherkins

STEPS

1. In a small bowl add lemon juice, yoghurt, parsley and chilli (if using). Season to taste with salt and pepper and set aside.
2. In a separate bowl add mince, onion, egg, crushed garlic, spices, coriander and salt. Mix vigorously until all the ingredients are well combined.
3. Use your hands to make small patties and set aside.
4. Heat oil in a medium-sized frying pan on medium-high heat then add patties and cook in batches until golden brown, placing on a plate as they get cooked.
5. Divide patties onto cos lettuce leaves placed on plates and serve with dollops of yoghurt sauce and gherkins.

SERVES 4 | PREP + COOK TIME: 25 MINS | VEG | GLUTEN FREE | DAIRY FREE |

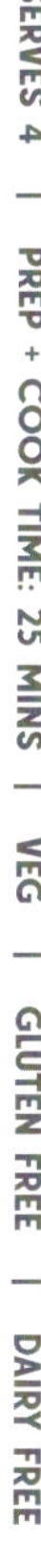

CRUNCHY QUINOA SALAD

1¼ cups (210g) white quinoa

2 cups (500ml) water

1 cucumber, diced

½ cup (110g) cherry tomatoes, halved

1 large yellow capsicum, sliced

4 cups (120g) baby spinach, chopped

½ cup (20g) parsley, roughly chopped

½ cup (20g) dill, roughly chopped

1 spring onion, finely sliced

Salt and pepper to taste

1½ tbsps olive oil

STEPS

1. Rinse quinoa in cold water. Pour into a medium-sized pot with the water. Bring to a boil then reduce heat and simmer, covered, for 15 minutes. Drain and set aside.

2. Toss all the ingredients together in a salad bowl with salt and pepper and drizzle olive oil over the top.

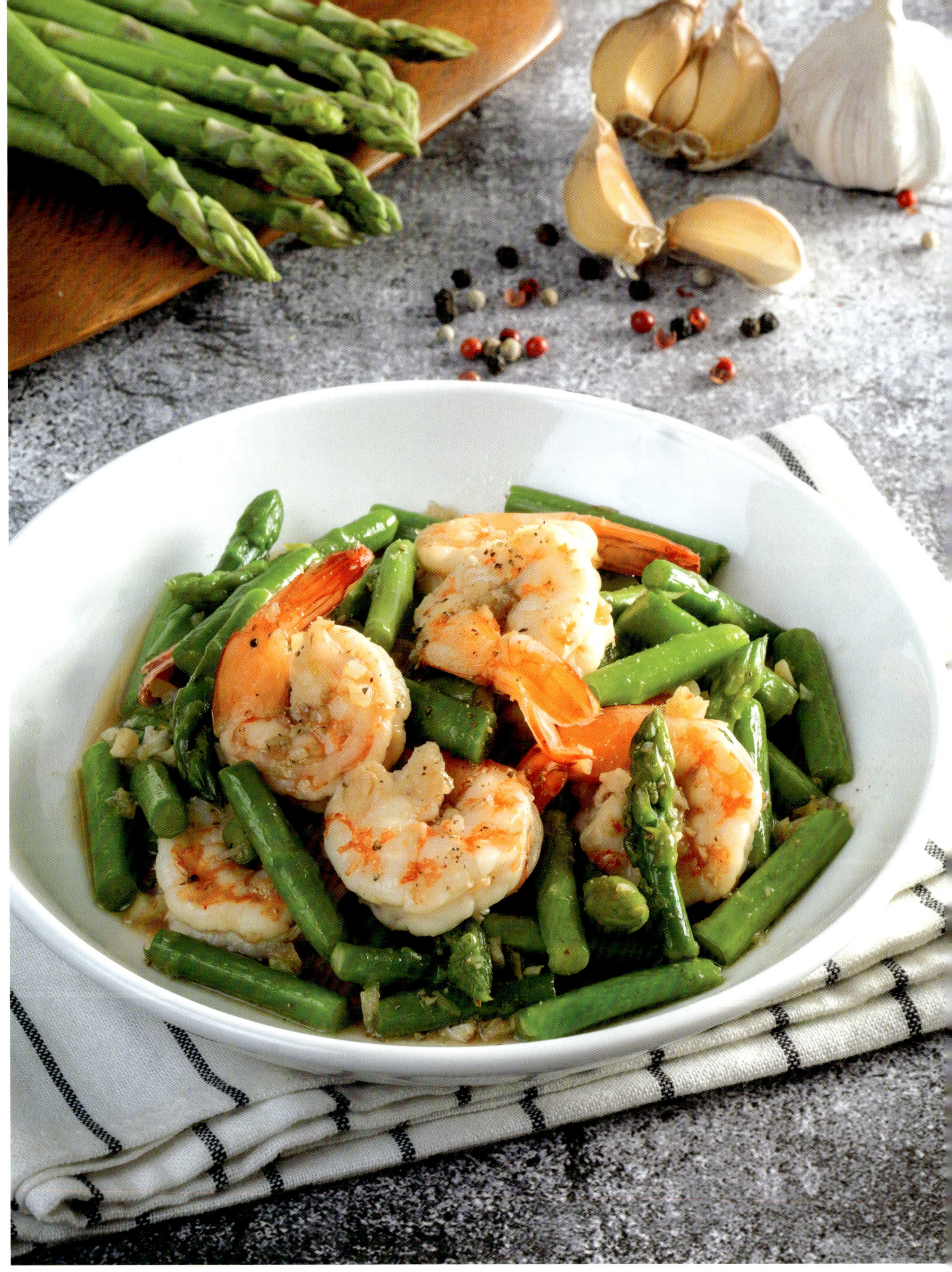

PRAWN & ASPARAGUS STIR-FRY

2 cloves garlic, minced

Small piece ginger, grated

2 tbsps soy sauce

1 tbsp oyster sauce

1 tbsp sesame oil

½ tsp sugar

1 tbsp vegetable oil

450g prawns, peeled and deveined

1 bunch asparagus, trimmed and cut into 4cm pieces

Salt and pepper to taste

STEPS

1. In a medium bowl, combine the minced garlic, grated ginger, soy sauce, oyster sauce, sesame oil and sugar. Stir well to combine.
2. Heat the vegetable oil in a large frying pan or wok over medium-high heat. Add the prawns and stir-fry for 2-3 minutes until they turn pink and are cooked through. Remove the prawns from the pan and set aside.
3. In the same pan, add the asparagus and stir-fry for 2-3 minutes until tender-crisp. Return the cooked prawns to the pan with the asparagus.
4. Pour the sauce mixture over the prawns and asparagus. Stir-fry for another minute or until everything is well coated and heated through. Season with salt and pepper to taste.
5. Remove from heat and serve the stir-fry hot on its own or with rice noodles.

SERVES 4 | PREP + COOK TIME: 20 MINS | DAIRY FREE |

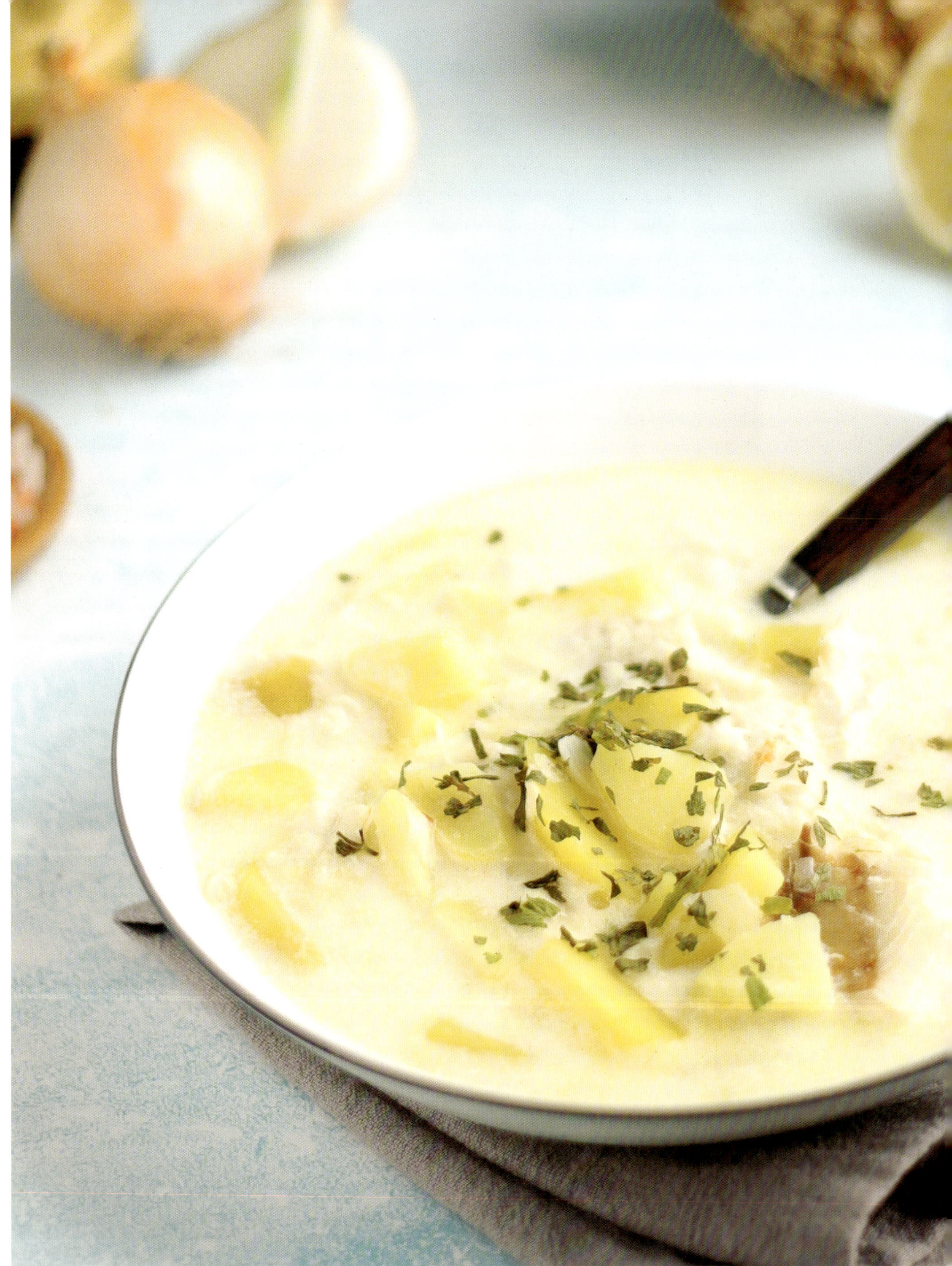

CREAMY FISH CHOWDER

1½ tbsps butter

1 leek, sliced

2 cloves garlic, minced

2 cups (500ml) fish stock (or vegetable stock)

1 head cauliflower, cut into florets

1 medium potato, cubed (optional)

1⅔ cups (400ml) milk

1 bay leaf

400g smoked cod (or smoked mackerel or smoked trout)

⅓ cup (100ml) thickened cream

Salt and pepper to taste

1 tbsp chopped chives

STEPS

1. Heat butter in a saucepan over medium heat. Add leek and garlic; cook for 5-10 minutes. Add the stock and bring to a simmer, then add the cauliflower and potato and continue to simmer for 10 minutes.

2. Meanwhile in a separate pan heat milk and bay leaf. Add fish, cover with a lid, then turn off the heat. Allow the fish to poach in the milk for 5 minutes or until cooked through.

3. Retrieve some potato pieces to serve, then blend the cauliflower and the rest of the potato and stock with a stick blender.

4. Using a slotted spoon, remove fish and bay leaf from poaching milk and flake the fish into large chunks. Discard bay leaf.

5. Add poaching milk to the soup along with the cream. Blend once more. Spoon into bowls and top with the flaked fish and potato pieces and scatter with chopped chives.

SERVES 4 | PREP + COOK TIME: 45 MINS | GLUTEN FREE |

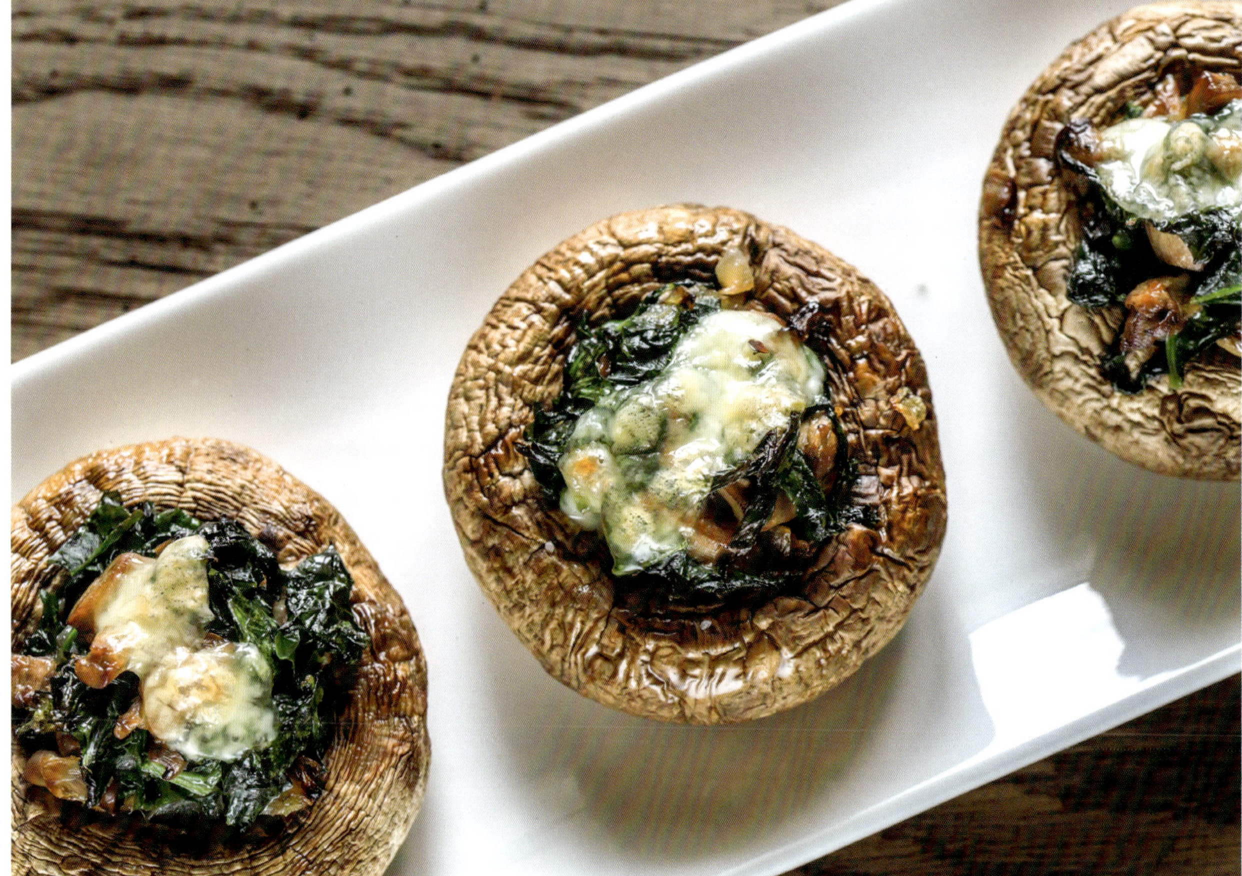

SPINACH-STUFFED MUSHROOMS

12 flat white mushrooms

2 tbsps olive oil

2 cloves garlic, minced

4 cups (120g) fresh spinach leaves

Salt and pepper to taste

½ cup (60g) shredded mozzarella cheese

¼ cup (25g) grated Parmesan cheese

STEPS

Preheat oven to 180°C.

1. Remove the stems from the mushrooms and gently scrape out the gills to create space for the stuffing.
2. In a large frying pan, heat oil over medium heat. Add garlic and saute for about 1 minute until fragrant. Add the spinach and cook until wilted, about 2-3 minutes. Season with salt and pepper to taste.
3. Remove from the pan and chop the spinach into small pieces. Add the spinach to a mixing bowl and combine with mozzarella, Parmesan, salt and pepper. Mix well to combine.
4. Stuff each mushroom cap with the spinach and cheese mixture. Place the stuffed mushrooms on a lined baking tray and bake for 30 minutes or until cheese has melted.

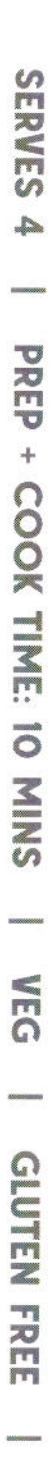

GREEK SALAD

1 cup (225g) cherry tomatoes, halved

1 tsp dried thyme + extra to serve

1 red onion, thinly sliced

½ cup (75g) pitted Kalamata olives, sliced

½ cup (125ml) olive oil

200g Greek feta, cubed

2 Lebanese cucumbers

STEPS

1. Trim the ends from the cucumbers, then cut in half lengthways. Using a spiraliser with the thinnest attachment, spiralise the cucumber into long, thin strands. (See note).
2. Combine tomatoes, thyme, onion, olives and half the oil in a serving bowl and toss gently to combine.
3. To assemble the salad divide cucumber into bowls and layer the tomato mixture on top.
4. Sprinkle over the feta and extra thyme leaves then drizzle with remaining oil. Serve immediately.

NOTE: If you don't have a spiraliser, use a potato peeler to create cucumber strips.

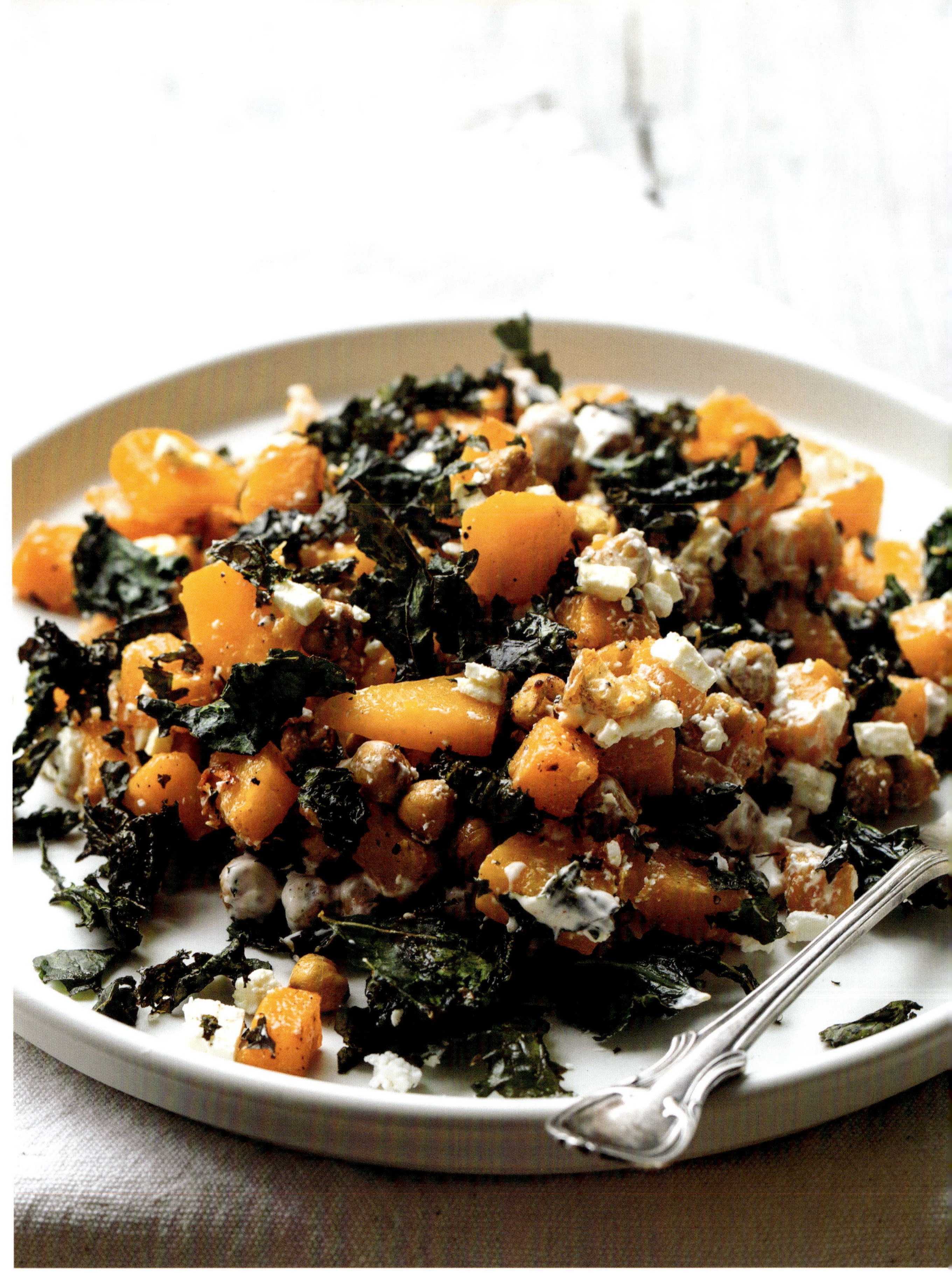

WARM PUMPKIN, KALE & FETA SALAD

2 cups (270g) diced pumpkin

1 bunch Tuscan kale, stems removed and leaves torn into bite-size pieces

1 x 400g can chickpeas

2 tbsps olive oil

2 tbsps balsamic vinegar

1 tbsp honey (optional, for added sweetness)

Salt and pepper to taste

½ cup (60g) pecans, roughly chopped

¼ cup (60g) crumbled feta cheese

STEPS

Preheat oven to 200°C.

1. Place the diced pumpkin, Tuscan kale and chickpeas on a lined baking tray, drizzle with 1 tablespoon of olive oil, and season with salt and pepper. Toss to coat, making sure all the ingredients are well coated.
2. Roast the pumpkin mixture in the preheated oven for about 20-25 minutes or until it is tender and lightly caramelised.
3. While the pumpkin is roasting, make the dressing. In a small bowl, whisk together the balsamic vinegar, the rest of the olive oil and honey (if using).
4. Once the pumpkin, kale and chickpeas are cooked, remove from the oven and let cool slightly.
5. In a large salad bowl, combine the roasted pumpkin, kale, chickpeas, chopped pecans and crumbled feta, then drizzle the dressing over the salad and toss gently to combine.

SERVES 4 | PREP + COOK TIME: 40 MINS | VEG | GLUTEN FREE |

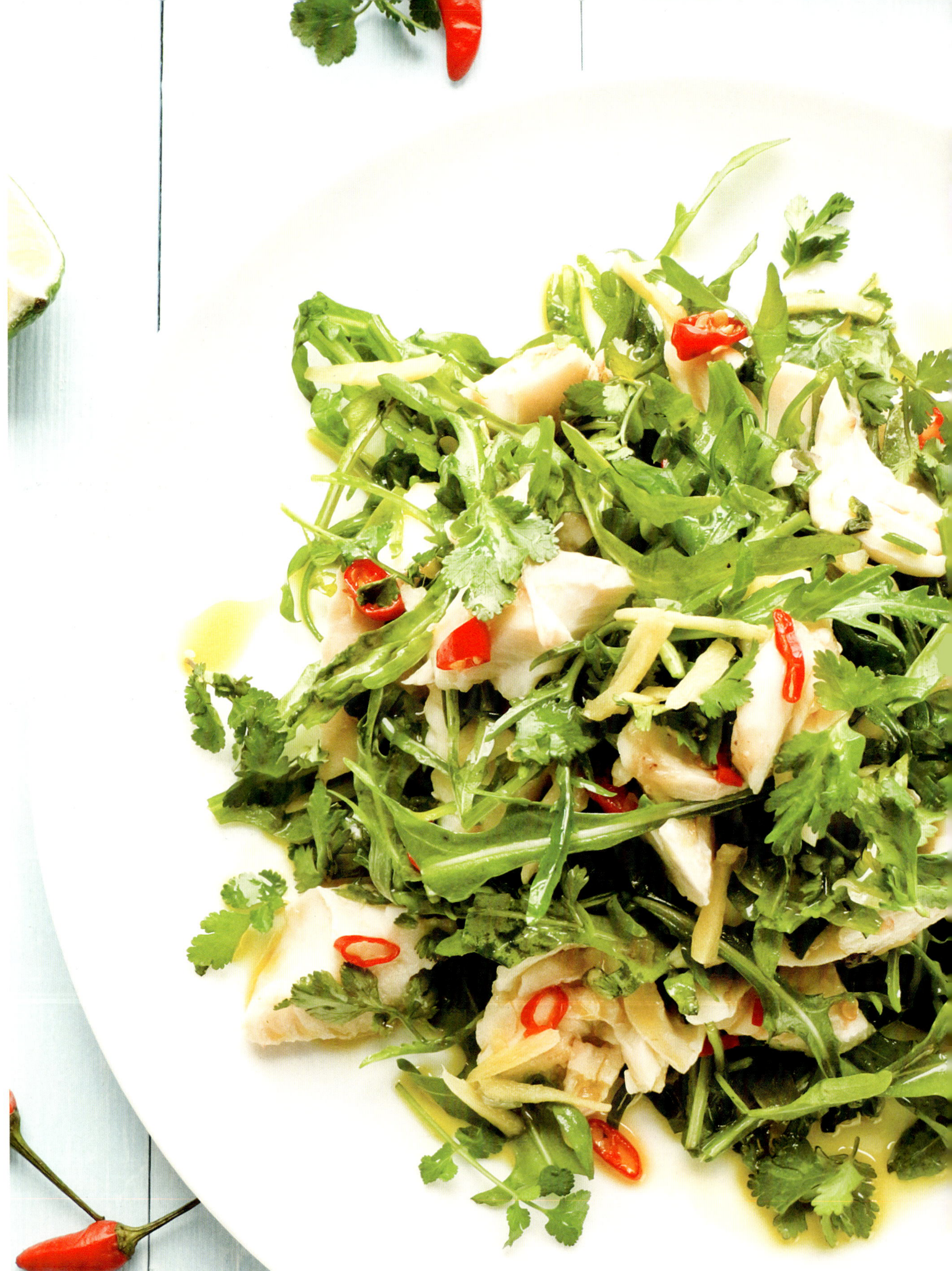

ASIAN-STYLE SNAPPER SALAD

700g snapper fillets, deboned, skin removed

1 tbsp minced fresh ginger + small piece ginger, sliced into thin matchsticks

1 large lemon, zested and juiced

⅓ cup (75ml) olive oil

300g rocket leaves

3 small red chillies, deseeded and sliced

¼ cup (10g) fresh coriander leaves, roughly chopped

¼ cup (60ml) flaxseed oil

Salt and pepper to taste

STEPS

Preheat oven to 180°C.

1. Place the snapper fillets in large squares of baking paper.
2. Mix together the minced ginger, ½ tablespoon lemon zest and 1 tablespoon of the olive oil and drizzle over the snapper. Fold up the baking paper into parcels and wrap the parcels in foil.
3. Bake for 15 minutes until the snapper is cooked through. Set aside to cool, then flake into bite-size pieces.
4. Place the rocket, chillies, sliced ginger, coriander and snapper in a large bowl.
5. Whisk together the remaining olive oil, the flaxseed oil and 1 tablespoon lemon juice along with a couple of grinds of salt and pepper. Drizzle the dressing over the top and serve.

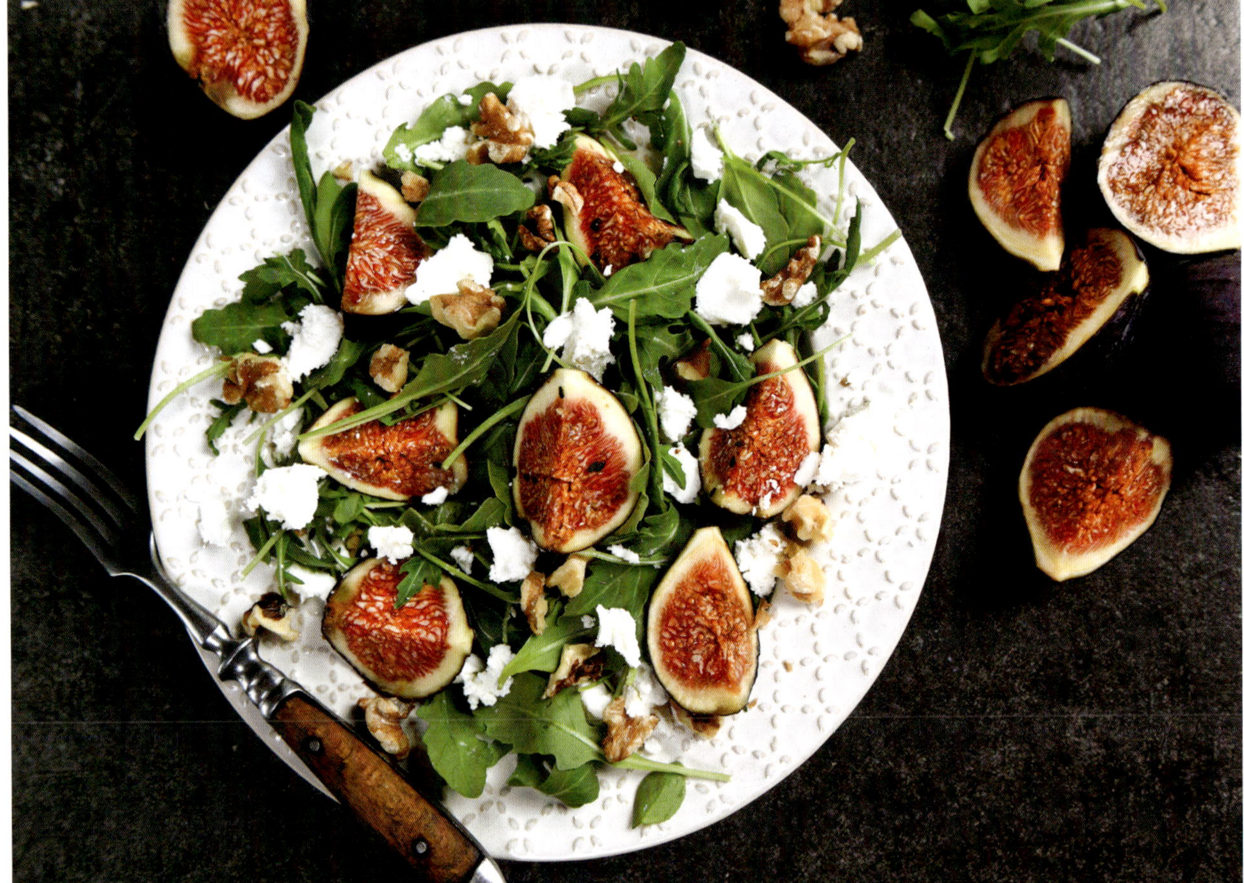

ROCKET, FIG & FETA SALAD

¾ cup (90g) pecans

3 cups (90g) rocket leaves

2 large green figs, cut into quarters

¾ cup (180g) feta

GLAZE

1 cup (250ml) balsamic vinegar

2 tbsps brown sugar

Pinch of salt

STEPS

1. Dry fry the pecans in a small frying pan over medium heat for 2 minutes until just starting to brown. Remove immediately from the pan and set aside.
2. To make the glaze, heat the vinegar in a medium frying pan over medium heat until simmering. Cook for 10 minutes until reduced by about half. Add the sugar and salt and stir until dissolved. Remove from heat into a pouring jug.
3. Arrange the rocket, figs, feta and pecans on your serving plates.
4. Drizzle over the glaze and serve.

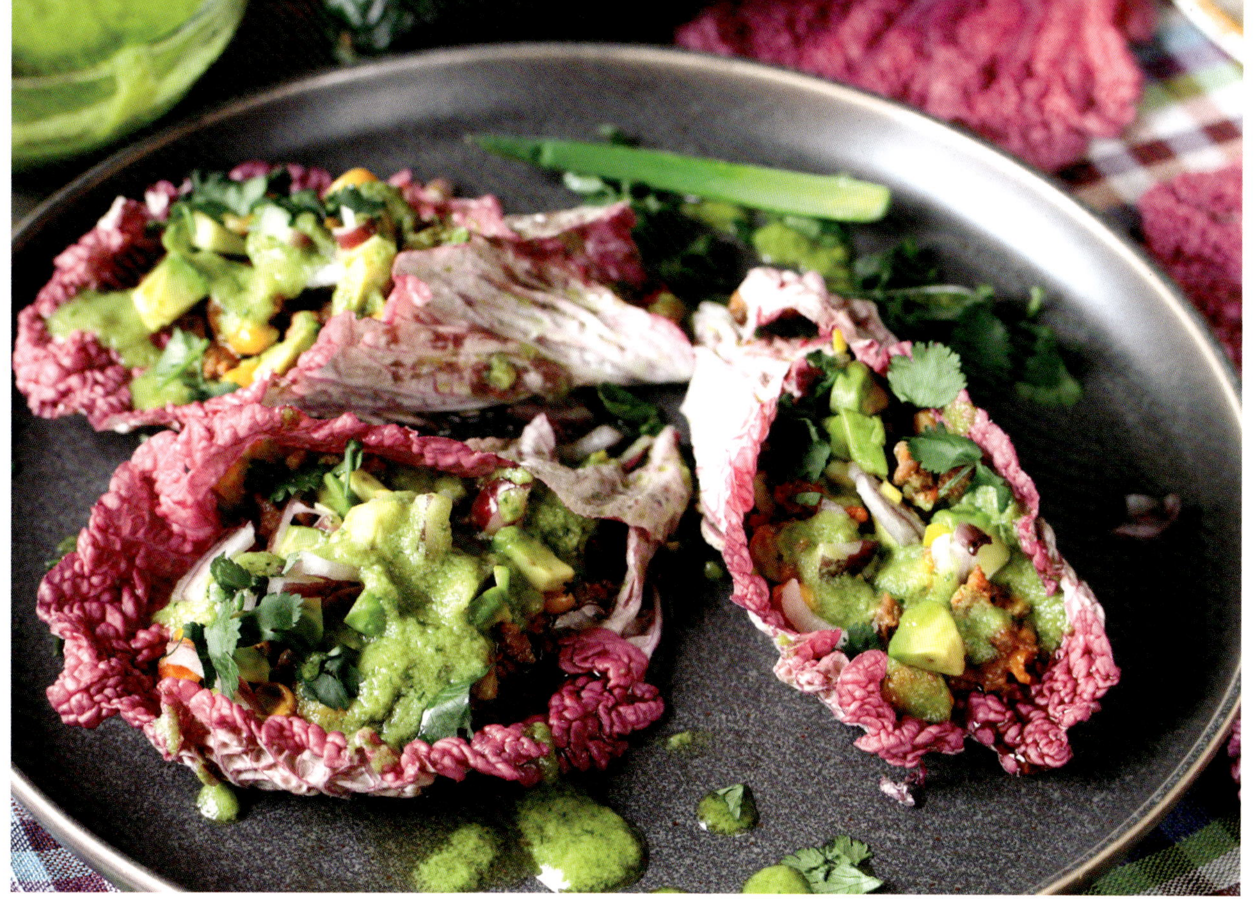

SERVES 4 | PREP + COOK TIME: 30 MINS | GLUTEN FREE | DAIRY FREE |

WOMBOK WRAPS WITH AVOCADO MAYO

3 large avocados, diced
2 tsps lemon juice
2 tbsps coconut oil
2 tsps apple cider vinegar
¼ cup (60ml) water
Salt and pepper to taste
1 tbsp olive oil
½ medium red onion, chopped
500g beef mince
½ cup (85g) corn kernels
¼ cup (60ml) tamari
1 large wombok (Chinese cabbage; red or white)

STEPS

1. To make the mayo, place ⅔ cup of the diced avocado, the lemon juice, coconut oil, vinegar, water and a pinch each of salt and pepper in a blender and puree until smooth. Season further to taste and set aside.
2. Heat the olive oil in a medium frying pan over medium heat. Fry the onion for 2 minutes, then add the beef and fry for 5 more minutes until browned. Add the corn, tamari and a couple of grinds of salt and pepper and cook for another 5 minutes.
3. To serve, separate the wombok leaves and fill with portions of the warm beef mince, top with avocado and drizzle the avocado mayonnaise over the top.

NOTE: Wombok comes in a red variety (pictured) and more commonly in pale green. Either variety is fine to use for this recipe.

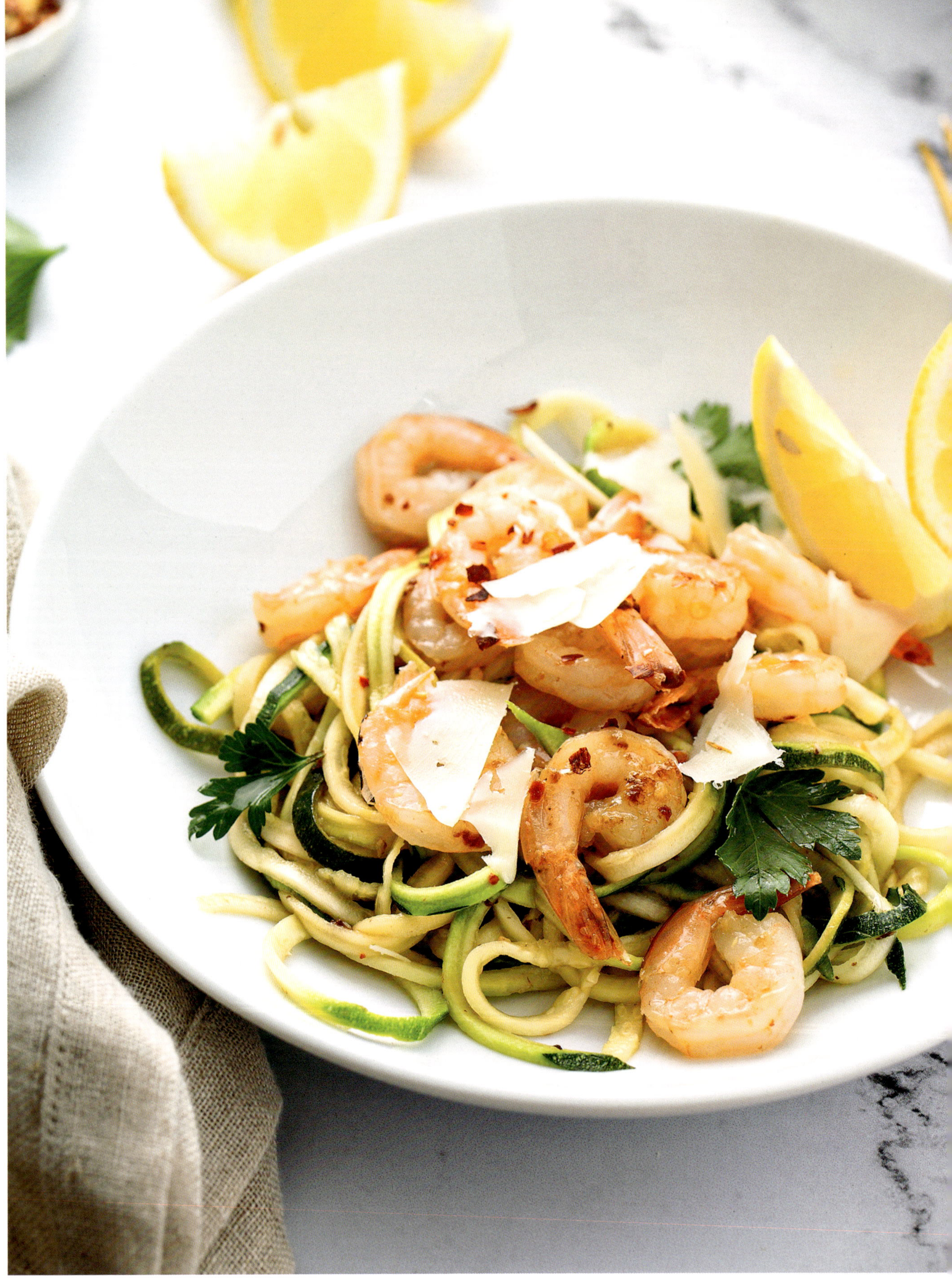

SPICY PRAWNS WITH ZOODLES

2 cloves garlic, minced

1 tsp chilli flakes

1 tbsp olive oil

Salt and pepper to taste

450g large prawns, peeled and deveined

1 cup (250ml) chicken or vegetable stock

3-4 medium zucchinis, spiralised into noodles

Handful of fresh parsley, chopped

Lemon wedges to serve

Shaved Parmesan cheese to serve

STEPS

1. Mix the garlic, chilli flakes, oil and a couple of grinds of salt and pepper and toss with the prawns.
2. Heat a large nonstick frying pan over medium-high heat. Fry the prawns for 2 minutes on each side until cooked through. Set aside.
3. Add the stock to the pan, bring to a simmer then add the zucchini and stir for 3 minutes until the zucchini is cooked through. Drain off any excess liquid.
4. Toss the prawns with the zucchini noodles and parsley.
5. Season to taste and serve with lemon wedges and shaved Parmesan cheese.

SERVES 4 | PREP + COOK TIME: 30 MINS | GLUTEN FREE |

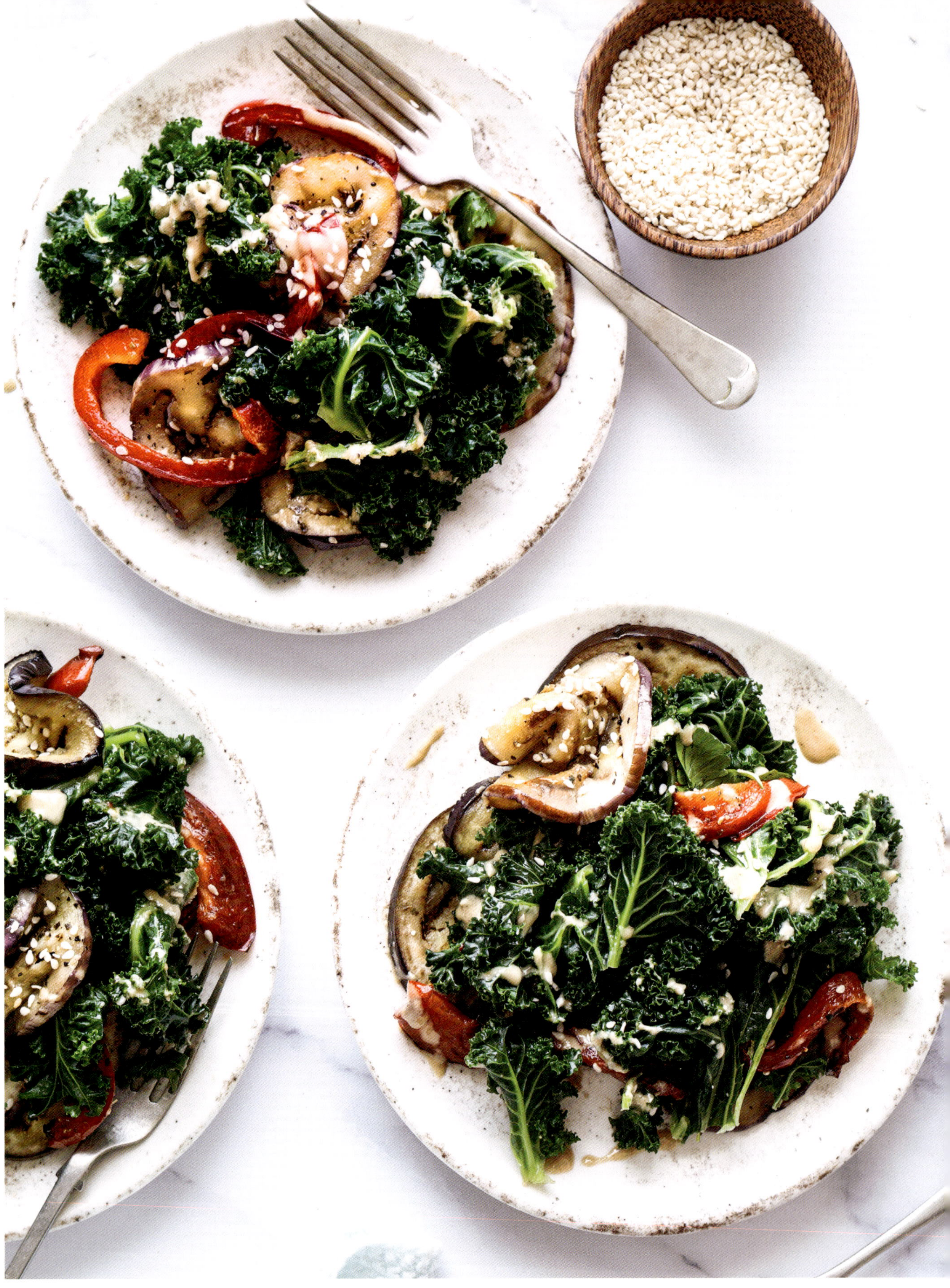

EGGPLANT & KALE SALAD WITH TAHINI DRESSING

DRESSING

⅓ cup (80ml) olive oil

6 tbsps tahini paste

1 tsp lemon juice

1 small clove garlic, crushed

1 tbsp water

Salt and pepper to taste

SALAD

2 tbsps olive oil

2 large eggplants, thinly sliced

1 bunch curly kale, roughly chopped

Salt and pepper to taste

1 cup (240g) store-bought roasted capsicums strips, drained

¼ cup (10g) parsley, roughly chopped (retain a few sprigs to garnish)

1 tbsp sesame seeds

STEPS

1. To make the dressing, combine all the dressing ingredients in a small bowl. Set aside.
2. Heat a grill pan or barbecue over high heat. Brush eggplant slices with half the oil. Cook eggplant, in batches, for 4-5 minutes each side, or until browned and tender.
3. Massage chopped kale with remaining olive oil and salt and pepper and divide into bowls.
4. Add eggplant, capsicums and the parsley to the bowls and then drizzle a generous amount of dressing in each.
5. Garnish with a sprinkling of sesame seeds and parsley sprigs.

SERVES 4 | PREP + COOK TIME: 40 MINS | VEG | GLUTEN FREE | DAIRY FREE |

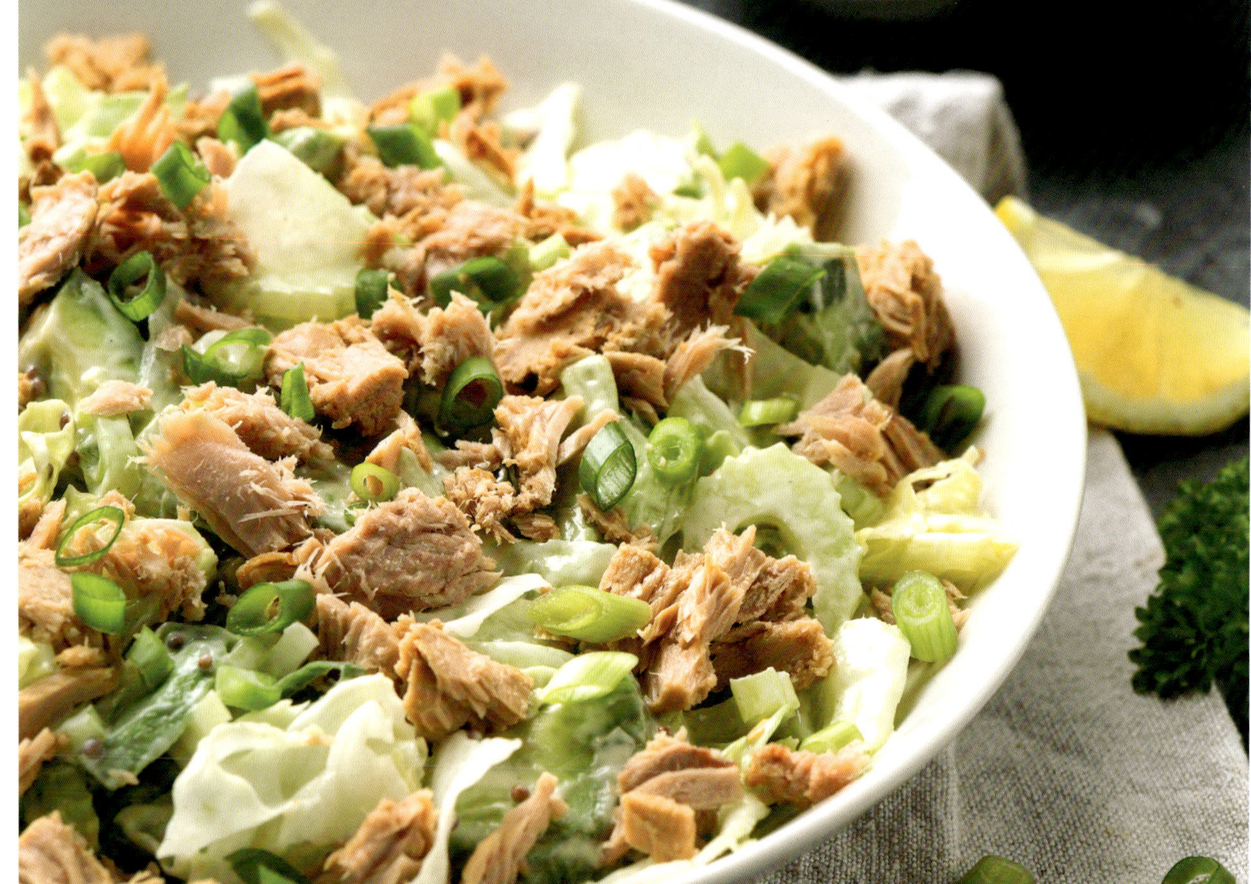

SMOKED TUNA & CELERY SALAD

2 x 95g cans smoked tuna, drained and flaked

2 stalks celery, thinly sliced

¼ cup (10g) chopped fresh parsley

½ head iceberg lettuce, roughly chopped

2 spring onions, finely sliced + extra for garnish

2 tbsps capers, drained

2 tbsps lemon juice

2 tbsps olive oil

Salt and pepper to taste

STEPS

1. In a large bowl, combine the smoked tuna, celery, chopped parsley, lettuce, spring onions and capers.
2. For the dressing, in a separate small bowl, whisk together the lemon juice, olive oil, salt and pepper.
3. Pour the dressing over the tuna mixture and toss gently to coat all the ingredients.
4. Let the salad sit for a few minutes to allow the flavours to meld together. Garnish with some extra cracked pepper and sliced spring onions.

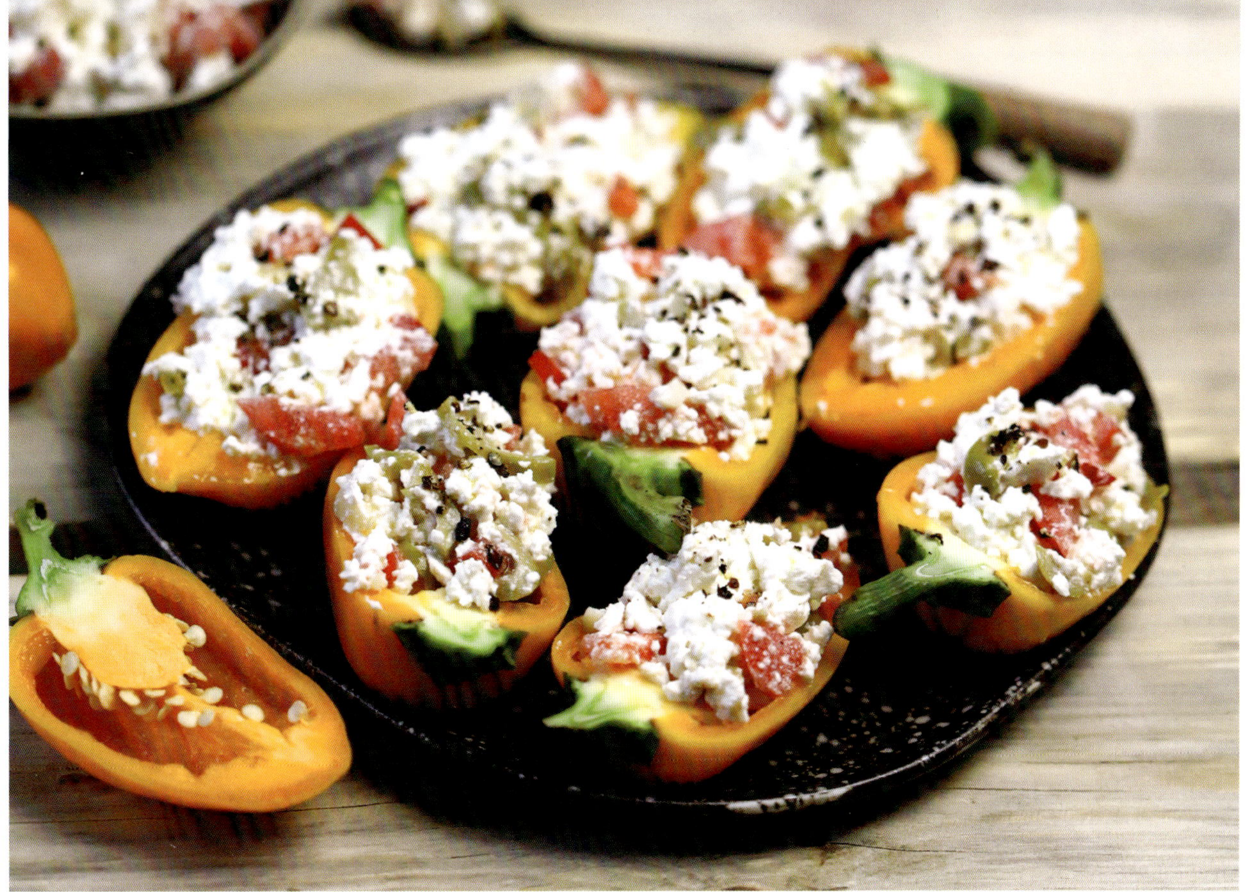

RICOTTA-STUFFED CAPSICUM

500g ripe tomatoes, diced

½ cup (70g) green olives, sliced

¼ red onion, finely chopped

¼ cup (10g) chopped basil leaves

1 tbsp chopped oregano leaves

2 tbsps olive oil

1 tbsp balsamic vinegar

Salt and pepper to taste

1 cup (250g) ricotta cheese

4 yellow capsicums (or sweet baby vine capsicums)

STEPS

1. Place tomatoes, olives, red onion, basil and oregano in a large bowl. Drizzle with olive oil and balsamic vinegar. Season generously with salt and pepper. Toss to coat.
2. Crumble in the ricotta. Carefully toss once more.
3. Cut the capsicums in half lengthways.
4. Spoon the tomato-ricotta salad into the capsicum halves.
5. Season once more with salt and pepper. Serve immediately.

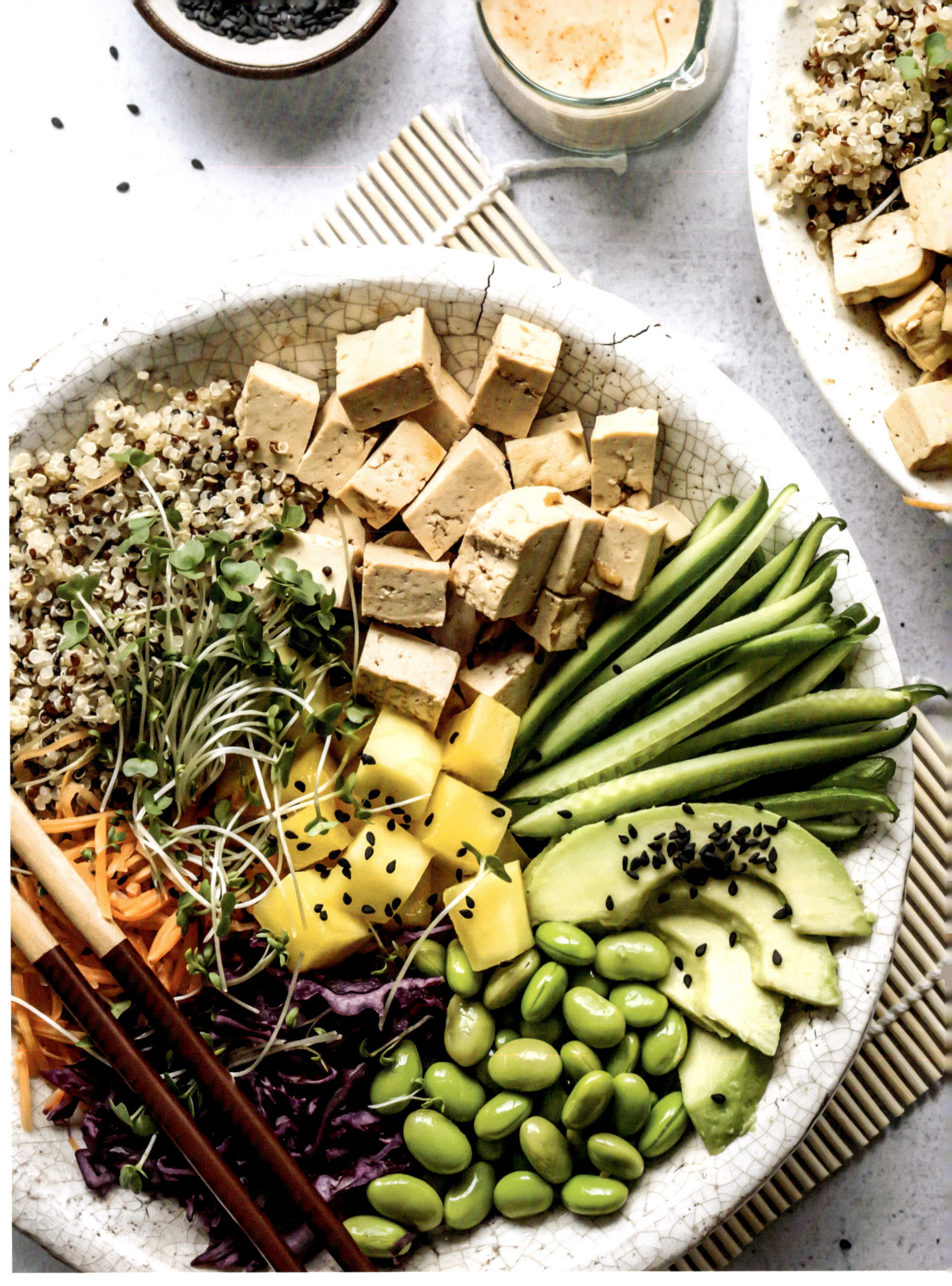

TOFU NOURISH BOWL

DRESSING

2 cloves garlic, crushed

1 tbsp minced fresh ginger

2 tbsps tamari sauce

2 tbsps fish sauce

2 tbsps lime juice

2 tbsps agave syrup

1 tsp lemon juice

1 tsp chilli sauce

BOWL

300g firm tofu, cut into 3cm cubes

1 tbsp oil

1 avocado, sliced

½ small Lebanese cucumber, julienned

1 cup (100g) shredded red cabbage

1 mango, cut into cubes

1 carrot, julienned

½ cup (90g) edamame

2 cups (370g) cooked quinoa

GARNISH

1 tsp black sesame seeds

2 tbsps micro herbs

STEPS

1. Whisk all the dressing ingredients together in a small bowl and set aside.
2. Pour 1 tablespoon of the dressing over the tofu and toss to coat.
3. Heat the oil in a wok over high heat. Add the tofu and stir-fry for 4 minutes or until it starts to brown.
4. To assemble the salad divide prepared vegetables and quinoa into bowls, arranging each ingredient in neat sections.
5. Spoon warm tofu on top, then pour dressing over the salad. Sprinkle with black sesame seeds and micro herbs.

SERVES 2 | PREP + COOK TIME: 40 MINS | GLUTEN FREE | DAIRY FREE |

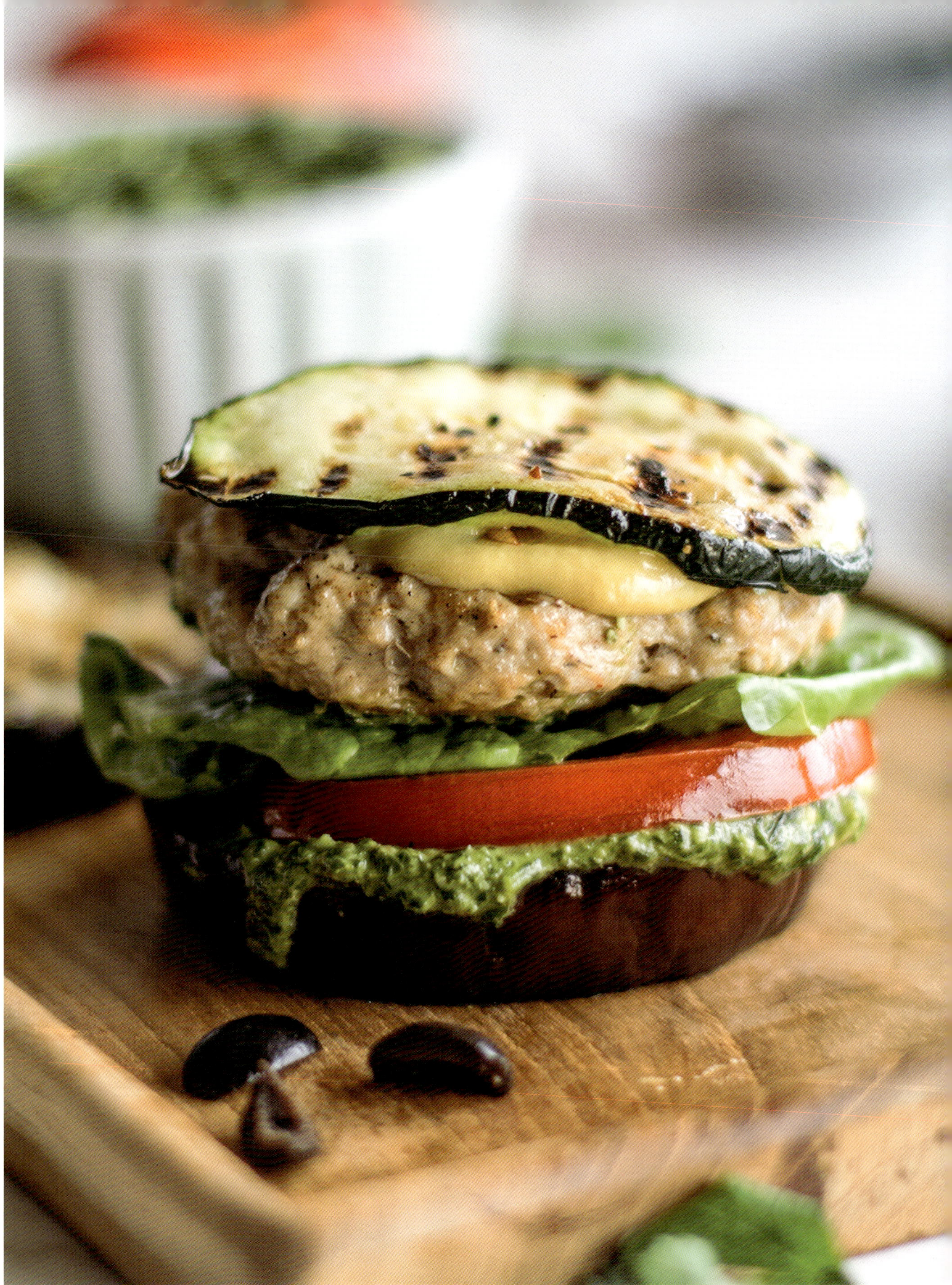

EGGPLANT PORK BURGERS

1 large eggplant, cut into 2½ cm-thick slices

1 large zucchini, thinly sliced

2 tbsps olive oil

½ tsp salt

500g pork mince

¼ cup (25g) almond flour

¼ cup (25g) grated Parmesan cheese

¼ cup (10g) chopped fresh parsley

2 cloves garlic, minced

1 tsp onion powder

½ tsp dried oregano

½ tsp salt

¼ tsp pepper

TO SERVE

¼ cup (60g) pesto (store-bought or see recipe page 69)

1 large tomato, sliced

8 lettuce leaves

2 tbsps Dijon mustard

STEPS

1. Brush the eggplant and zucchini slices with half the olive oil and salt both sides. Heat a grill pan to medium-high heat and cook in batches until browned and softened slightly, approximately 3-4 minutes per side. Set aside.

2. To make the pork patties combine the mince, almond flour, Parmesan cheese, parsley, garlic, onion powder, oregano, salt and pepper in a medium bowl. Mix well to combine.

3. Divide the mixture into equal portions and shape into eight patties, about 2½ cm thick.

4. Heat remaining oil in a frying pan and cook patties for 4-5 minutes per side until cooked through. Allow to rest for a few minutes.

5. To assemble, spread pesto onto an eggplant slice, followed by a slice of tomato, lettuce leaf, patty, mustard and zucchini, then top the burger with another slice of eggplant.

SERVES 4 | PREP + COOK TIME: 50 MINS | GLUTEN FREE | DAIRY FREE |

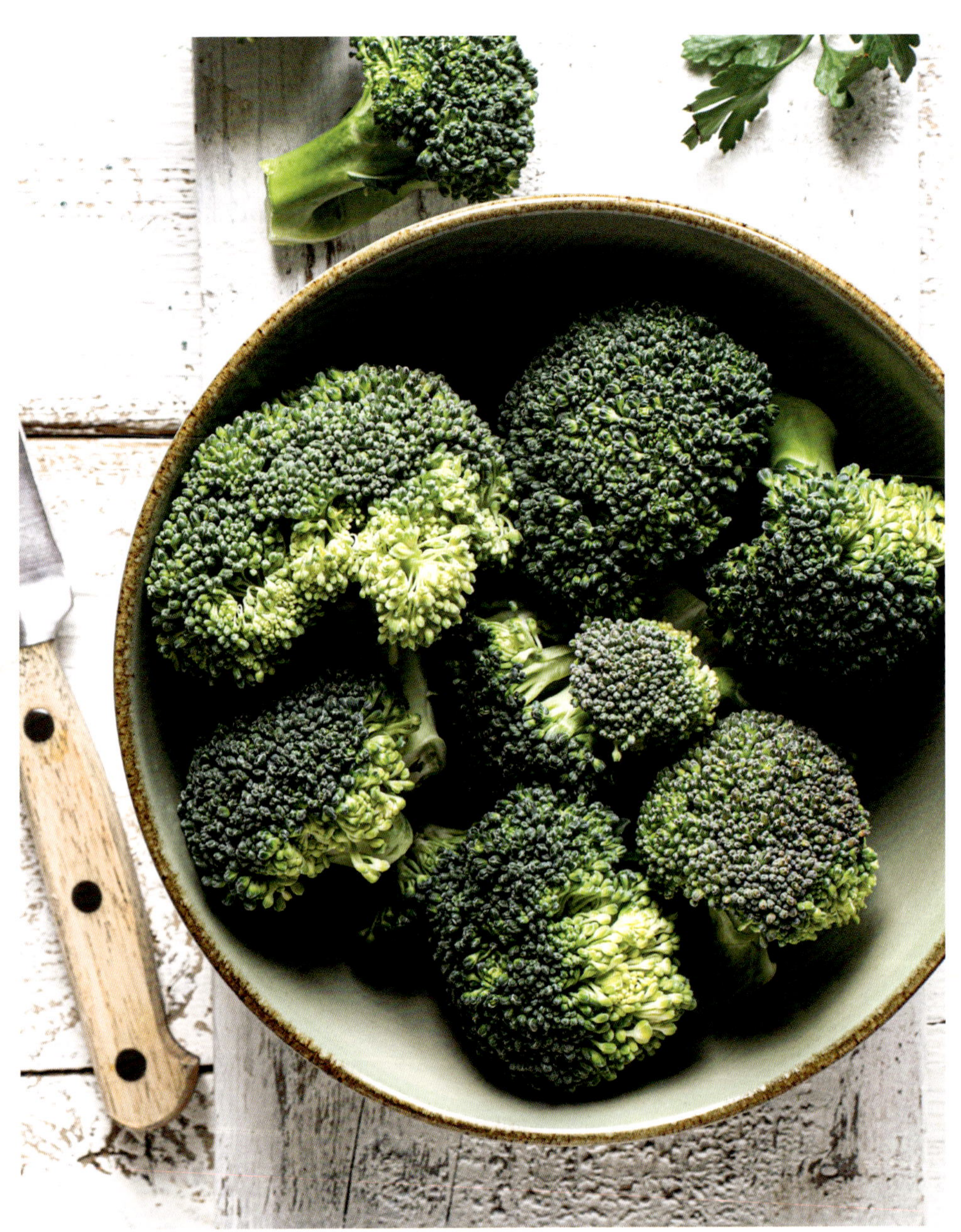

VEGGIE SIDES & MAINS

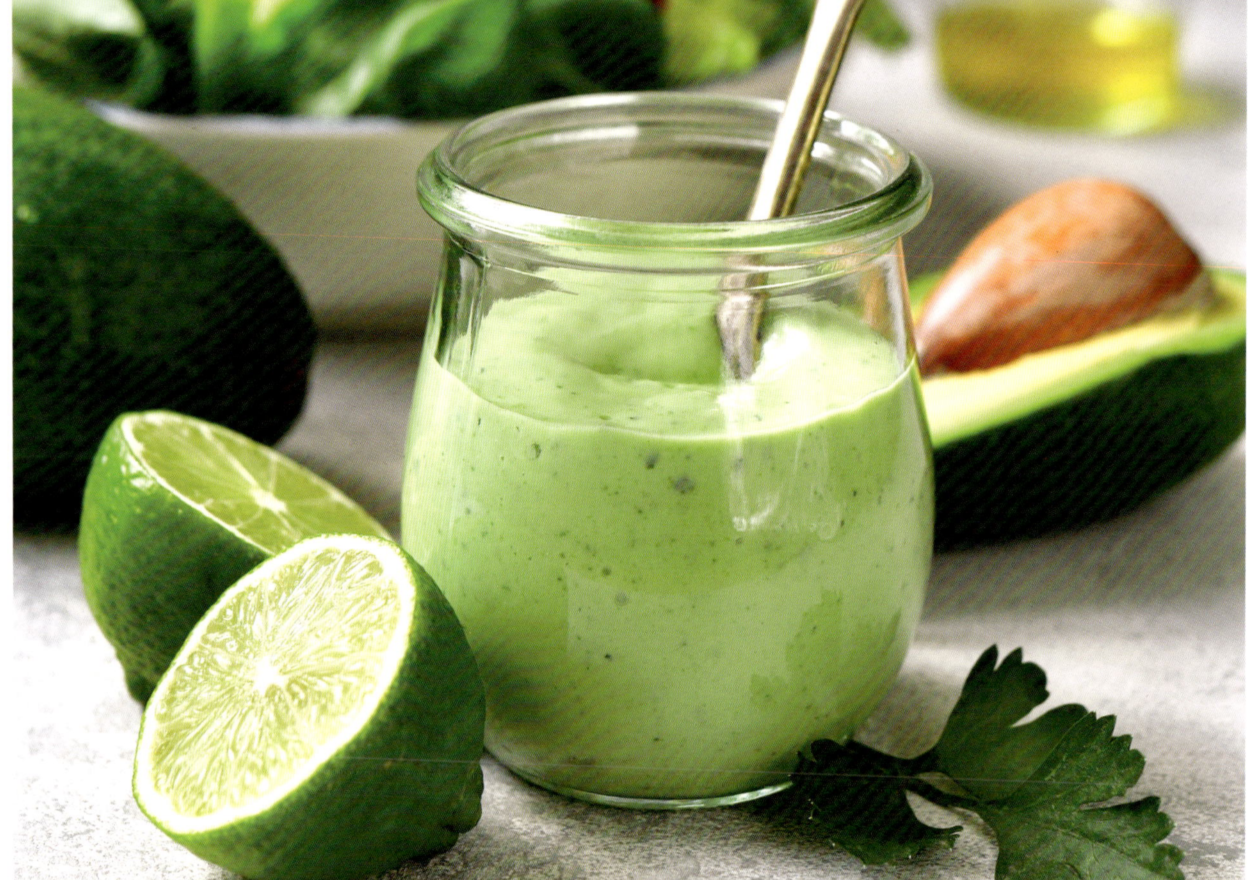

AVOCADO YOGHURT DRESSING

1 avocado

⅔ cup (160ml) Greek yoghurt

Juice of 1 lime

¼ cup (5g) loosely packed fresh coriander

Pinch of salt

STEPS

1. In a food processor or blender, add the avocado flesh, yoghurt, lime juice and coriander.
2. Blend until smooth, then add salt to taste.
3. Use as a dressing for salads or serve with chicken or fish.

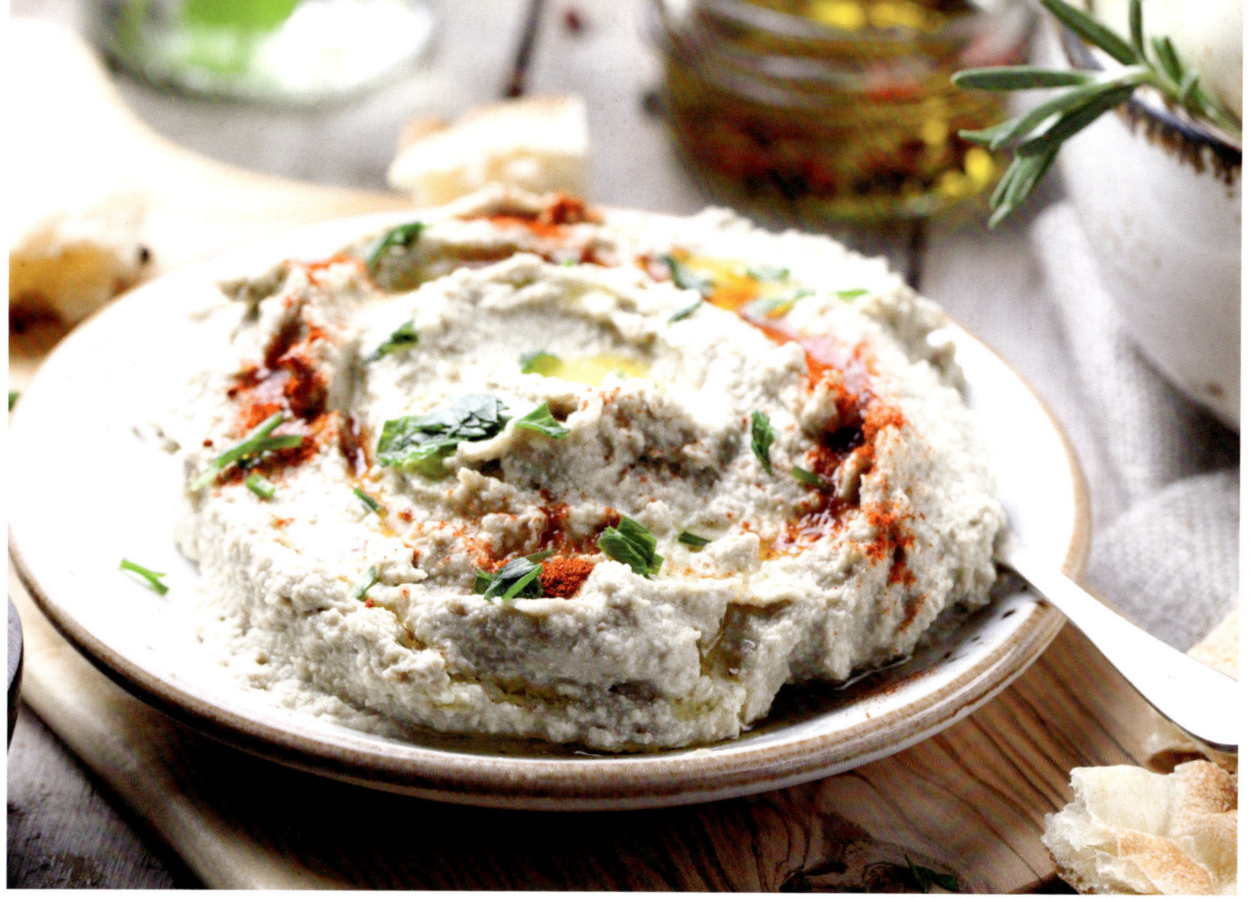

SERVES 4 | PREP + COOK TIME: 45 MINS | VEG | GLUTEN FREE | DAIRY FREE |

BABA GANOUSH

2 medium eggplants, halved lengthways
1 sprig rosemary
2 tbsps olive oil
2 cloves garlic, crushed
1 tsp salt
2 tbsps lemon juice
3 tbsps tahini
Pepper to taste
2 sprigs parsley, chopped
½ tsp smoky paprika
Sumac (or more paprika) to serve

STEPS

Preheat the oven to 200°C.

1. Place the eggplants on a lined baking tray cut-side down with a sprig of rosemary and drizzle with half the olive oil. Bake for 30 minutes or until softened.
2. Scoop out the eggplant flesh and put in a medium bowl with the baked rosemary leaves. Add the garlic, salt, lemon juice, tahini a couple of good grinds of pepper, half the parsley and the paprika.
3. Blend the mixture with a stick blender until nearly smooth. Season to taste.
4. Serve with the remaining parsley, a sprinkle of sumac or paprika and the rest of the olive oil drizzled on top.

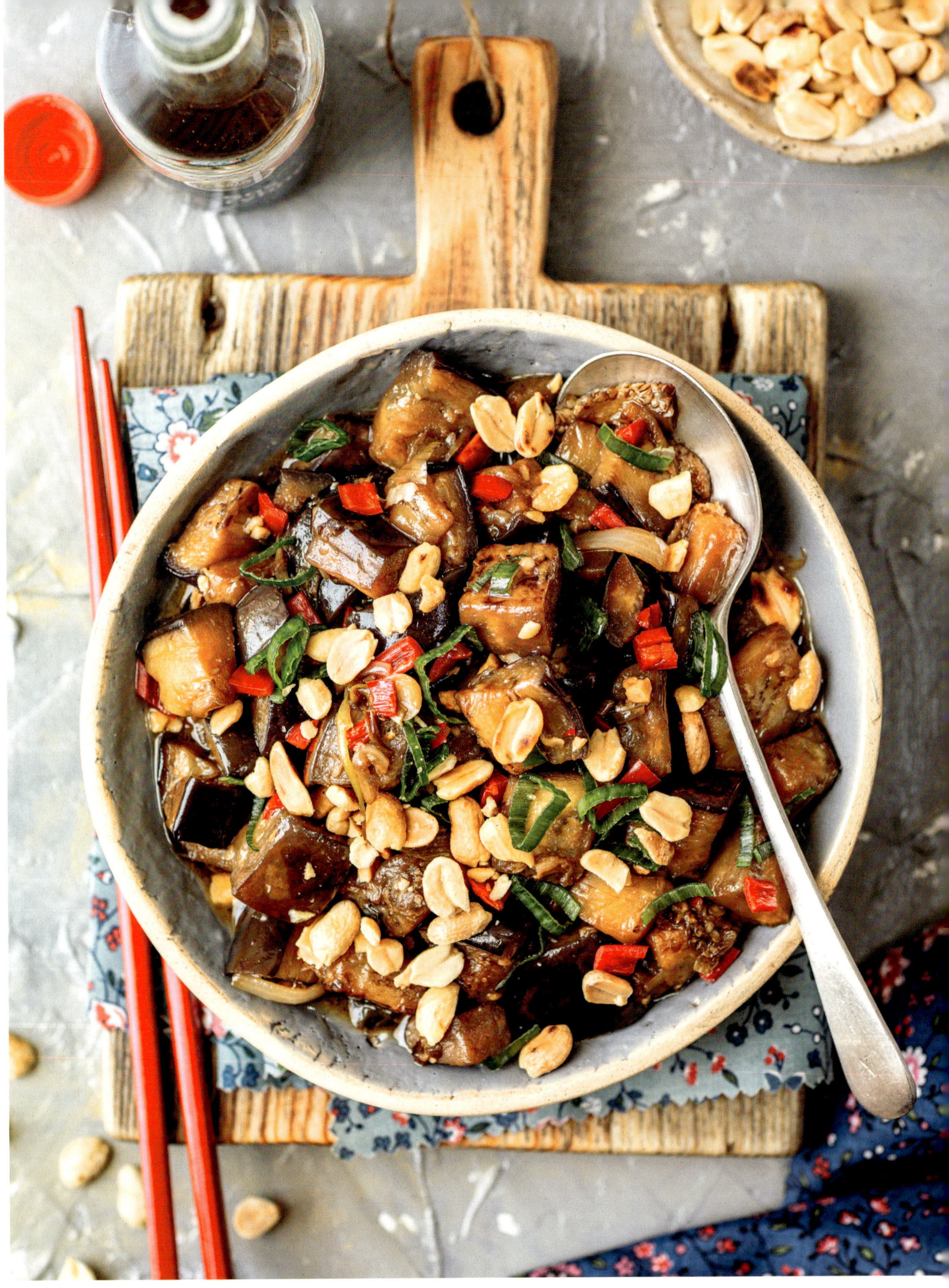

EGGPLANT & PEANUT STIR-FRY

2 tbsps soy sauce
1 tbsp oyster sauce
1 tbsp rice wine vinegar
1 tsp sesame oil
1 tsp sugar
Salt and pepper to taste
2 tbsps vegetable oil
3 cloves garlic, crushed
Small piece ginger, grated
2 spring onions, chopped (reserve some for garnish)
1 large red chilli, deseeded and chopped
2 eggplants, cut into bite-sized pieces
¼ cup (30g) peanuts, chopped
Cauliflower rice to serve
Fresh coriander, chopped, to garnish

STEPS

1. In a small bowl, whisk together the soy sauce, oyster sauce, rice wine vinegar, sesame oil, sugar and a pinch of salt and pepper. Set aside.
2. Heat the vegetable oil in a large frying pan or wok over medium-high heat. Add the garlic, grated ginger, chopped spring onions and fresh chilli to the pan then stir-fry for about 1 minute until fragrant.
3. Add the eggplant pieces to the pan and stir-fry for about 5-6 minutes until they are tender and slightly browned.
4. Pour the soy mixture over the eggplant in the pan and stir-fry for another 2-3 minutes to coat the eggplant evenly.
5. Add the chopped peanuts to the pan and stir-fry for an additional minute. Serve with cauliflower rice and fresh coriander and spring onions.

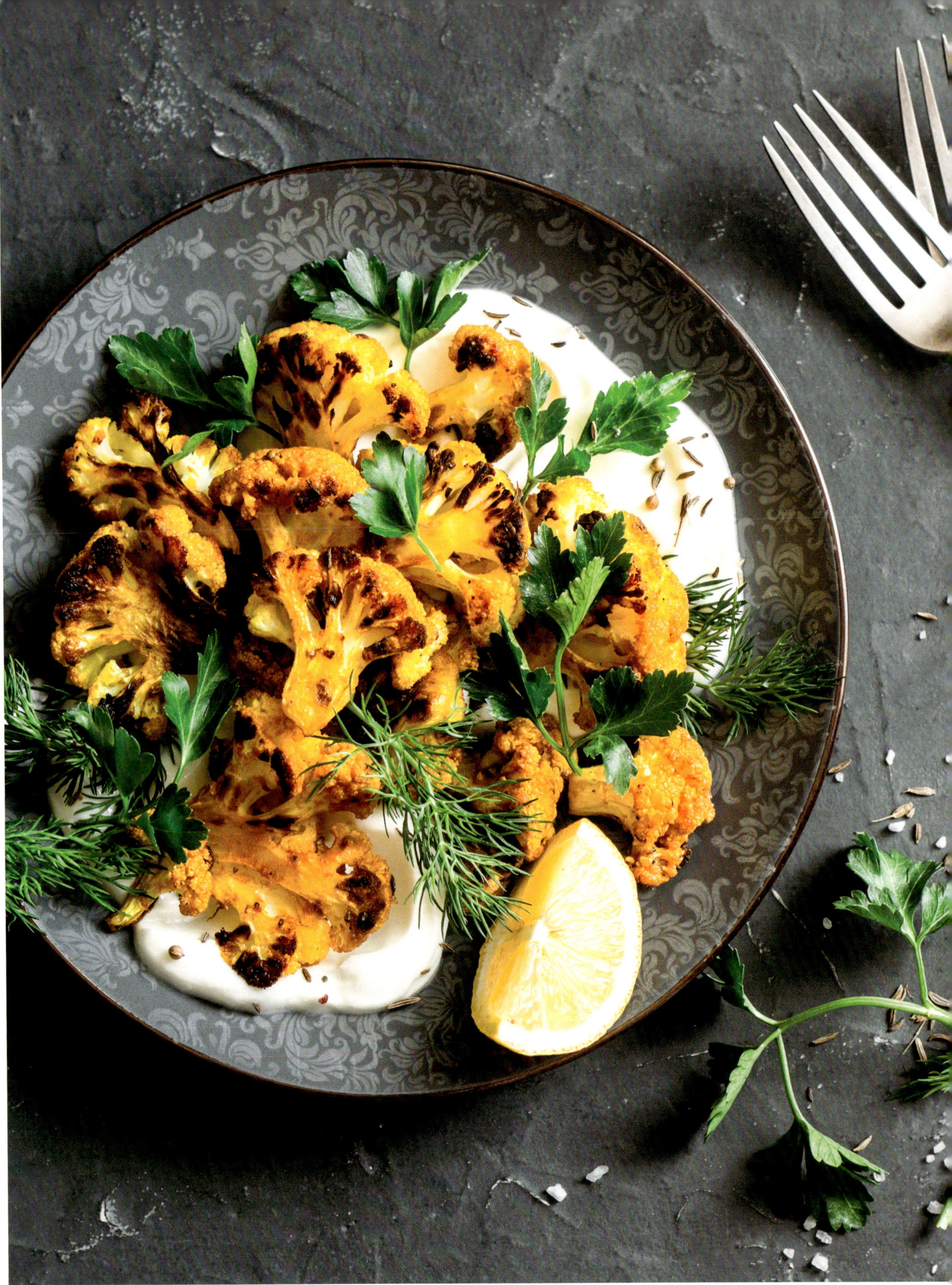

ROASTED TURMERIC CAULIFLOWER WITH GREEK YOGHURT DRESSING

SERVES 4 | PREP + COOK TIME: 45 MINS + CHILLING | VEG | GLUTEN FREE |

2 cups (500ml) Greek yoghurt

4 large cloves garlic, crushed

2 small lemons; 1 juiced, 1 cut into wedges for garnish

3 tbsps olive oil

Salt and pepper

1 medium head cauliflower, cut into small florets

½ tbsp harissa

1 tsp ground turmeric

¼ cup (10g) fresh parsley and dill, to garnish (optional)

STEPS

1. Whisk together the yoghurt, half the garlic, 2 teaspoons lemon juice, 1 tablespoon olive oil and ½ teaspoon each of salt and pepper until thoroughly combined. If time allows, chill for 1 hour in the refrigerator before serving.
2. Preheat oven to 220°C and grease and line a large, flat baking tray with baking paper.
3. Toss the cauliflower with the remaining garlic and oil, harissa, turmeric and 1 teaspoon each of salt and pepper.
4. Roast for 30 minutes until the cauliflower is cooked through and blackened in places.
5. Serve hot with the yoghurt dressing and lemon wedges on the side. Add fresh herbs if desired.

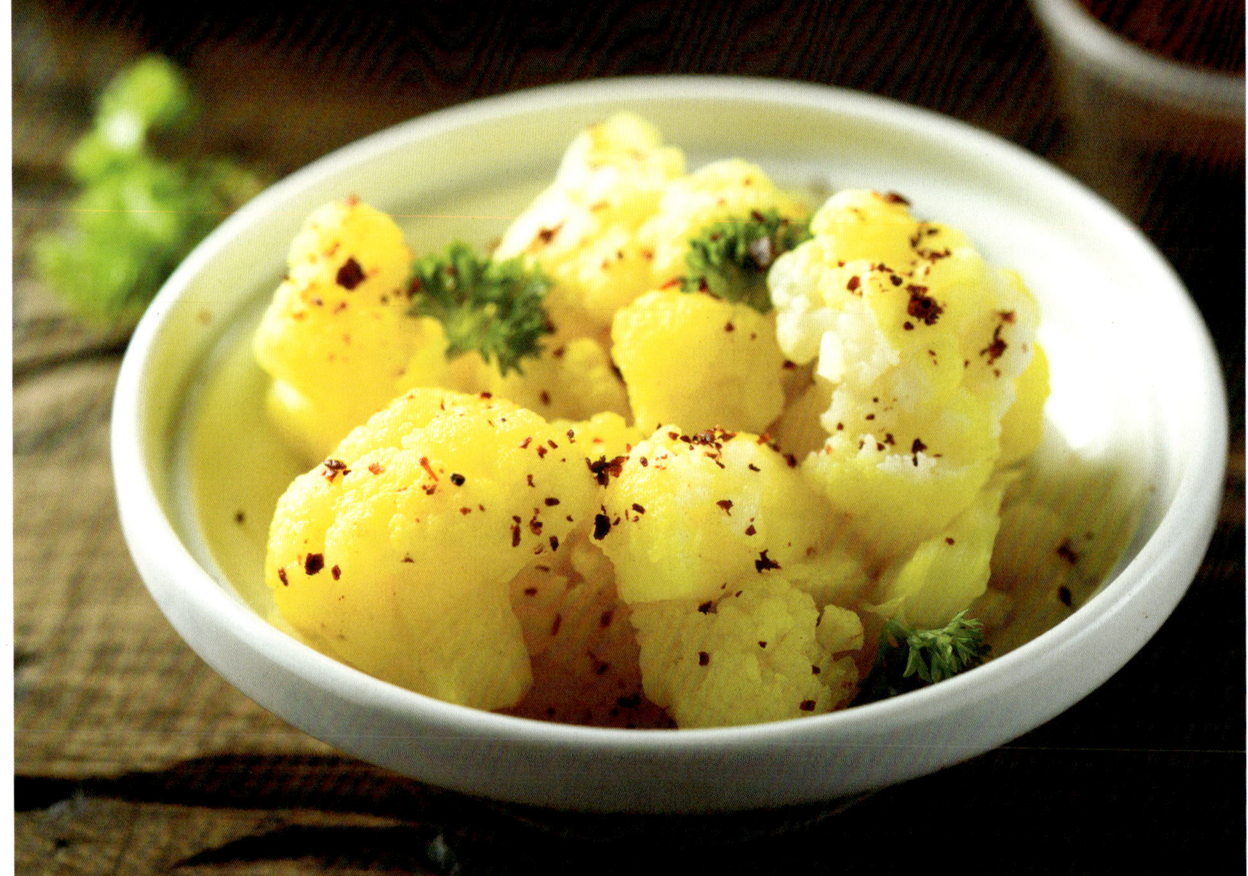

PICKLED CAULIFLOWER

¼ cup (55g) sugar

2 cups (500ml) white vinegar

1 cup (250ml) water

1 tsp ground turmeric

1 tbsp mustard seeds

1 tbsp whole black peppercorns

4 cloves garlic, peeled and smashed

2 tbsps salt

1 bay leaf

1 head cauliflower, cut into bite-size pieces

Pinch of dried chilli flakes to serve (optional)

STEPS

1. Combine the sugar, vinegar, water and turmeric in a saucepan and place over medium heat. Whisk until sugar has dissolved.

2. Allow to cool, then combine the pickling liquid, mustard seeds, peppercorns, garlic, bay leaf and salt with the cauliflower in a large bowl.

3. Transfer to sterilised glass jars, seal and store in the fridge for up to a month.

4. Sprinkle with dried chilli flakes, if desired, to serve.

NOTE: You can eat these pickles straight away, but they taste best after a few days in the fridge.

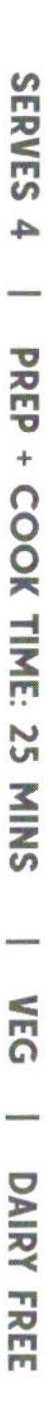

WAKAME SEAWEED SALAD

30g dried wakame seaweed
1 cup (250ml) water
2 tbsps rice wine vinegar
3 tbsps light soy sauce
1 tbsp sesame oil
1¼ tbsps sugar
1 tsp grated ginger
2 cloves garlic, crushed
2 tsps sesame seeds
1 tsp cornflour
1 tbsp cold water

STEPS

1. In a bowl rinse the seaweed and let soak for about 10 minutes until re-hydrated and tender.
2. Drain and gently squeeze the seaweed to remove excess water. Chop or use kitchen scissors to form small strips of seaweed.
3. In a small salad bowl combine rice wine vinegar, light soy sauce, sesame oil, sugar, grated ginger, garlic, cornflour and cold water and whisk to combine. Set aside.
4. Add seaweed to the dressing and toss gently to combine, making sure the seaweed is evenly coated. Sprinkle salad with sesame seeds and serve.

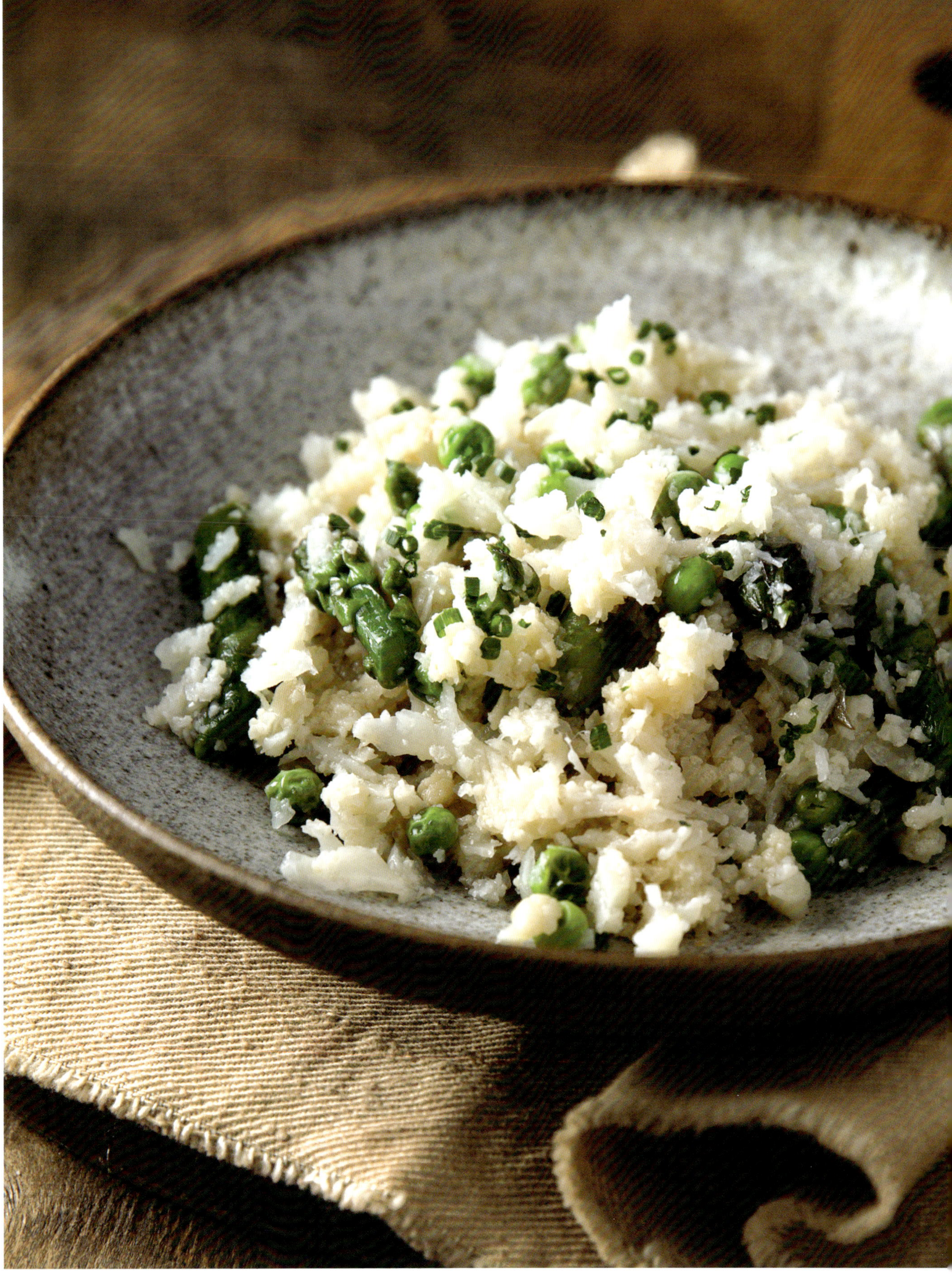

CAULIFLOWER COUSCOUS WITH PEA & ASPARAGUS

1 medium head cauliflower, cut into florets

½ cup (125ml) water

Salt and pepper to taste

1 cup (170g) frozen peas, thawed

2 tbsps olive oil

1 Asian shallot, minced

1 bunch asparagus, trimmed and cut into 5cm lengths

Zest and juice of 1 lemon

1 tsp chopped thyme leaves

1 tbsp chopped chives

STEPS

1. Place the cauliflower florets in a food processor and pulse until the cauliflower is very finely chopped and resembles rice or couscous.

2. Place water and a pinch of salt in a large frying pan. Bring to a simmer then add the cauliflower in a single layer. Bring back to a simmer, reduce heat, cover and cook for 5 minutes, until the cauliflower is tender-crisp. Remove the cauliflower from the pan and drain. Transfer to a serving bowl.

3. Meanwhile bring a pan of water to a boil. Add the peas and cook for 1 minute until tender, but still bright green. Drain and add to the cauliflower.

4. Heat olive oil in a frying pan over medium heat. Add the shallot and saute for 2-3 minutes, until soft and translucent. Add the asparagus and continue cooking for 3-4 minutes, stirring regularly, until the asparagus is al dente. Add the lemon zest, juice and thyme. Season with salt and pepper and cook another 30 seconds.

5. Add the shallot-asparagus mixture to the cauliflower. Drizzle with a little olive oil and toss gently to combine. Adjust the salt and pepper and lemon juice to taste then scatter with chopped chives to serve.

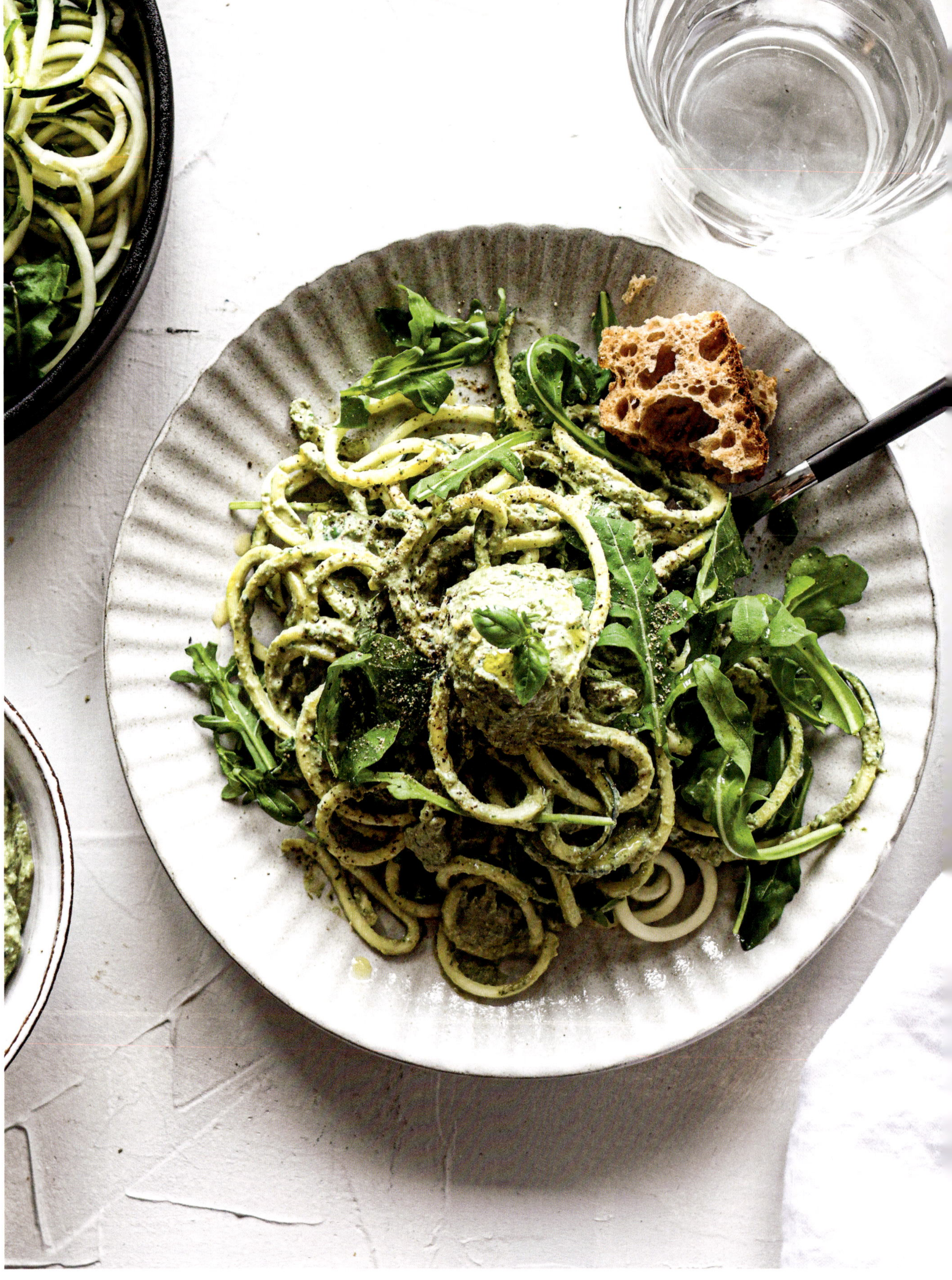

GREEN PESTO ZOODLES

2 cups (30g) fresh basil leaves

1 cup (30g) fresh spinach leaves

¼ cup (35g) pine nuts

2 cloves garlic

Juice of 1 lemon

Salt and pepper to taste

¼ cup (60ml) olive oil

1 cup (250ml) chicken or vegetable stock

3-4 medium zucchinis, spiralised into noodles

¼ cup (25g) grated Parmesan cheese

1 cup (30g) rocket leaves to serve

STEPS

1. Place basil leaves, spinach leaves, pine nuts, garlic and lemon juice in a food processor with salt and pepper to taste. With the motor running, add oil gradually, until the pesto forms a smooth paste. Set aside.
2. In a frying pan add the stock, bring to a simmer then add the zucchini and stir for 3 minutes until the zucchini is cooked through. Drain off any excess liquid.
3. Add the drained zucchini back to the pan and pour in the pesto and grated Parmesan cheese.
4. Toss well to combine and serve with cracked pepper and rocket leaves.

SERVES 2 | PREP + COOK TIME: 25 MINS | VEG | GLUTEN FREE |

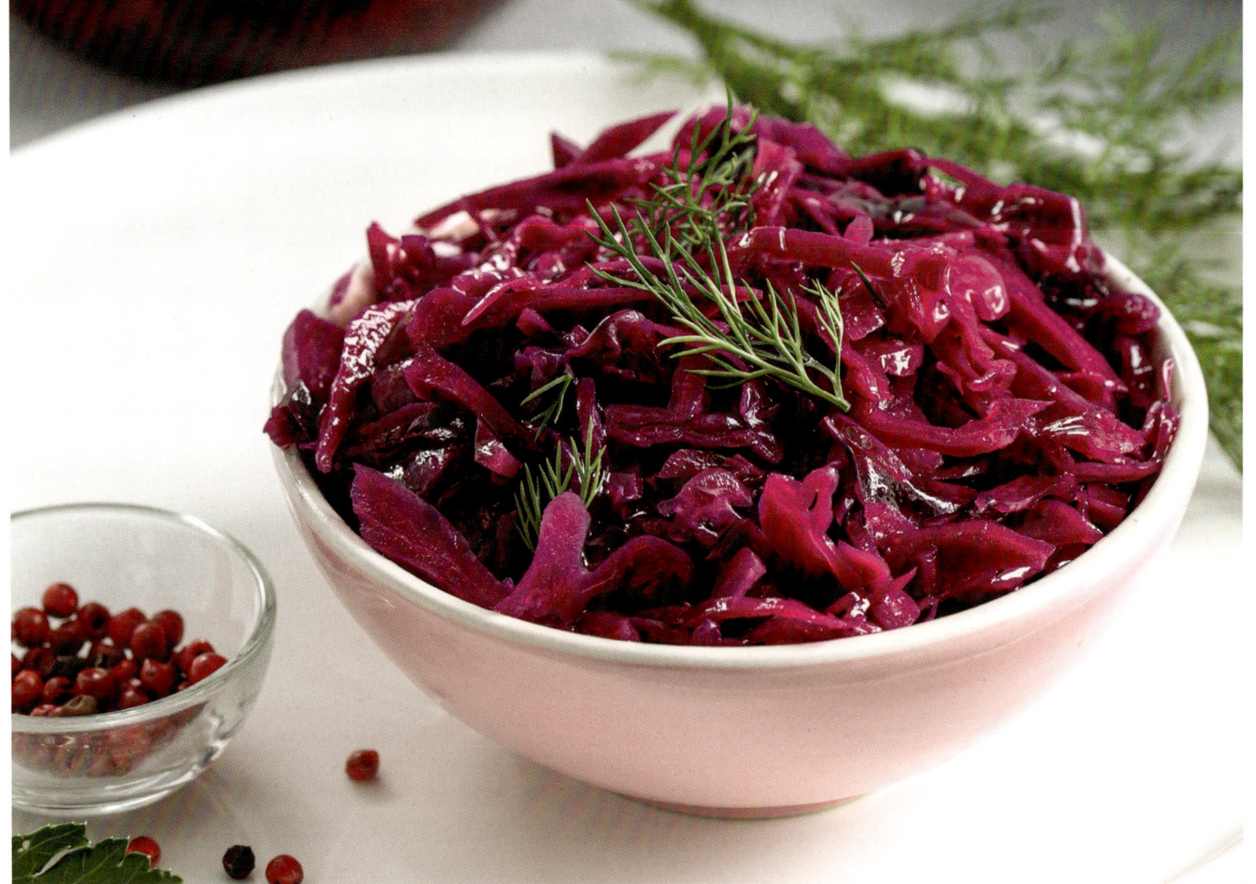

QUICK PICKLED RED CABBAGE

1 cup (250ml) apple cider vinegar

½ cup (125ml) water

¼ cup (55g) sugar

1 tsp salt

1 tsp whole black peppercorns

1 small head red cabbage, finely sliced

STEPS

1. In a medium saucepan, combine apple cider vinegar, water, sugar, salt and peppercorns. Bring the mixture to a simmer over medium heat, stirring until the sugar and salt are dissolved.
2. Add the sliced red cabbage to the simmering liquid. Cook for 2-3 minutes, just until the cabbage starts to soften slightly but still retains some crunch.
3. Remove the saucepan from heat and let the pickling liquid and cabbage cool to room temperature.
4. Once cooled, transfer the pickled red cabbage and the liquid to a clean jar or airtight container.

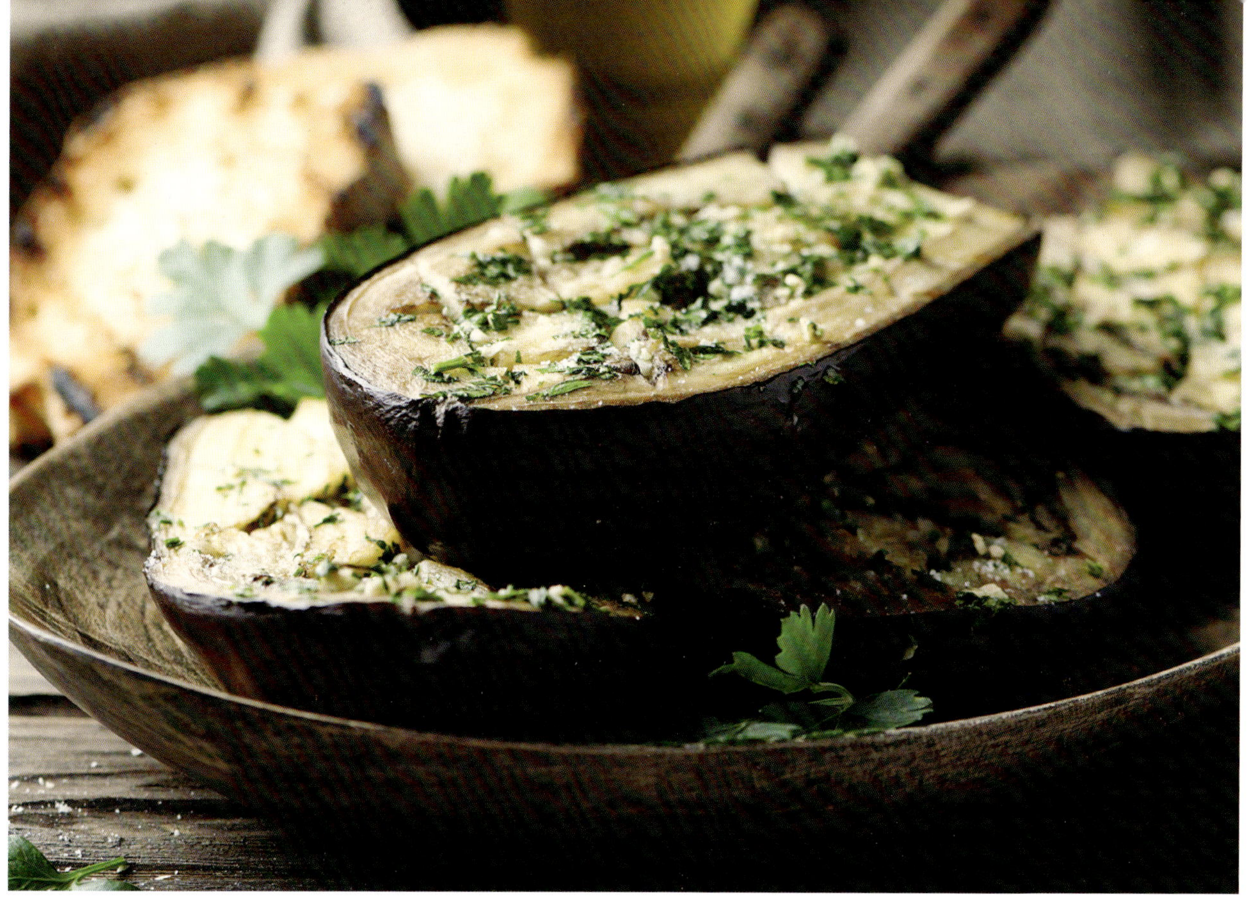

ITALIAN ROASTED EGGPLANT

2 medium eggplants, rinsed
3 tbsps olive oil
2 cloves garlic, crushed
1 tsp dried oregano
½ tsp dried basil
½ tsp dried thyme
Salt and pepper to taste
¼ cup (25g) grated Parmesan cheese
Fresh parsley leaves, for garnish

STEPS

Preheat oven to 180°C.

1. Cut each eggplant in half lengthwise, then score the flesh to create a cross-hatch pattern about 2cm deep, being careful not to pierce the skin.
2. In a small bowl, combine the olive oil, garlic, oregano, basil, thyme, salt and pepper. Mix well to combine.
3. On a lined baking tray, place the eggplant slices skin-side down and brush generously with the infused oil.
4. Roast the eggplant slices in the oven for about 20-25 minutes or until they become tender and golden brown, flipping halfway through.
5. Remove from oven and sprinkle with Parmesan and fresh parsley.

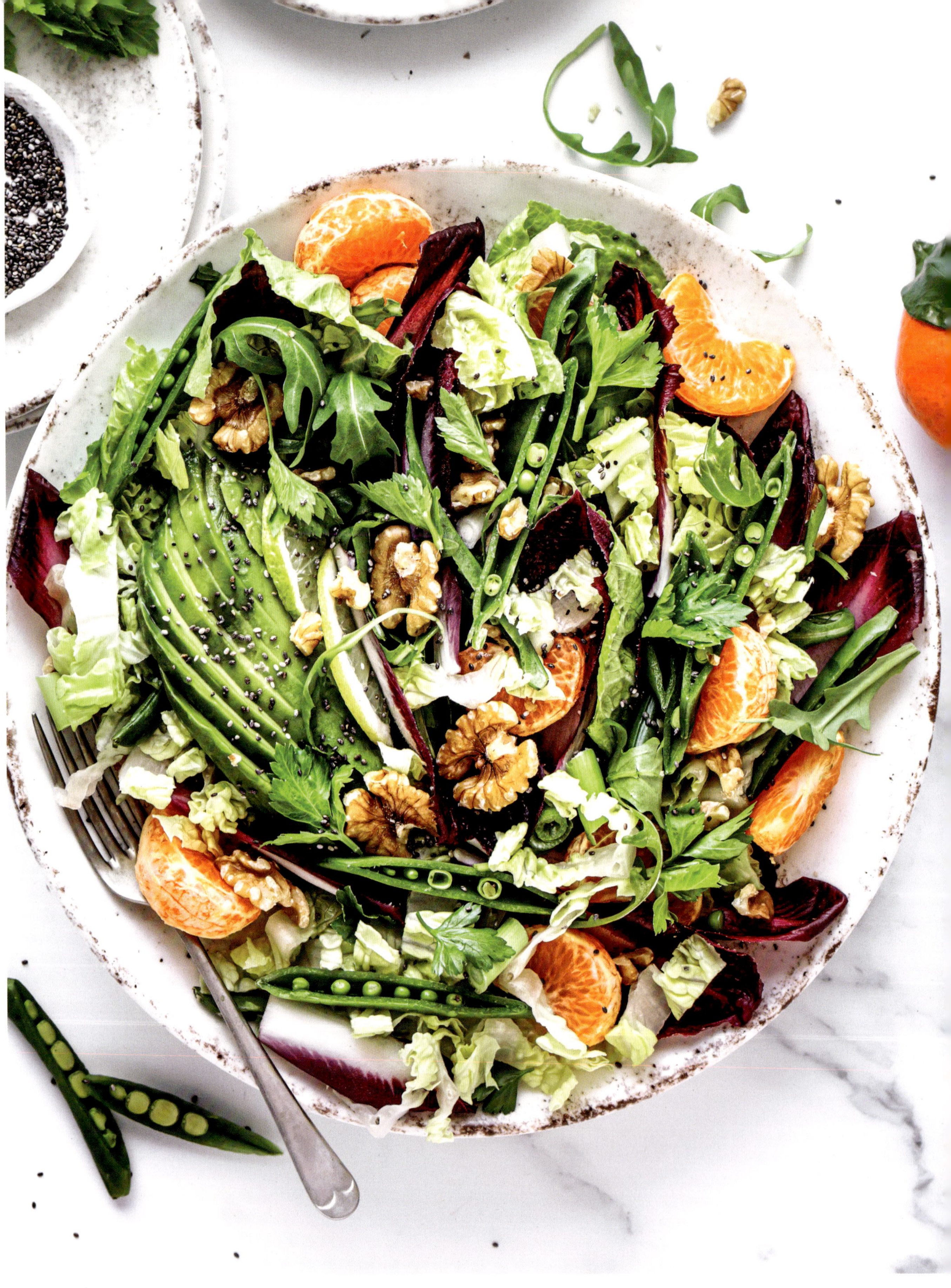

MANDARIN, AVOCADO & WALNUT SALAD

4 cups (300g) mixed lettuce leaves

300g sugar snap peas, sliced in half lengthways

2 small mandarins, segmented

½ cup (20g) fresh parsley

½ cup (60g) walnuts, chopped

2 avocados, sliced

2 tbsps poppy seeds to serve

Lemon wedges to serve

DRESSING

¼ cup (60ml) fresh orange juice

2 tbsps fresh lemon juice

1 tsp honey or maple syrup (optional, for sweetness)

¼ cup (60ml) olive oil

1 clove garlic, minced

½ tsp Dijon mustard

Salt and pepper to taste

STEPS

1. In a large salad bowl add mixed lettuce leaves, sugar snap peas, mandarin segments, parsley and walnuts. Toss to combine and set aside until ready to serve.

2. For the dressing, in a small bowl add juices, honey (if using), oil, garlic, Dijon mustard and salt and pepper and whisk thoroughly to combine.

3. To assemble, drizzle the dressing over the salad mix and place the sliced avocado on top, sprinkle with poppy seeds and serve with lemon wedges.

SERVES 4 | PREP + COOK TIME: 15 MINS | VEG | GLUTEN FREE | DAIRY FREE |

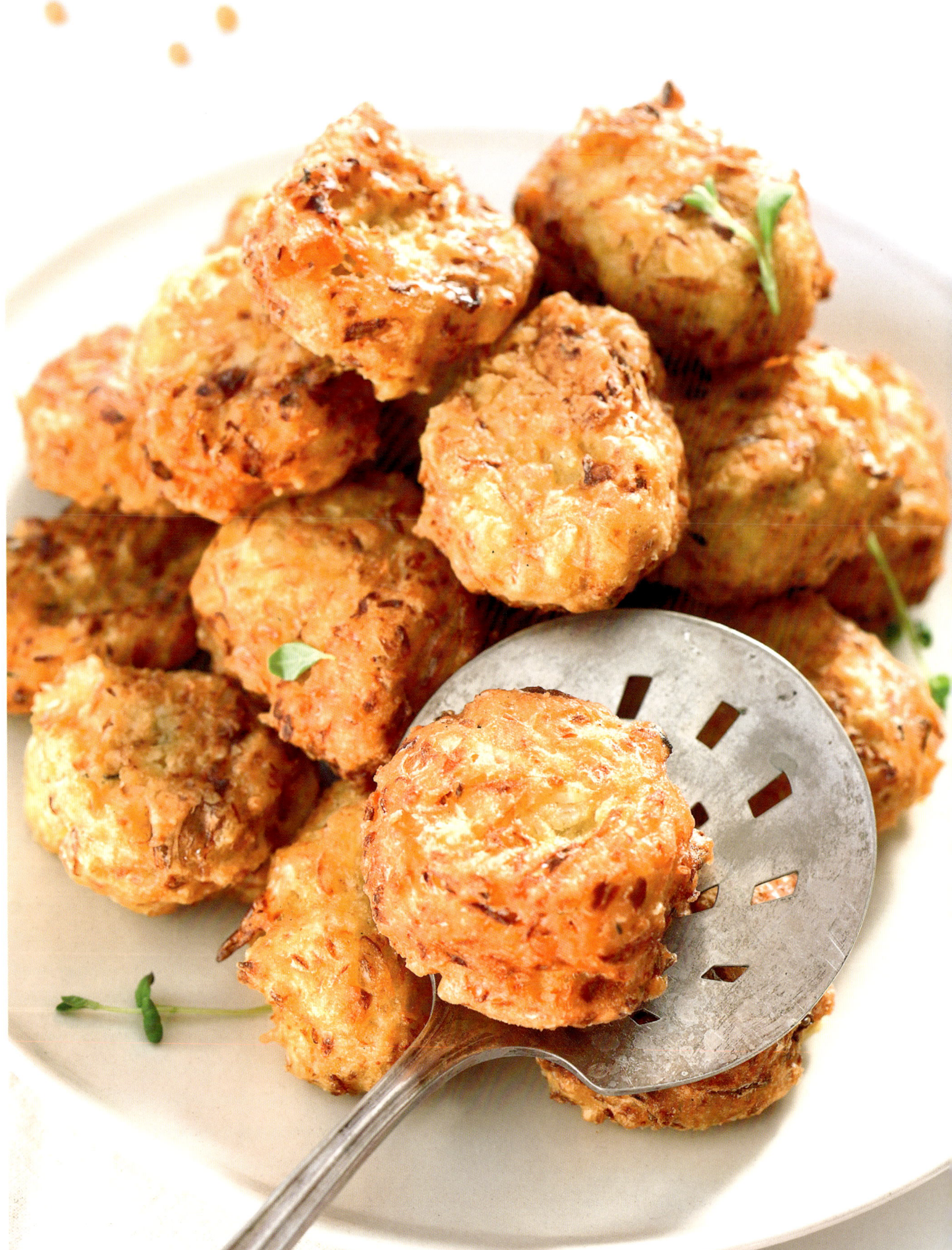

FRIED CABBAGE KOFTES

1 cup (95g) besan (chickpea flour)

½ cabbage, finely shredded

1 carrot, finely grated

½ cup (20g) finely chopped coriander

Small piece ginger, grated

½ tsp chilli powder

½ tsp garam masala

½ tsp salt

2 cups (500ml) vegetable or canola oil for frying

STEPS

1. In a large bowl, combine the besan, shredded cabbage, grated carrot, chopped coriander, ginger, spices and salt. Mix well until all the ingredients are evenly combined.
2. Take small portions of the mixture and shape them into small round or oval-shaped koftes.
3. Heat vegetable oil in a deep pan or saucepan over medium heat. Fry the koftes in batches until golden brown and crispy.
4. Remove them from the oil and drain on a paper towel-lined tray. Set aside to cool slightly.
5. Serve warm with preferred dipping sauce.

SERVES 2 | PREP + COOK TIME: 30 MINS | VEG | GLUTEN FREE | DAIRY FREE |

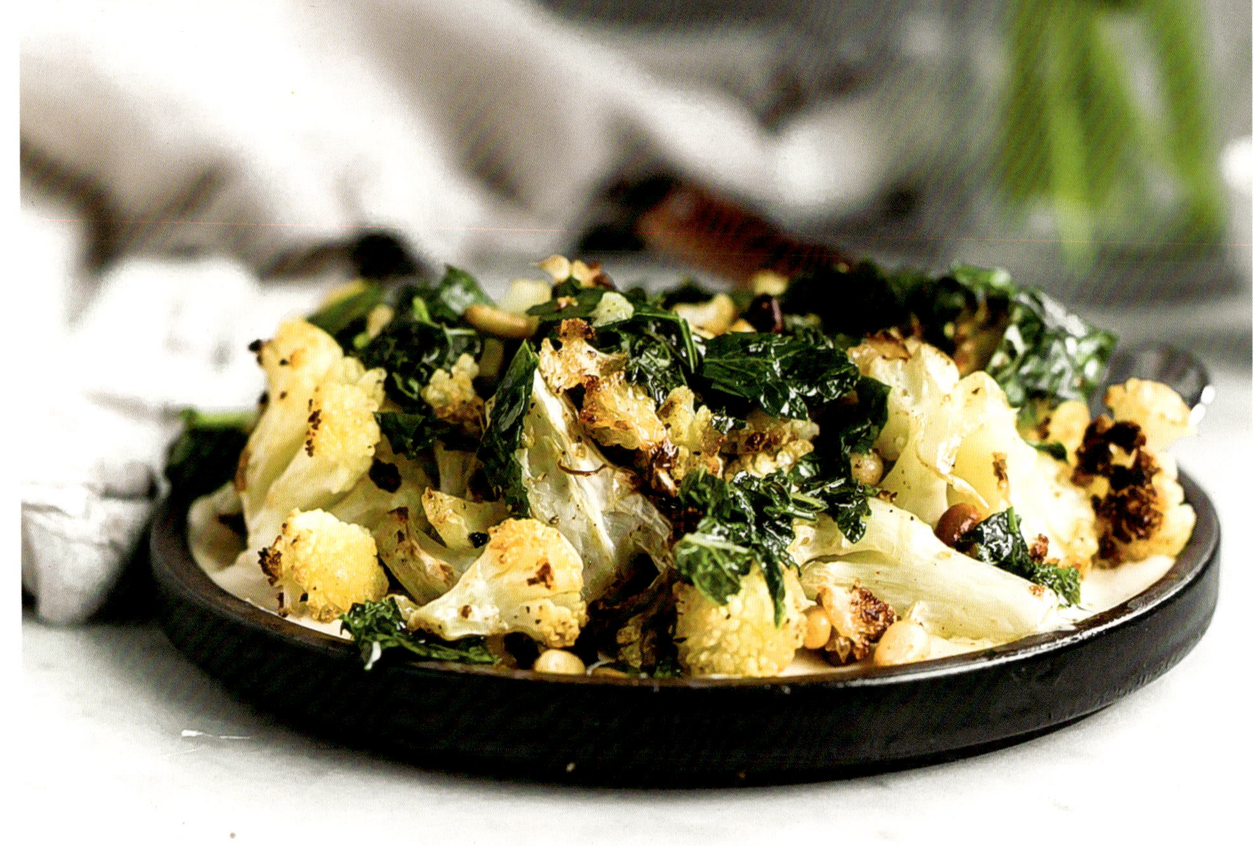

SERVES 4 | PREP + COOK TIME: 40 MINS | VEG | GLUTEN FREE | DAIRY FREE |

ROASTED CAULIFLOWER WITH TAHINI

1 large or 2 small heads cauliflower, cut into florets

2 tbsps olive oil

¼ tsp salt

2 pinches dried chilli flakes

¼ cup (35g) pine nuts

1 cup (15g) fresh mint leaves, roughly torn

TAHINI SAUCE

3 tbsps tahini

2 tbsps lemon juice

1 tsp olive oil

1 small clove garlic, grated

Pinch of salt

Pepper to taste

STEPS

Preheat oven to 230°C.

1. Place cauliflower florets into a large bowl. Drizzle with olive oil and sprinkle with salt and chilli flakes. Toss gently to coat.
2. Roast for 25-30 minutes, flipping halfway through, until just fork-tender.
3. Meanwhile place the sauce ingredients in a small bowl. Whisk until well combined. Refrigerate until ready to use.
4. Place a dry frying pan over a medium-low heat. Add the pine nuts and cook for 2-5 minutes, shaking the pan regularly, until the nuts are fragrant and slightly browned.
5. Divide the tahini sauce evenly between four plates. Toss the cauliflower with the pine nuts and torn mint and spoon on top of the sauce to serve.

SERVES 6 | PREP + COOK TIME: 15 MINS | VEG | GLUTEN FREE | DAIRY FREE |

APPLE & CABBAGE SLAW

1 cup (245g) mayonnaise

1 tbsp Dijon mustard

1 tbsp honey (optional, for added sweetness)

2 tbsps apple cider vinegar

Salt and pepper to taste

3 cups (300g) finely shredded red cabbage

3 cups (300g) finely shredded wombok (Chinese cabbage)

1 apple, julienned

2 carrots, julienned

½ red onion, sliced

1 cup (45g) roughly chopped fresh parsley

STEPS

1. In a small bowl whisk together mayonnaise, mustard, honey, cider vinegar and salt and pepper and set aside.
2. In a large salad bowl place cabbages, apple, carrots, onion and fresh parsley; toss to combine.
3. Drizzle the prepared dressing over the salad and coat the vegetables evenly.
4. Season to taste and serve immediately.

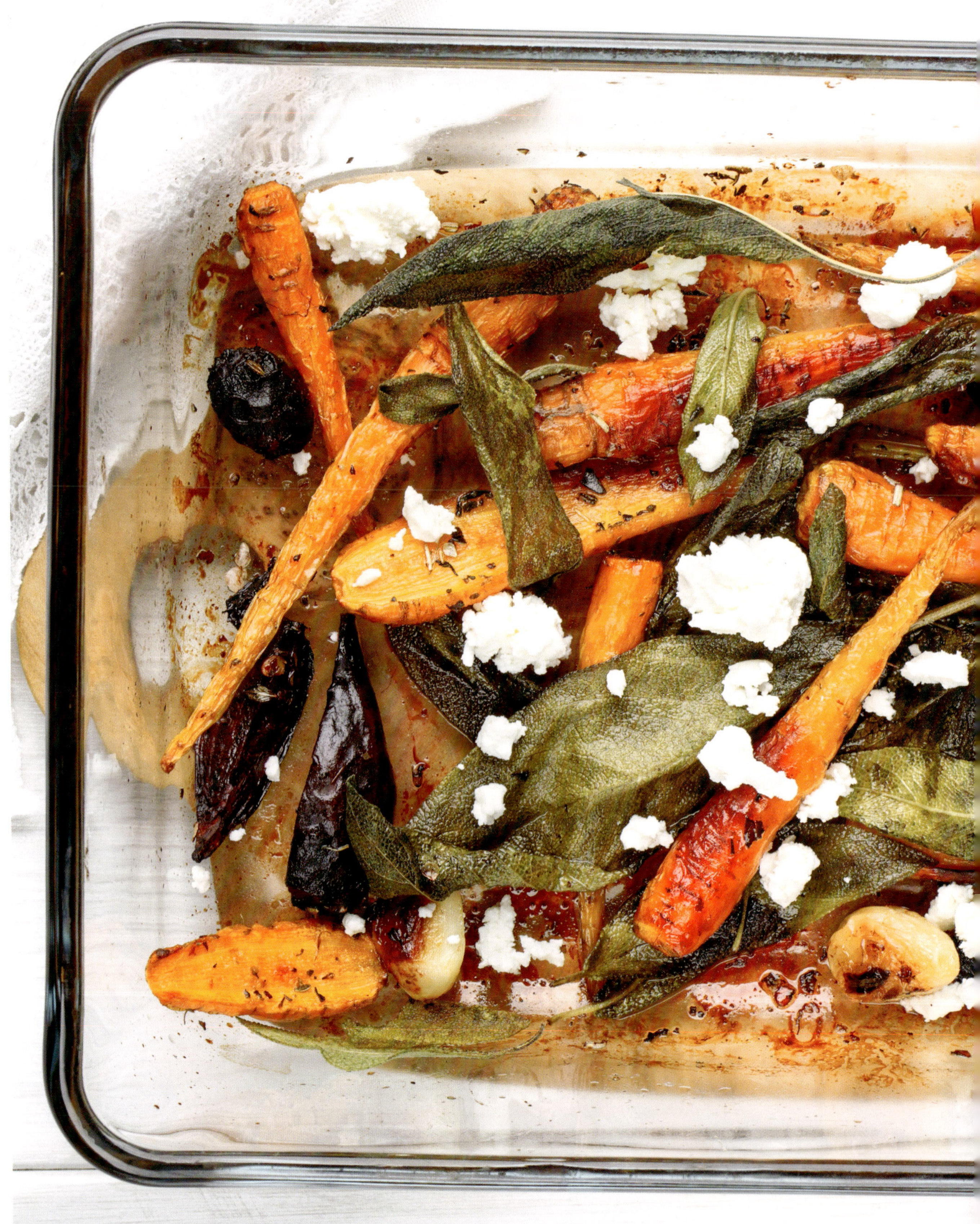

SAGE ROASTED VEGETABLES

300g beetroots, peeled and cut into wedges

700g carrots

6-8 cloves garlic, peeled and trimmed

3 tbsps olive oil

Salt and pepper to taste

2 tbsps butter

1 bunch sage leaves, picked

½ cup (100g) crumbled feta cheese

STEPS

Preheat the oven to 220°C.

1. Place beetroots, carrots and whole garlic cloves into a large roasting tin. Drizzle with olive oil and season with salt and pepper. Toss to coat.
2. Transfer to the oven and roast for 30-40 minutes until tender. Timing depends on the size of the vegetables.
3. When the vegetables are ready, melt butter in a saucepan over medium-high heat until the butter stops foaming and begins to turn a very light brown. Add sage leaves and fry for 30 seconds until crispy.
4. Drizzle the contents of the pan over the vegetables and toss to coat.
5. Scatter with crumbled feta and serve.

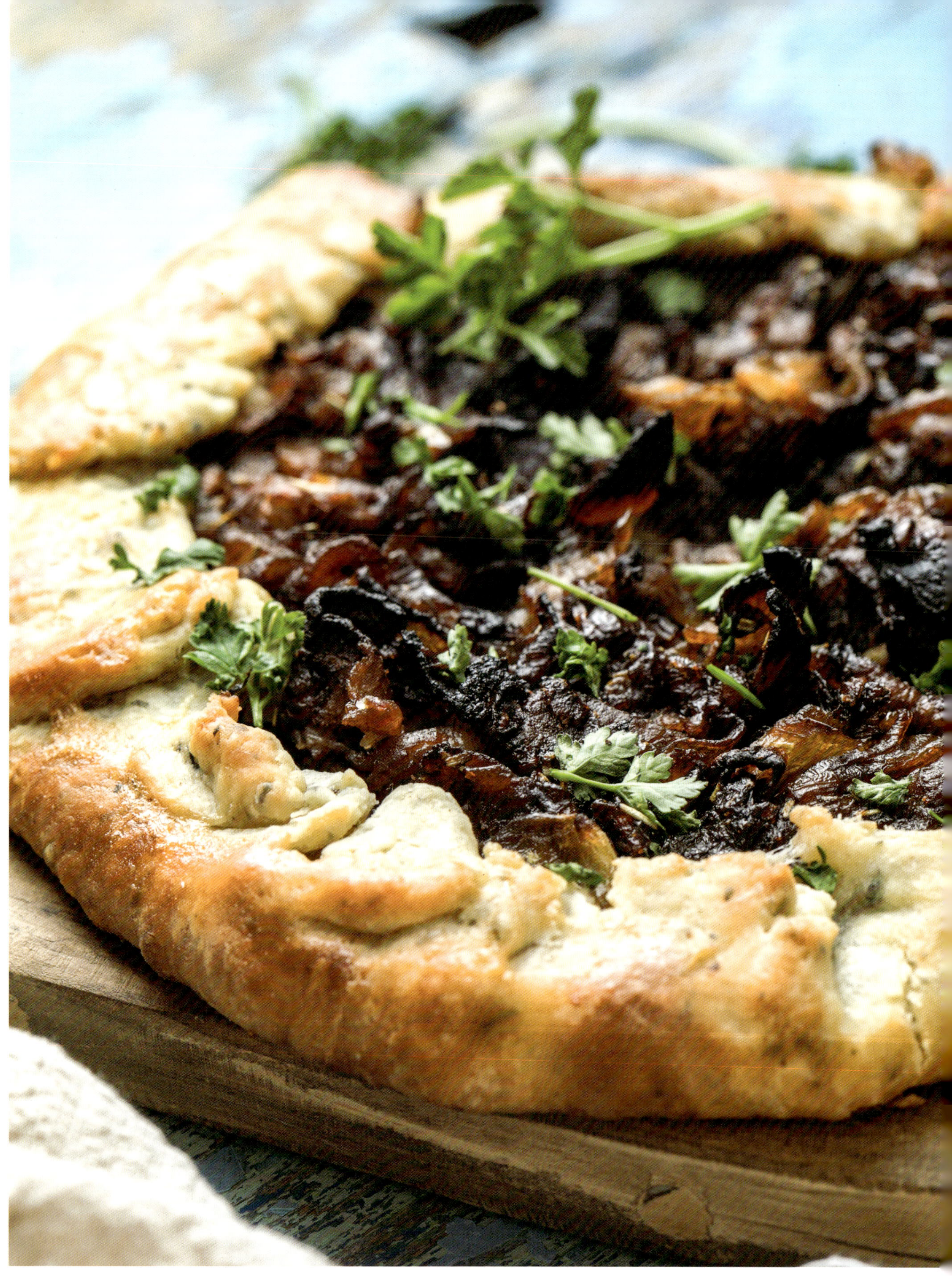

CARAMELISED ONION & MOZZARELLA GALETTE

CARAMELISED ONIONS

2 tbsps unsalted butter

1 tbsp olive oil

4 large onions, thinly sliced

1 tbsp brown sugar (optional, for added sweetness)

Salt and pepper to taste

GALETTE DOUGH (SEE NOTE)

1 tsp onion powder

1 cup (100g) almond flour

1 large egg, room temperature

Salt and pepper to taste

¼ cup iced water

FOR ASSEMBLY

200g mozzarella, sliced

1 egg, lightly beaten

Sprigs of thyme and parsley, to garnish

STEPS

Preheat oven to 200°C.

1. In a large saucepan, melt the butter and olive oil over medium-low heat. Add the onions and cook slowly, stirring occasionally, until they become soft and golden brown. This process can take 30-40 minutes. Sprinkle the brown sugar (if using) over the onions and continue cooking for an additional 5 minutes to enhance the caramelisation. Season with salt and pepper to taste. Set aside to cool slightly.
2. Meanwhile, in a food processor, combine the onion powder, almond flour, egg and a pinch each of salt and pepper. Gradually add the ice water, 1 tablespoon at a time, and pulse until the dough comes together.
3. Transfer the dough onto a flat surface and shape it into a disk. Wrap it in plastic wrap and refrigerate for at least 30 minutes. Once the dough has rested roll out to a large circle of 3mm thickness on a large sheet of baking paper. Transfer the baking paper with the dough to a baking tray.
4. Leaving a 4cm border, add the mozarella cheese to the centre of the dough, and spread caramelised onions evenly over the top. Fold the edges of the dough over the filling, pleating as you go, to create a rustic galette shape.
5. Brush the edges of the dough with beaten egg and bake the galette in the oven for about 30-35 minutes, or until the crust is golden brown and crisp. Serve warm with a garnish of fresh thyme and parsley leaves.

NOTE: Low-carb pastry mix is available to purchase from most supermarkets, and can be used in place of the pastry recipe in this book if preferred.

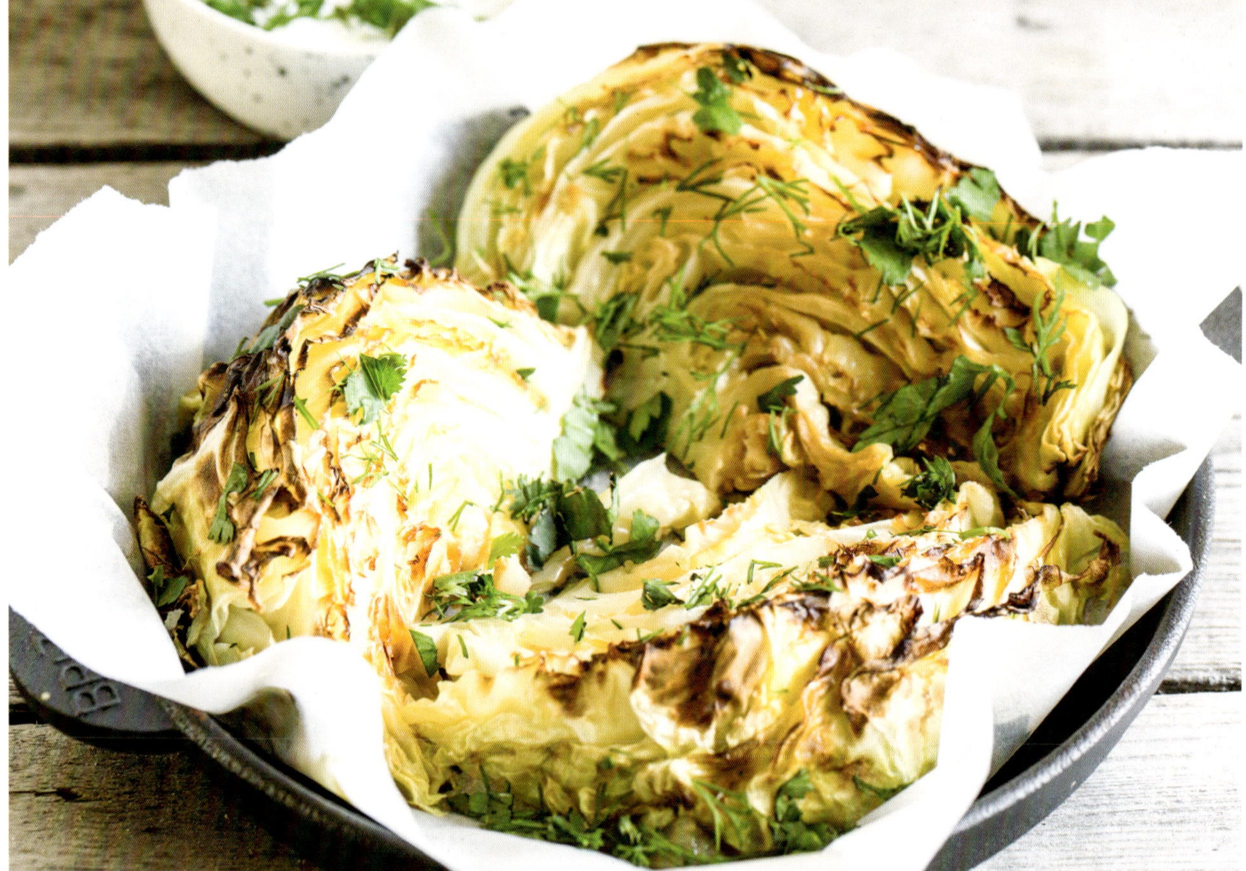

ROASTED CABBAGE WEDGES

1 x 1kg cabbage

2 tbsps olive oil

1 tsp salt

1 tsp garlic powder

½ tsp chilli flakes

Pepper to taste

½ cup (125ml) sour cream

1 tbsp horseradish cream

Fresh herbs, finely chopped (such as parsley and dill)

STEPS

Preheat oven to 200°C.

1. Remove the outer leaves from the cabbage. Cut in half, then into 3cm-wide wedges, leaving the core intact.
2. Place the wedges in a single layer in a lined roasting tin. Drizzle with olive oil. Season with salt, garlic powder, chilli flakes and pepper.
3. Roast the cabbage wedges for 20-25 minutes until golden brown and fork-tender.
4. Combine the sour cream with the horseradish and season with a little salt and pepper.
5. Drizzle the horseradish cream over the cabbage wedges and scatter with herbs to serve.

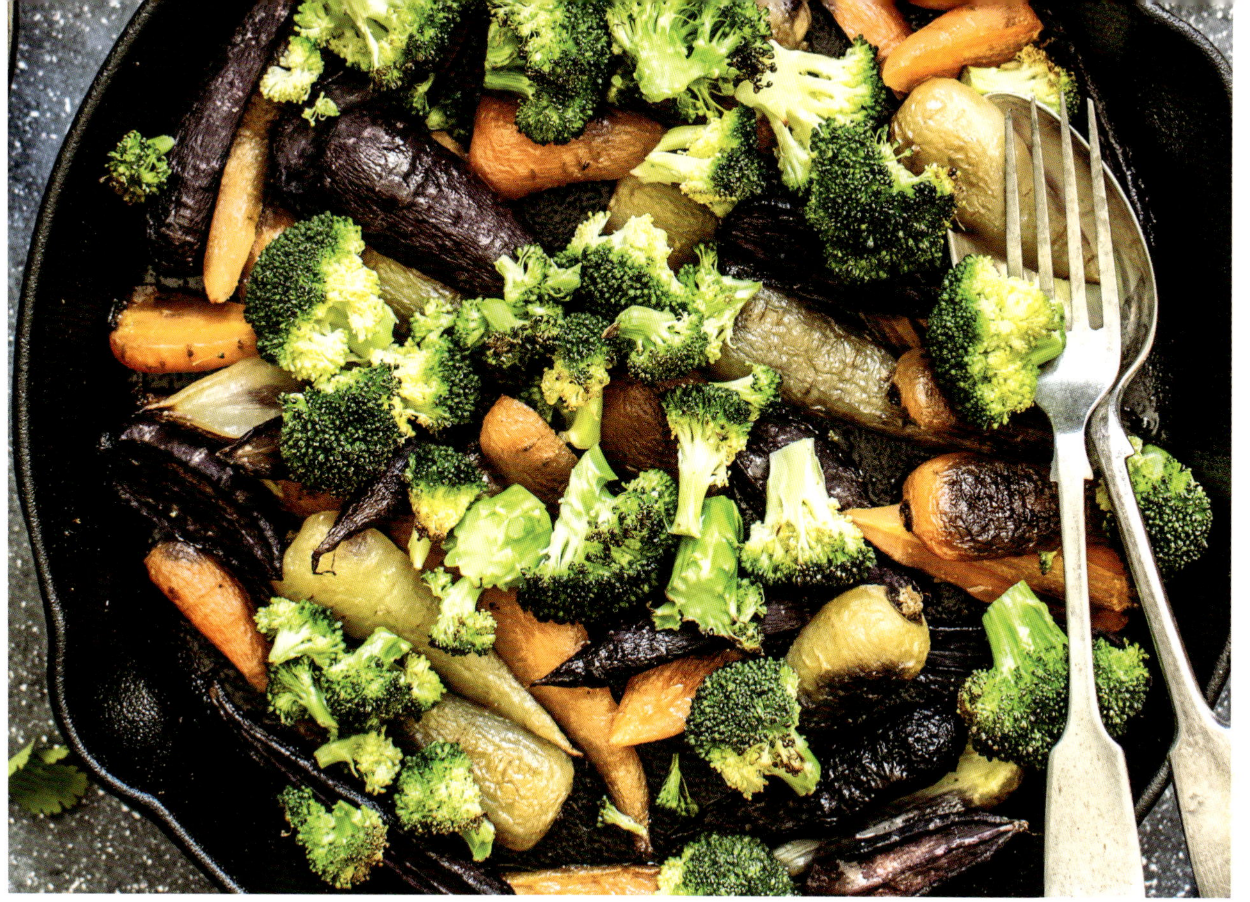

OVEN-ROASTED CARROTS & BROCCOLI

SERVES 4 | PREP + COOK TIME: 40 MINS | VEG | GLUTEN FREE | DAIRY FREE |

500g small carrots, trimmed

1 head broccoli, cut into florets

2 tbsps olive oil

2 cloves garlic, minced

1 tsp dried thyme

½ tsp paprika

Salt and pepper to taste

STEPS

Preheat oven to 180°C.

1. In a large bowl, combine the prepared carrot and broccoli florets.
2. In a small bowl, whisk together the olive oil, minced garlic, dried thyme, paprika, salt and pepper.
3. Pour the olive oil mixture over the carrots and broccoli. Toss well to ensure all the vegetables are coated with the seasoned oil.
4. Spread the carrots and broccoli in a single layer on a lined baking tray and roast in the oven for about 20-25 minutes, or until the vegetables are tender and slightly caramelised, stirring once halfway through the cooking time for even browning.
5. Remove from oven and serve immediately.

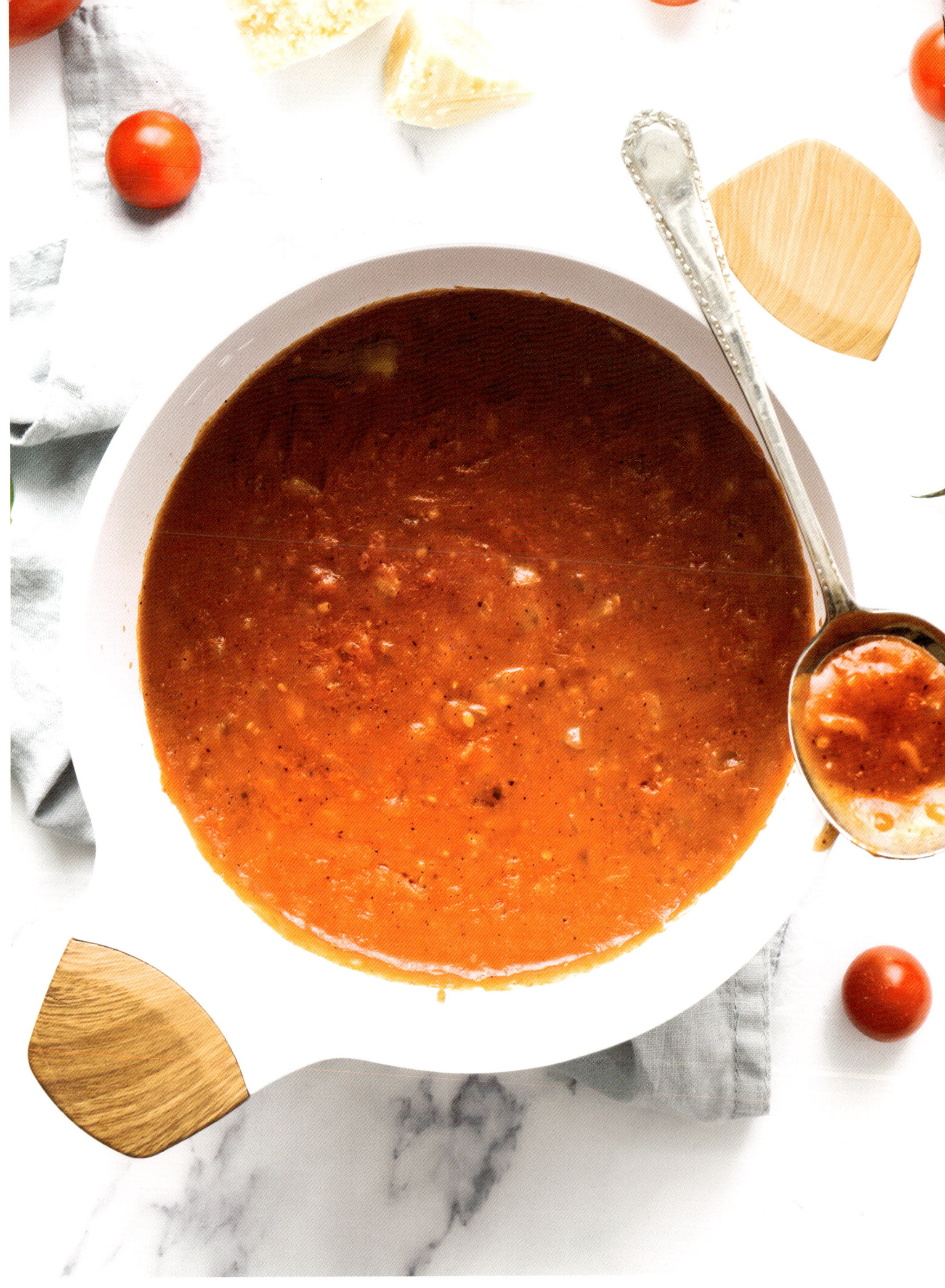

HOMEMADE TOMATO SOUP

2 tbsps olive oil

1 medium onion, chopped

3 cloves garlic, crushed

1 tbsp tomato paste

½ red capsicum, chopped

2 x 400g cans diced tomatoes

2 cups (500ml) vegetable stock

1 cup (250ml) cream

1 tbsp finely chopped rosemary + 1 sprig rosemary leaves, to garnish

Salt and pepper to taste

STEPS

1. Heat the oil in a large pot over medium heat. Fry the onion for 5 minutes until softened and browned. Add the garlic and fry for 1 further minute.
2. Mix in the tomato paste and capsicum and cook for another 1 minute. Add the tomatoes, stock, cream and chopped rosemary and bring to the boil.
3. Reduce the heat to low and simmer, covered, for 30 minutes. Remove from heat and let cool for 10 minutes.
4. Use a stick blender to puree the soup until smooth.
5. Season to taste with salt and pepper and serve garnished with rosemary leaves.

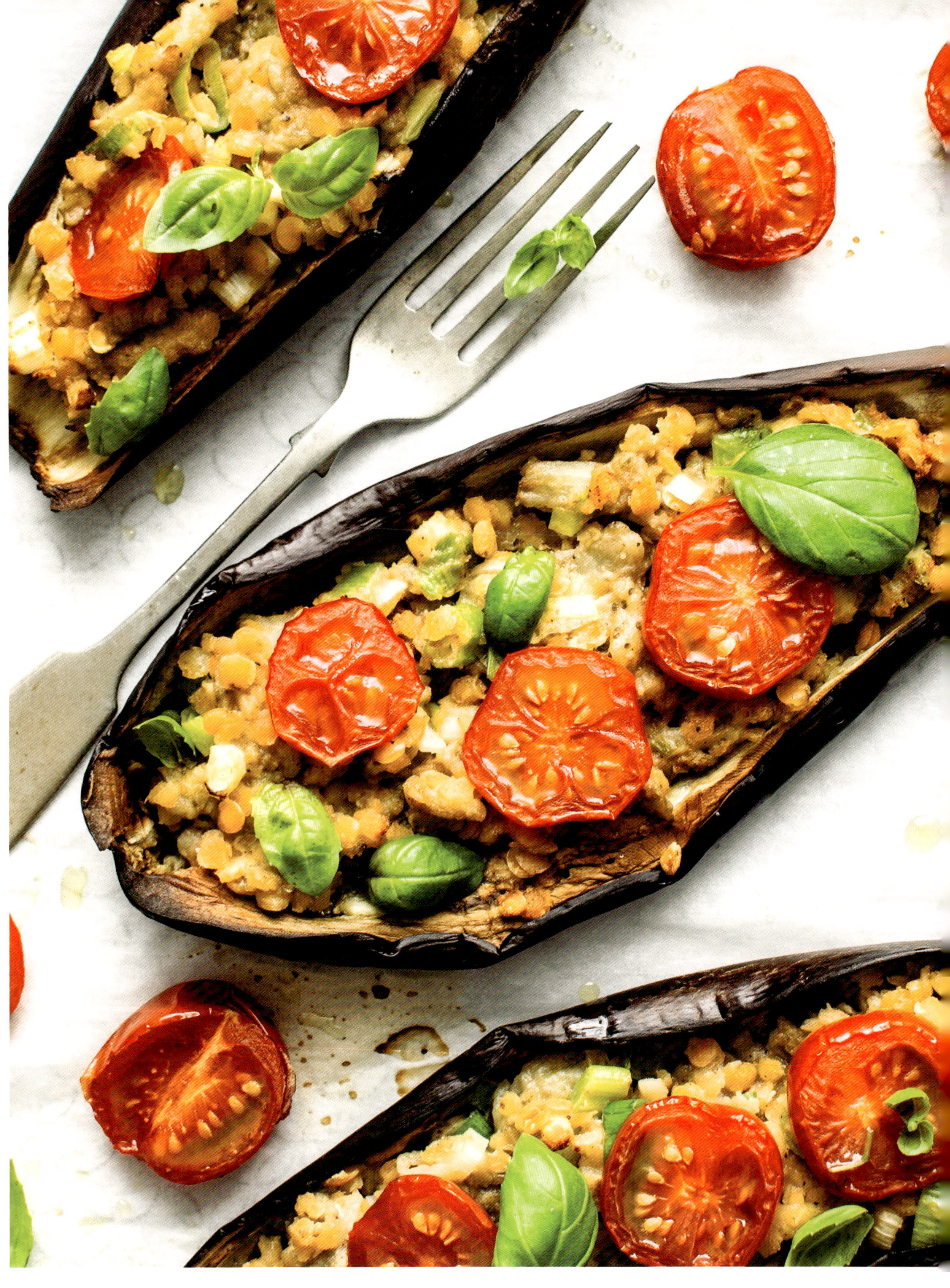

SPLIT PEA STUFFED EGGPLANT

4 large eggplants, halved lengthways
¼ cup (60ml) olive oil
Salt and pepper to taste
1 large onion, quartered and sliced
3 cloves garlic, crushed
1 x 400g can crushed tomatoes
1 tbsp tomato passata
2 cups (500ml) vegetable stock
250g yellow split peas
2 cups (500ml) vegetable oil
Roasted cherry tomatoes
Basil leaves

STEPS

Preheat oven to 150°C.

1. Brush the eggplant halves with half the oil and dust with salt and pepper. Bake them in the oven, cut-side down, for 15 minutes. Remove and let cool.
2. Scoop out the filling, leaving 1cm of flesh attached to the skin. Roughly chop the scooped-out flesh and set aside.
3. Heat the remaining oil in a large frying pan over medium heat. Fry the onion for 5 minutes, then add the garlic and fry for another 2 minutes.
4. Add the canned tomatoes and passata, eggplant flesh, stock and split peas to the pan then simmer uncovered for 45 minutes or until split peas are tender and liquid has reduced. Season with salt and pepper.
5. Stuff the eggplants with the filling and place them snugly in a shallow baking dish. Cover with foil and bake for 45 minutes. Serve warm with roasted tomatoes and basil leaves.

SERVES 4 | PREP + COOK TIME: 2 HOURS | VEG | GLUTEN FREE | DAIRY FREE |

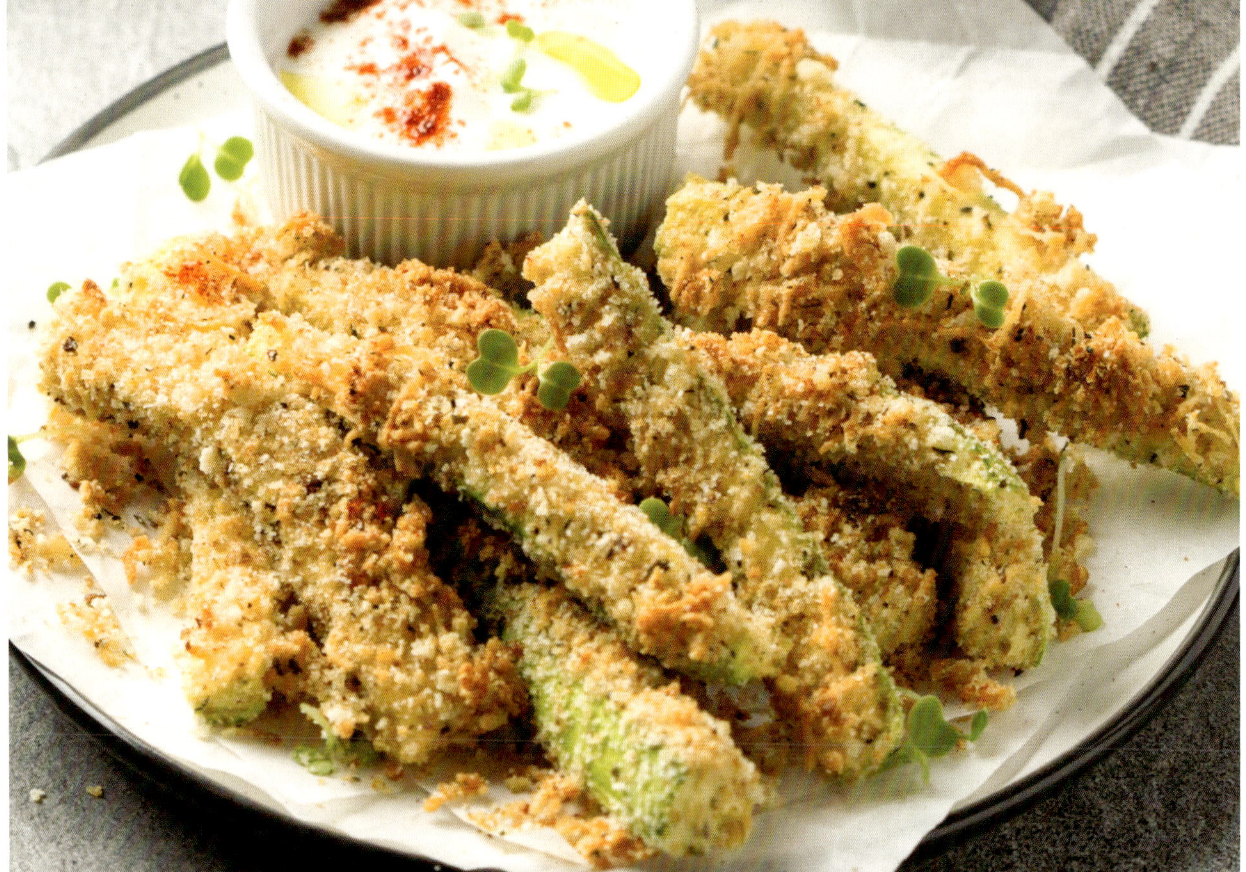

ZUCCHINI FRIES

½ cup (50g) almond flour

¼ cup (25g) grated Parmesan cheese

1 tsp garlic powder

1 tsp paprika

½ tsp salt

¼ tsp pepper

2 large eggs

2 large zucchinis, cut into long chip shapes

STEPS

Preheat oven to 220°C.

1. In a shallow bowl, combine the almond flour, grated Parmesan cheese, garlic powder, paprika, salt and pepper. Mix well.
2. In a separate bowl, whisk the eggs until well combined. Dip each zucchini stick into the beaten eggs, allowing any excess to drip off.
3. Roll the zucchini stick in the almond flour mixture, pressing gently to adhere the coating evenly. Then place the coated zucchini sticks on a lined baking tray in a single layer, making sure they are not touching.
4. Bake in the preheated oven for about 15-20 minutes, or until the zucchini fries are golden brown and crispy. Flip them halfway through the baking time for even browning.

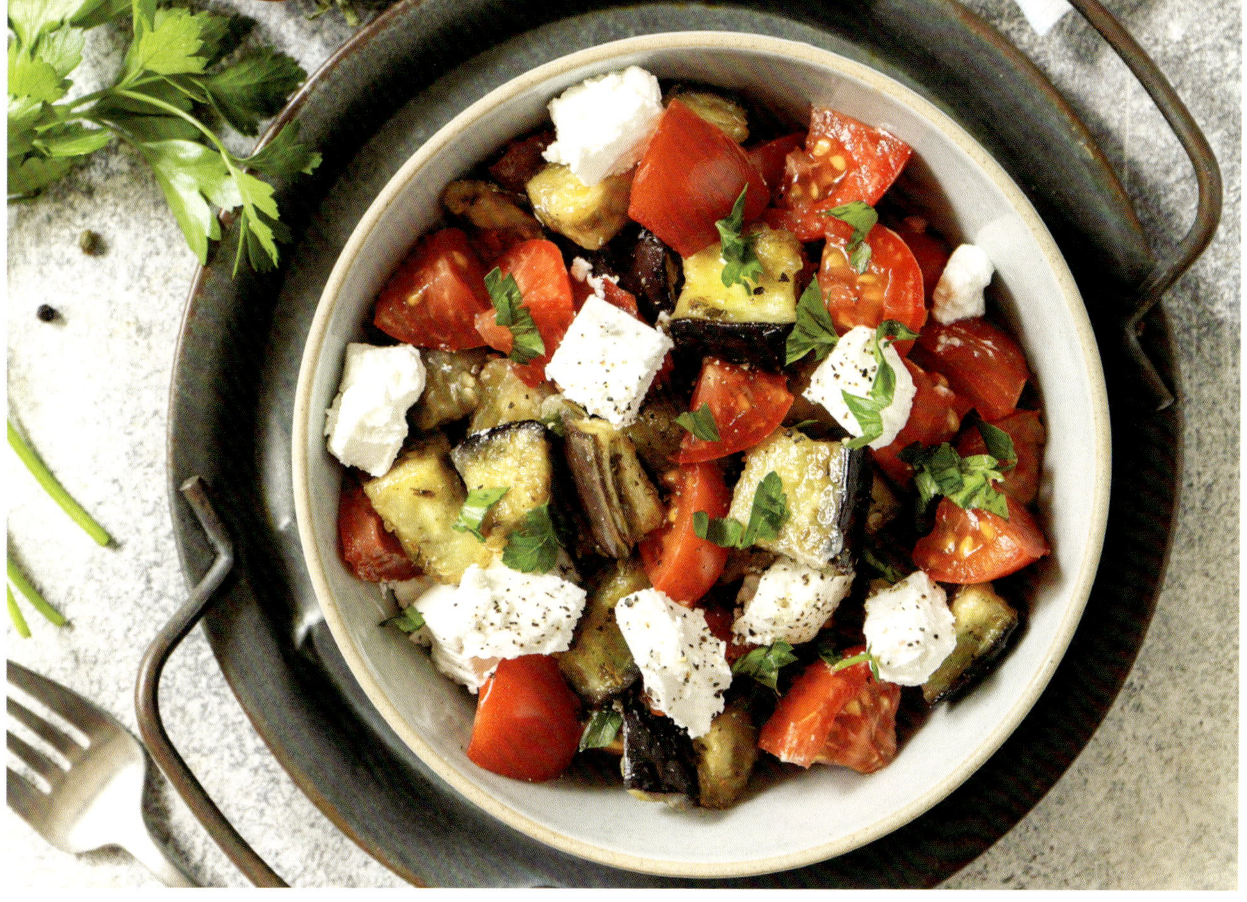

GRILLED EGGPLANT SALAD

2 medium eggplants, cut in 2cm thick slices

4 tbsps olive oil

Salt and pepper to taste

2 large tomatoes, cubed

1 large ball mozzarella, torn

2 tbsps olive oil

2 tbsps balsamic vinegar

2 tbsps pesto (store-bought or see recipe page 69)

¼ cup (10g) fresh basil leaves

STEPS

1. Brush the eggplant slices with half the olive oil and a good couple of grinds of salt and pepper.
2. Heat a large grill pan over medium-high heat. Grill the eggplant for 5 minutes on each side until softened. Remove from the pan and cut into chunks.
3. To assemble the salad, in a serving bowl, add the warm eggplant chunks, the cubed tomato and mozzarella, toss gently to combine.
4. Drizzle over the oil, vinegar and pesto and garnish with basil leaves.

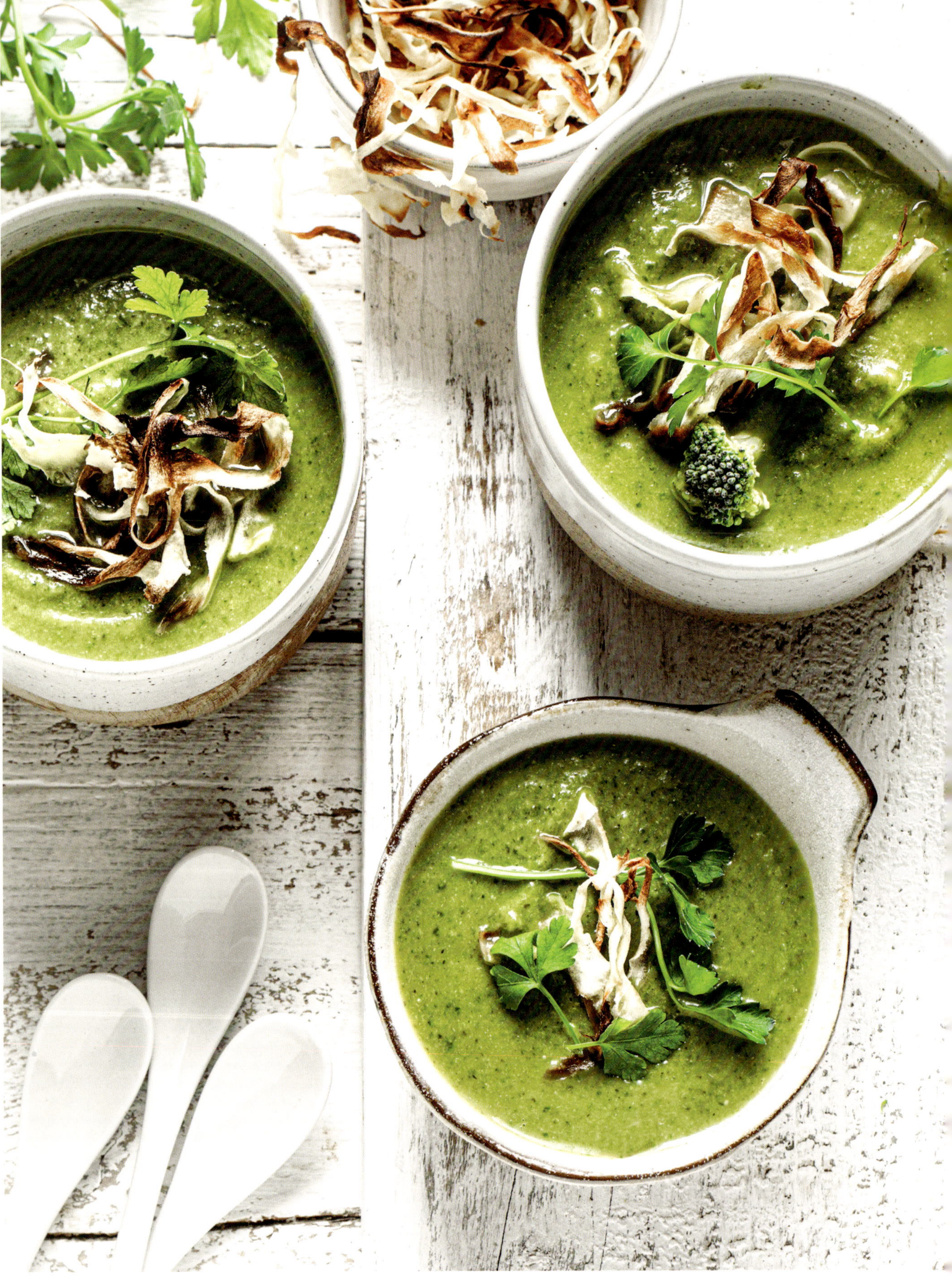

CREAMY BROCCOLI SOUP

SERVES 4 | PREP + COOK TIME: 1 HOUR | VEG | GLUTEN FREE |

1 head broccoli (about 800g)

2 tbsps olive oil

1 onion, finely chopped

2 cloves garlic, crushed

4 cups (1L) vegetable stock

50g baby spinach leaves

2 tbsps fresh thyme sprigs, chopped

1 tbsp Dijon mustard

1 cup (250ml) thickened cream

Salt and pepper to taste

OPTIONAL GARNISHES

Handful of parsnip crisps

Fresh parsley leaves

STEPS

1. Cut stems from broccoli and separate florets into small, bite-sized pieces.
2. In a heavy-based saucepan heat olive oil over high heat and add the onion and garlic, cooking and stirring for 2 minutes or until aromatic.
3. Add the broccoli stems and florets, stock, baby spinach leaves and thyme to the pan then cover and bring to the boil. Reduce heat to medium and simmer, partially covered, for 30 minutes or until the broccoli is tender. Cool slightly.
4. Transfer soup mixture to a blender, add the mustard and cream and process until smooth. Season with salt and plenty of pepper.
5. Divide soup into bowls and serve with fresh parsley and parsnip crisps, if desired.

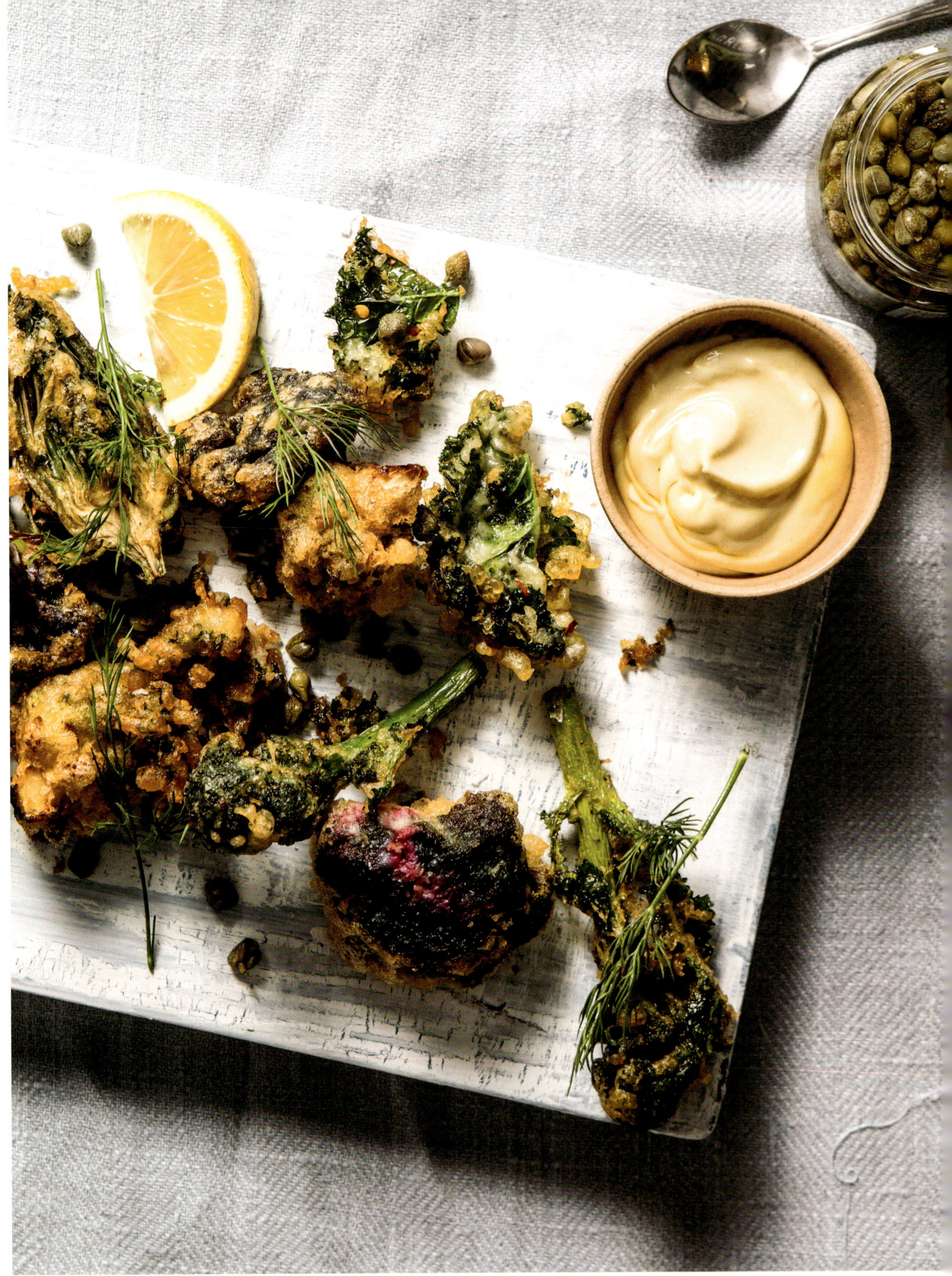

CRISPY SPICED VEGETABLES

2 cups (130g) curly kale, stemmed and roughly chopped

100g broccolini, separated

100g purple broccoli, cut into florets

1 tsp ground cumin

1 tsp ground coriander

½ tsp garam masala

½ tsp salt

1 cup (95g) besan (chickpea flour)

3 tbsps cornflour

1 tsp baking powder

¾ cup (185ml) + 1 tbsp cold sparkling water

3 cups (750ml) canola oil or grapeseed oil for frying

TO SERVE

Salt to taste

½ cup (120g) store-bought aioli

1 tbsp capers

Fresh dill leaves

STEPS

1. In a large bowl combine kale, broccolini, broccoli, spices and salt. Toss to combine.
2. In another bowl whisk together chickpea flour, cornflour and baking powder then whisk in the sparkling water. The batter should have consistency of thick cream.
3. Pour oil into a medium-sized saucepan with a depth of approximately 7cm and heat over medium-high heat, and prepare an oven tray with a few layers of paper towel and place near the cook top.
4. Using tongs, dip the vegetables into the batter. Carefully transfer coated vegetables into the hot oil. Fry in batches until golden, approximately 1 minute. Using a slotted spoon flip the pieces over or press them down into the oil so that all sides of the vegetables crisp up. Remove from the oil, allowing excess oil to drip back into the pan.
5. Drain on the towel-covered tray and allow to cool slightly. Sprinkle with salt and serve with garlic aioli, capers and fresh dill sprigs.

SERVES 2 | PREP + COOK TIME: 40 MINS | VEG | GLUTEN FREE | DAIRY FREE |

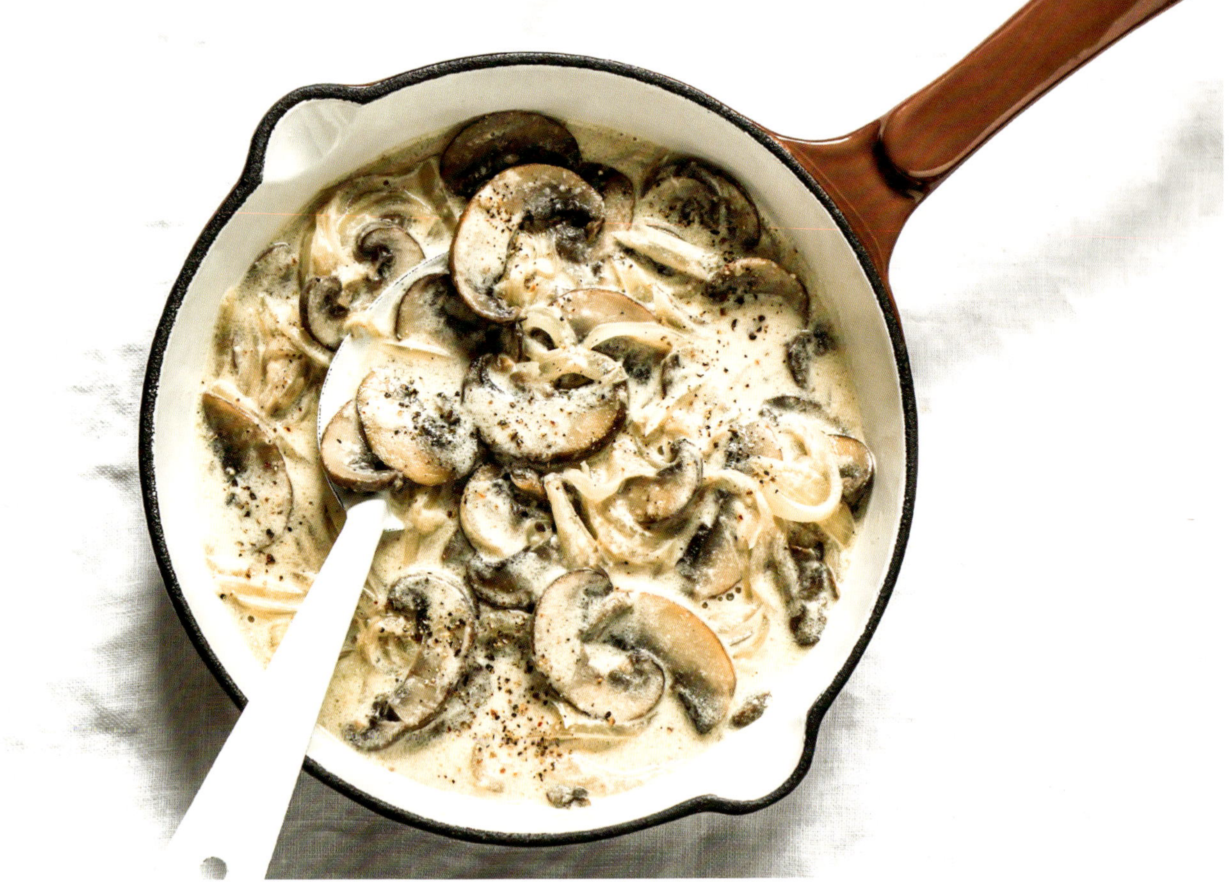

MUSHROOMS IN CREAM SAUCE

2 tbsps olive oil
1 onion, finely sliced
500g mushrooms, sliced
4 cloves garlic, minced
½ cup (125ml) cream
2 tbsps parsley, chopped
Salt and pepper to taste

STEPS

1. Heat olive oil in a large frying pan over medium heat. Add onion and cook for 3-4 minutes until starting to turn golden. Add mushrooms and cook, stirring regularly, for 7-8 minutes until the mushrooms release their liquid and become golden brown and tender.
2. Add the garlic and cook for another minute until fragrant.
3. Stir in the cream and parsley.
4. Season to taste with salt and pepper before serving.

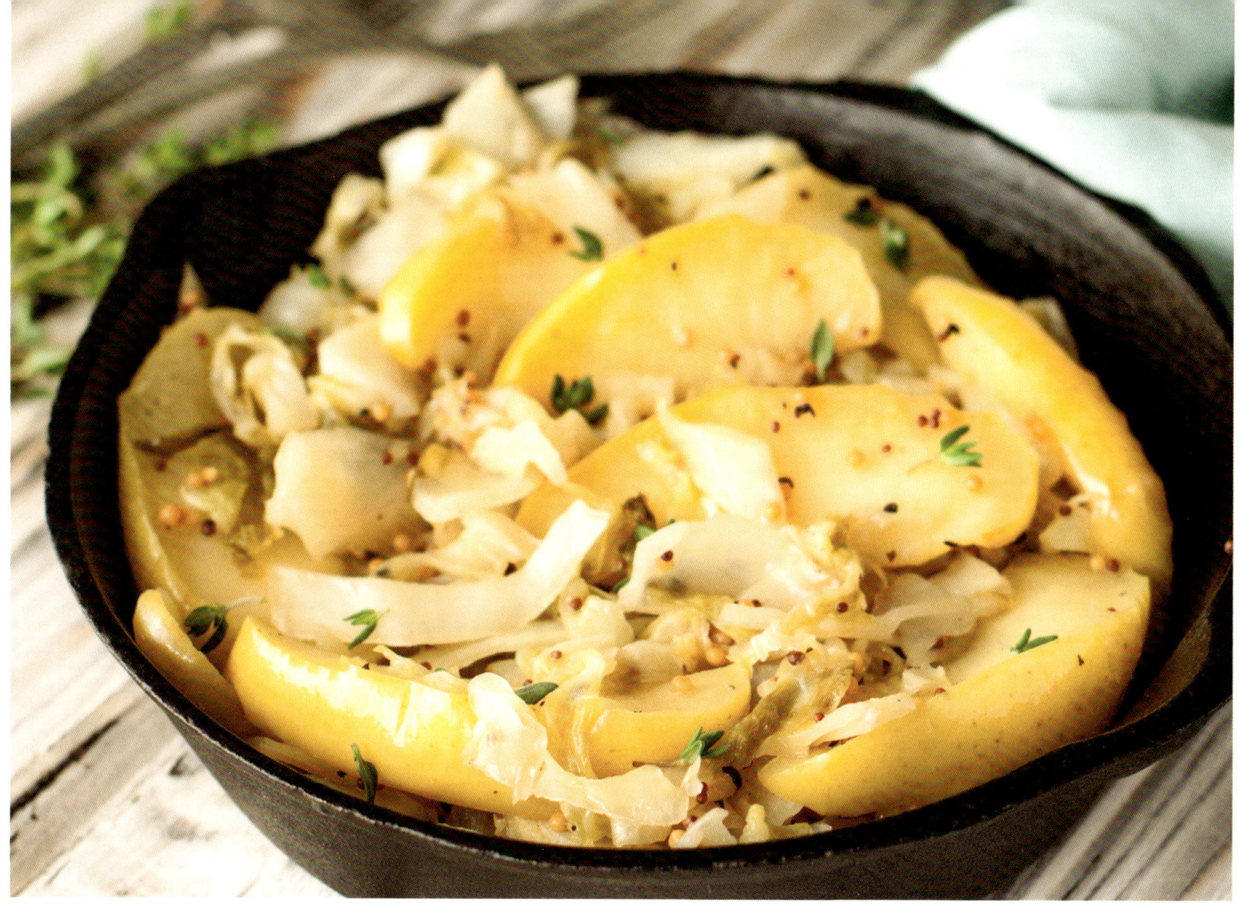

BRAISED CABBAGE WITH APPLE & THYME

2 tbsps olive oil

1 onion, thinly sliced

2 cloves garlic, crushed

1 small head cabbage, thinly sliced

1 large apple, cored and thinly sliced

1 tsp fresh thyme leaves + extra to garnish

1 tbsp seeded mustard

1 cup (250ml) vegetable stock

2 tbsps apple cider vinegar

Salt and pepper to taste

STEPS

1. Heat the olive oil in a large frying pan over medium heat. Add the sliced onion and garlic and saute for about 2-3 minutes or until the onion becomes translucent.

2. Add the cabbage to the pan and cook for about 5-7 minutes, stirring occasionally, until the cabbage begins to wilt. Stir in the sliced apple, thyme leaves and seeded mustard then continue cooking for another 2-3 minutes until the apple softens slightly.

3. Pour in stock and apple cider vinegar and then season with salt and pepper.

4. Reduce the heat to low, cover with a lid and let the cabbage mixture simmer for about 10-15 minutes until the cabbage is tender, stirring occasionally.

5. Serve warm with extra thyme leaves.

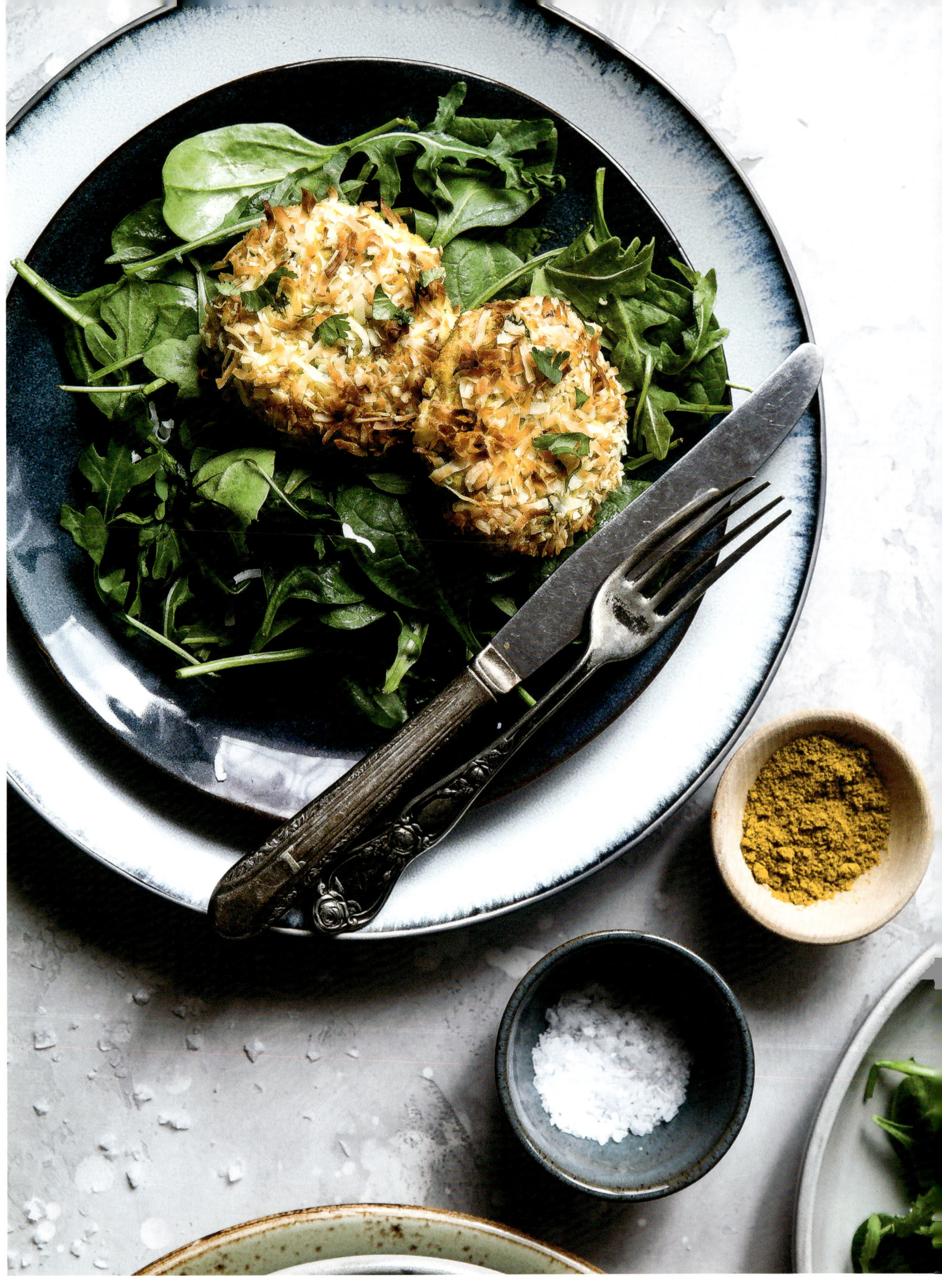

CAULIFLOWER PATTIES

1 tbsp olive oil

3½ cups (350g) cauliflower rice

2 eggs

¼ cup (30g) almond meal

3 tbsps grated onion

½ tsp garlic powder

½ tsp curry powder

1 tbsp fresh coriander leaves

¾ tsp salt or to taste

¼ tsp pepper

1 cup (90g) shredded coconut

2 tbsps avocado oil, ghee or butter

2 cups (70g) mixed salad leaves to serve

STEPS

1. Heat olive oil in large frying pan over medium heat. Add cauliflower rice and cook, stirring occasionally, for 5-8 minutes until tender.

2. Transfer to a clean tea towel and squeeze out excess liquid.

3. Transfer cauliflower rice to a large bowl with eggs, almond meal, onion, garlic powder, curry powder, coriander, salt and pepper. Mix to combine.

4. Scoop out about 1½ tablespoons of the mixture and shape into a patty with your hands. Roll in shredded coconut then set aside. Repeat with remaining mixture.

5. Add the avocado oil, ghee or butter to a pan and heat over medium-high heat. Cook patties in batches of four to six at a time, taking care not to overcrowd the pan. Cook for 5-6 minutes on one side, until crispy and browning. Flip and cook for another 3-4 minutes. Serve hot with salad leaves and your favourite dipping sauce.

MAKES 20 | PREP + COOK TIME: 45 MINS | VEG | GLUTEN FREE | DAIRY FREE |

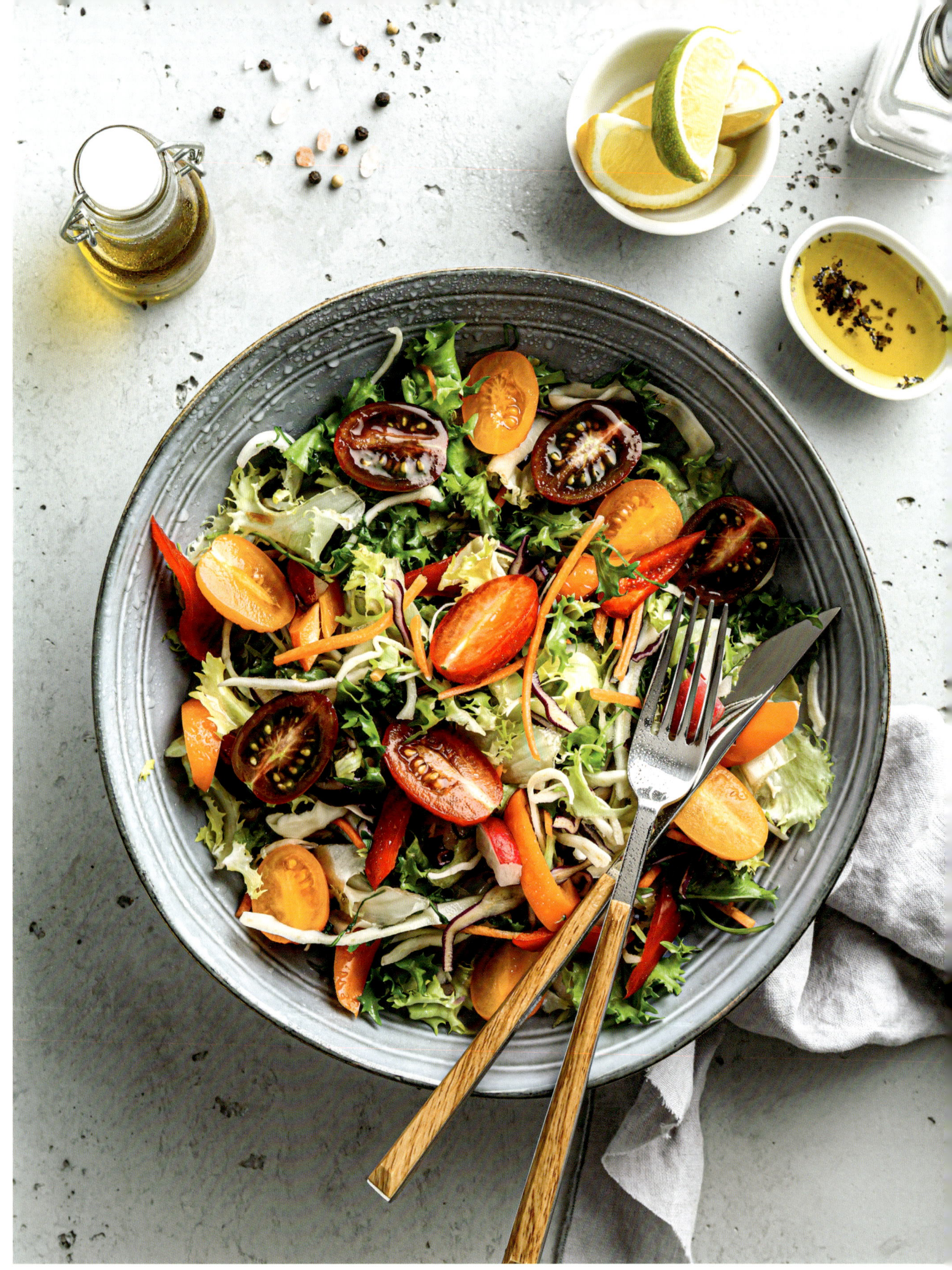

SIMPLE SALAD WITH THREE VINAIGRETTES

½ cup (110g) cherry tomatoes, halved

200g mixed lettuce leaves

1 carrot, julienned

4-5 radishes, julienned

1 cup (100g) shredded red cabbage

DRESSING SUGGESTIONS (SEE NOTE):

SIMPLE VINAIGRETTE

¼ cup (60ml) olive oil

2 tbsps red wine vinegar

1 tsp Dijon mustard

1 clove garlic, crushed (optional)

Salt and pepper to taste

HONEY SOY DRESSING

2 tbsps soy sauce

2 tbsps rice wine vinegar

1 tbsp sesame oil

1 tbsp honey or maple syrup

1 tsp grated fresh ginger

1 clove garlic, crushed

1 tbsp sesame seeds

TAHINI DRESSING

¼ cup (60g) tahini

2 tbsps fresh lemon juice

2 tbsps water

1 clove garlic, crushed

1 tbsp olive oil

1 tbsp maple syrup or honey

½ tsp ground cumin

Salt and pepper to taste

STEPS

1. For the salad, place the cherry tomatoes, lettuce leaves, carrot, radishes and cabbage and toss to combine. Set aside while you prepare your chosen dressing.
2. For the Simple Vinaigrette, in a small bowl combine the olive oil, vinegar, Dijon mustard, garlic (if using), salt and pepper. Whisk ingredients vigorously until they are well combined and emulsified.
3. For the Honey Soy Dressing, in a small bowl whisk together the soy sauce, rice wine vinegar, sesame oil, honey or maple syrup, grated ginger, garlic and sesame seeds.
4. For the Tahini Dressing, in a small bowl whisk together tahini, fresh lemon juice, water, garlic, olive oil, maple syrup or honey, ground cumin, salt and pepper. Whisk the ingredients together until well combined and the dressing is smooth. If the dressing is too thick, you can add more water, a tablespoon at a time, until you achieve the desired consistency.
5. Drizzle chosen dressing liberally over salad and toss to coat well.

NOTE: Three different styles of vinaigrette are included in this recipe. Don't use them all at once! Experiment with each one, and you will soon have learned three easy and tasty ways to liven up a simple salad.

SERVES 2 | PREP + COOK TIME: 15 MINS | VEG | GLUTEN FREE | DAIRY FREE |

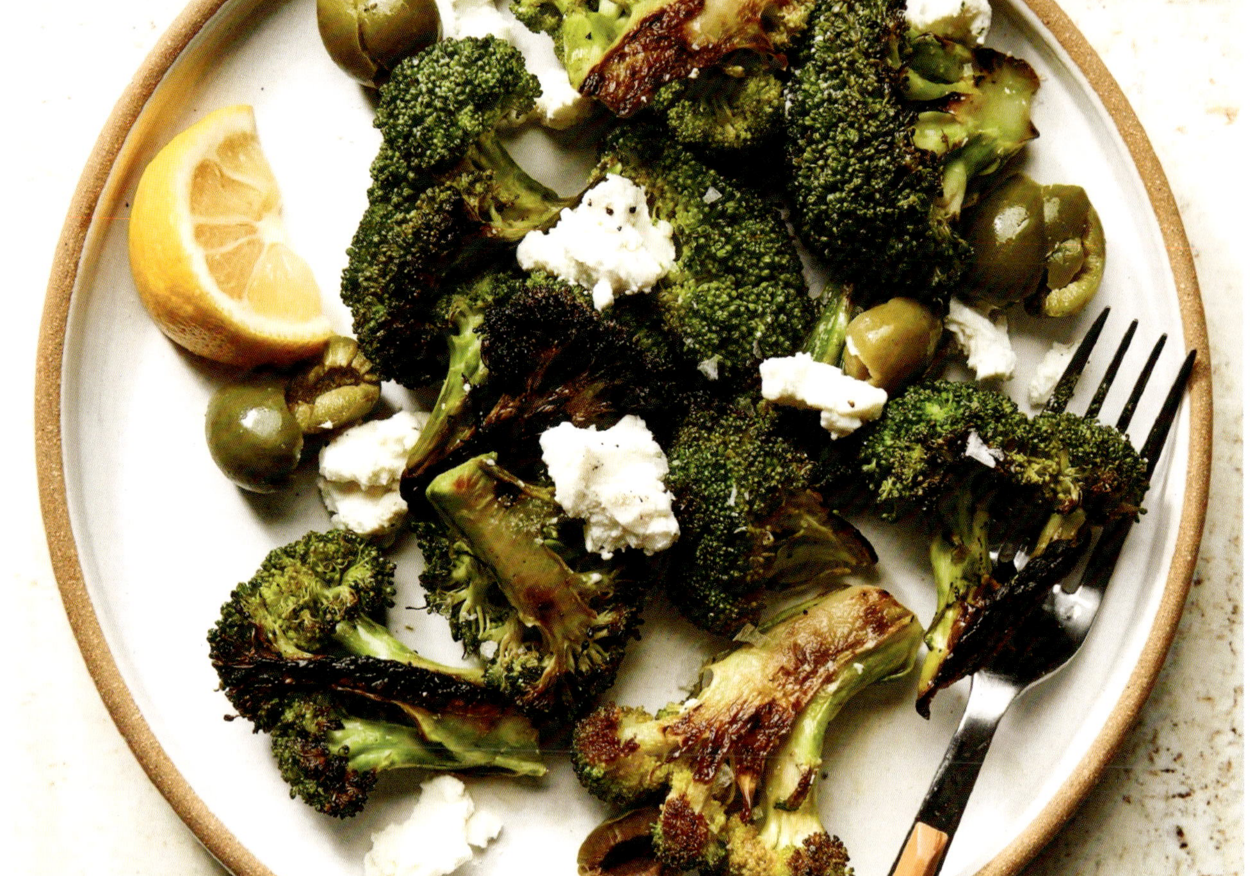

CHARRED BROCCOLI SALAD

3 tbsps olive oil

1 large head broccoli, cut into florets

¼ tsp salt

¼ tsp dried chilli flakes

½ cup (70g) green olives, crushed, pitted

60g fresh goat's cheese

1 lemon, cut into wedges

STEPS

1. Heat 2 tablespoons oil in a large frying pan over medium-high heat. Add the broccoli and season with salt and chilli flakes. Stir, then cook untouched for 3 minutes.
2. Turn over and cook for another 2-3 minutes until broccoli is browned on the other side and fork-tender.
3. Transfer to a serving plate. Scatter with olives and goat's cheese. Squeeze over lemon wedges to serve.

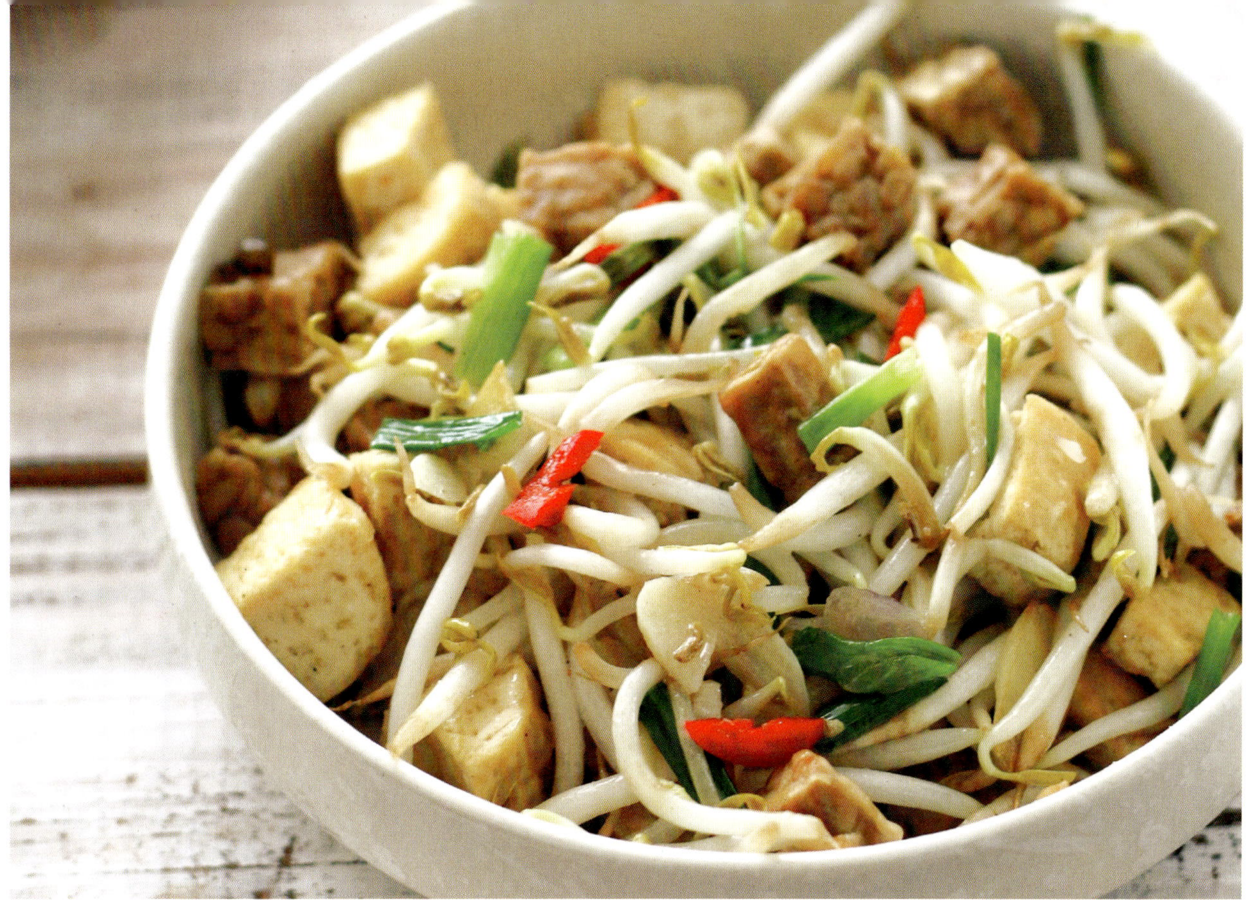

SERVES 2 | PREP + COOK TIME: 15 MINS | VEG | GLUTEN FREE | DAIRY FREE |

BEAN SPROUT & TOFU STIR-FRY

2 cups (225g) bean sprouts

3 tbsps peanut oil or other neutral-flavoured oil

200g firm tofu, diced

200g tempeh, diced

3 cloves garlic, thinly sliced

½ long red chilli, sliced

1 tbsp soy sauce

1 spring onion, cut into 2cm lengths

STEPS

1. Rinse the bean sprouts under cold water. Drain and set aside.
2. Heat 2 tablespoons oil in a wok or large frying pan over medium-high heat. Fry the tofu and tempeh for 3-4 minutes on each side until golden brown. Transfer to a plate lined with paper towel and set aside.
3. Heat another tablespoon of oil in the same wok or pan. Add the garlic and chilli and stir-fry for 30 seconds until fragrant.
4. Return the tofu and tempeh to the pan then add the bean sprouts, soy sauce and spring onion. Stir-fry for a minute or so until heated through.
5. Serve immediately.

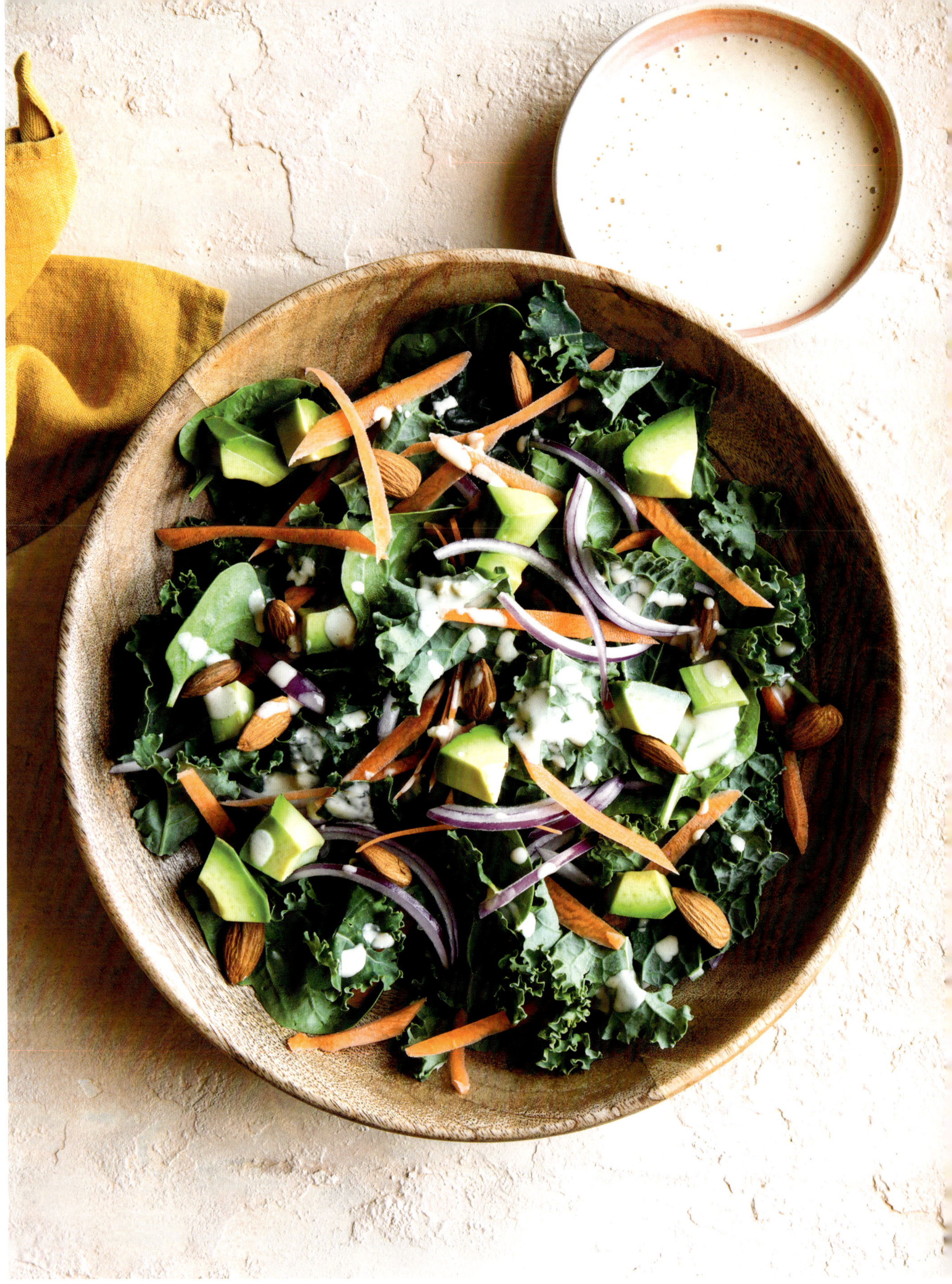

KALE SALAD WITH MAYONNAISE DRESSING

SERVES 2 | PREP + COOK TIME: 15 MINS | VEG | GLUTEN FREE | DAIRY FREE |

200g curly kale, torn into bite-size pieces

1 small red onion, finely sliced

2 carrots, julienned

1 avocado, cubed

¼ cup (30g) whole almonds

DRESSING

1 tsp Dijon mustard

2 tbsps mayonnaise

1 tbsp apple cider vinegar

Salt and pepper to taste

STEPS

1. For the salad place the kale, onion, carrot, avocado and whole almonds in a large serving bowl and toss well to combine.

2. For the dressing, in a small bowl or a jar place mustard, mayonnaise, cider vinegar and salt and pepper then shake vigorously until the dressing looks creamy and well combined. If it's too thick add small amounts of water until the desired consistency is achieved.

3. Drizzle the prepared salad with the dressing and serve immediately.

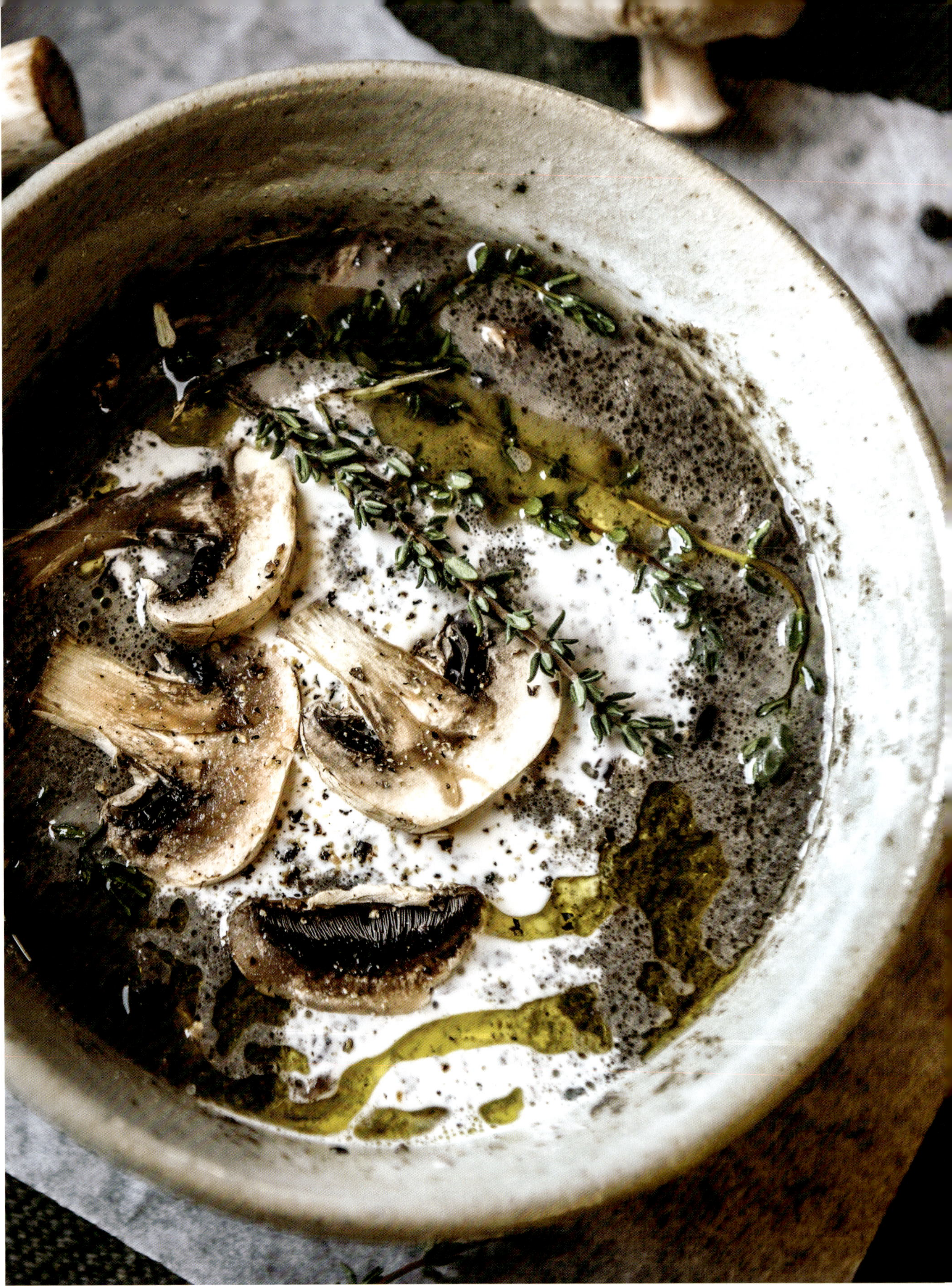

MUSHROOM & THYME SOUP

100g butter

1 leek, sliced

4 cloves garlic, roughly chopped

3 sprigs thyme; 2 whole, 1 broken into pieces

650g mushrooms, sliced

3 cups (750ml) chicken stock

1 cup (250ml) thickened cream + ¼ cup (60ml) to serve

Salt and pepper to taste

Olive oil for drizzling

STEPS

1. Melt butter in a large saucepan over medium heat. Add leek, garlic and whole thyme sprigs and saute for 5 minutes until leek is softened. Add mushrooms and stir; continue to cook for 3 minutes until tender. Remove about ¼ cup of mushrooms from the pan and set aside for garnish, if desired.

2. Add chicken stock to the pan and simmer for 15-20 minutes. Remove the pan from the heat and remove and discard thyme sprigs. Allow to cool slightly.

3. Transfer soup to a blender or use a stick blender to blend mushroom soup until smooth. Return soup to the pan and stir in cream. Season with salt and pepper to taste.

4. Ladle the soup between bowls and garnish with the reserved mushrooms pieces, cream, olive oil and thyme pieces. Season with salt and pepper once more to serve.

SERVES 4 | PREP + COOK TIME: 40 MINS | VEG | GLUTEN FREE |

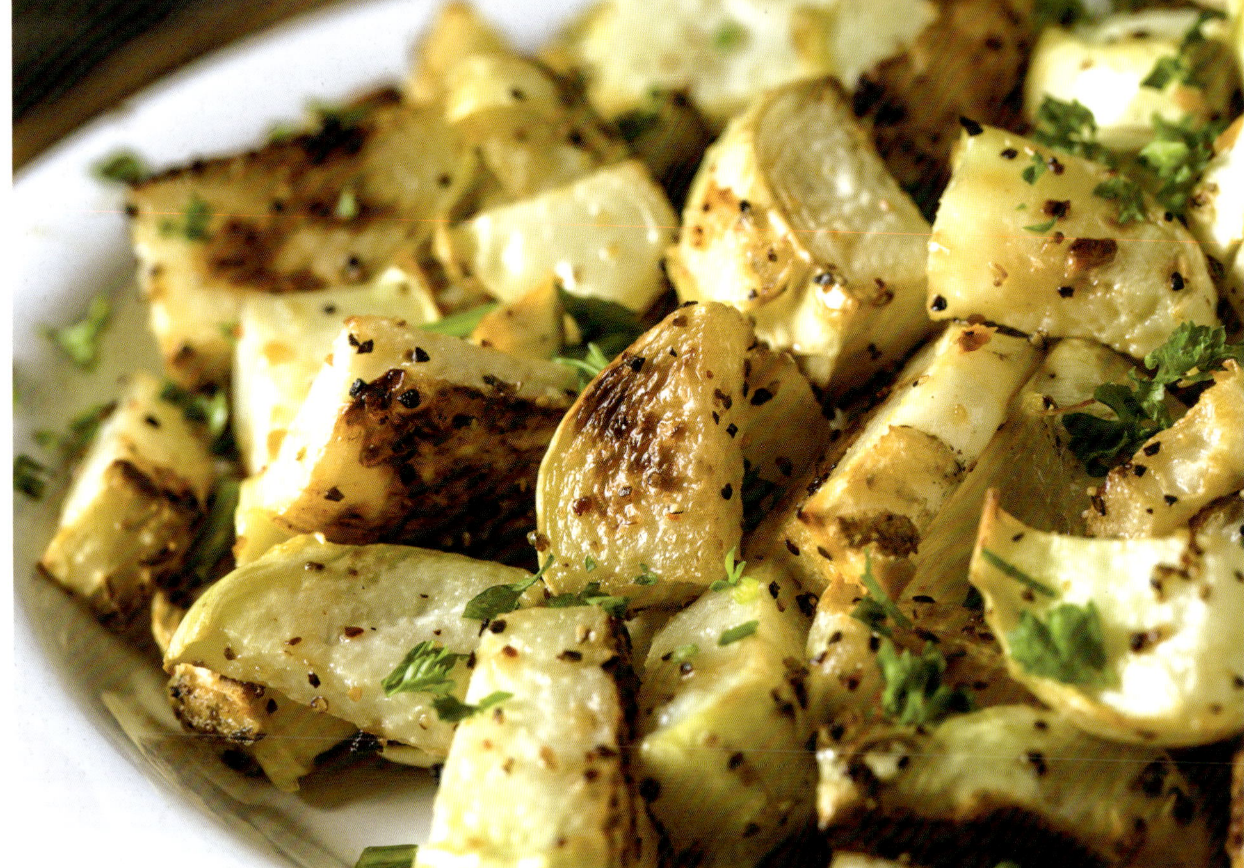

ROASTED KOHLRABI

2 kohlrabi bulbs

2 tbsps olive oil

1 tsp chilli flakes

½ tsp garlic powder

½ tsp dried thyme

½ tsp dried rosemary

Salt and pepper to taste

STEPS

Preheat oven to 200°C.

1. Peel the kohlrabi bulbs using a vegetable peeler. Cut off the tough ends and slice the bulbs into bite-sized pieces.
2. In a large bowl, whisk together the olive oil, chilli flakes, garlic powder, dried thyme, dried rosemary, salt and pepper. Add the kohlrabi pieces to the bowl and toss them in the marinade until they are evenly coated.
3. Transfer the coated kohlrabi pieces to a lined baking tray, spreading them out in a single layer.
4. Roast in the preheated oven for 25-30 minutes, or until the kohlrabi is tender and golden brown, stirring once or twice during cooking to ensure even browning.

SERVES 2 | PREP + COOK TIME: 30 MINS | VEG | GLUTEN FREE | DAIRY FREE |

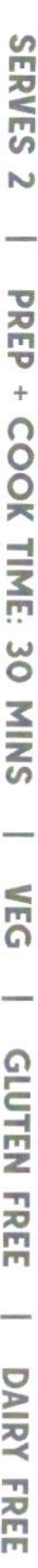

MUSHROOM BURGER WITH CASHEW CHEESE

CASHEW CHEESE SAUCE

½ cup (60g) cashews, soaked in ½ cup (125ml) water for at least 1 hour

1 tsp lemon juice

¼ tsp salt

2 tbsps water

TO ASSEMBLE

1 tbsp tamari

1 tbsp olive oil

Salt and pepper to taste

4 large portobello mushrooms, cleaned and stalks removed

¼ cup (55g) guacamole

1 beefsteak tomato, thickly sliced

½ cup (15g) mix of rocket and baby spinach

1 tsp sesame seeds (optional)

STEPS

1. To make the cashew cheese, drain and rinse the soaked cashews. Place in a food processor with lemon juice and salt. Blend for 1 minute to combine ingredients. Add water and process until completely smooth, about 3 minutes, and set aside.
2. Mix together tamari and olive oil, salt and pepper and lightly brush the mushrooms with the mix.
3. Heat a grill pan or barbecue to a medium-high heat. Grill the mushrooms for 3 minutes on each side until just cooked.
4. To assemble, stack guacamole, sliced tomato, salad leaves and cashew cheese on two of the mushroom buns. Top with the two remaining mushroom buns and sprinkle sesame seeds over the top.

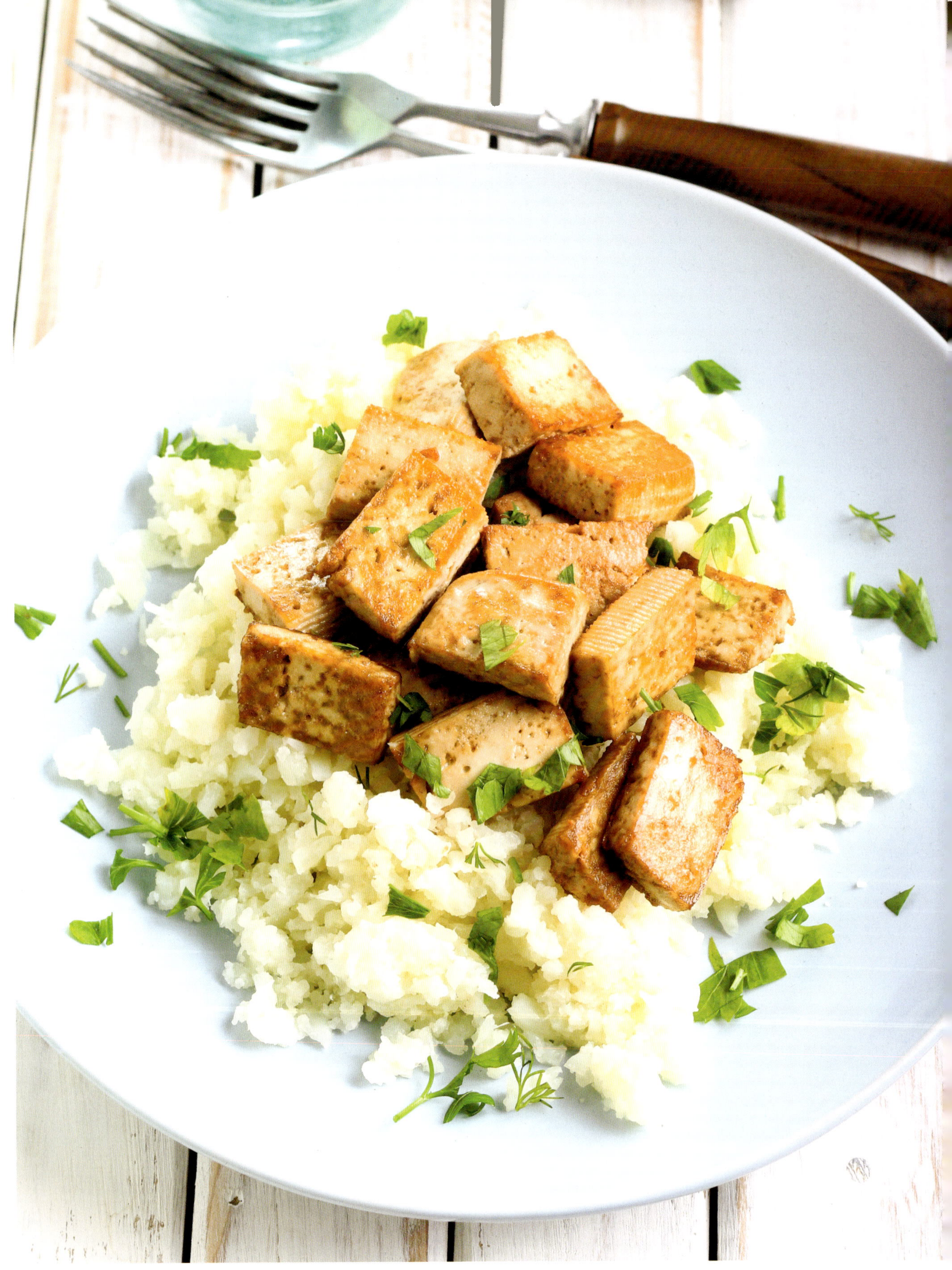

FRIED TOFU WITH CAULIFLOWER RICE

2 tbsps soy sauce
1 tbsp sesame oil
1 tbsp rice wine vinegar
2 cloves garlic, crushed
Small piece ginger, grated
300g firm tofu, drained and cubed
1 small head cauliflower
1 tbsp vegetable oil
Fresh coriander, chopped, to garnish

STEPS

1. In a small bowl, whisk together soy sauce, sesame oil, rice wine vinegar, crushed garlic and ginger, mixing well to combine. Add the tofu and let it marinate for 15-30 minutes.

2. For the cauliflower rice, remove the leaves and core of the cauliflower, then grate it using a box grater or pulse it in a food processor until it resembles rice.

3. Heat a nonstick frying pan on a low heat and add cauliflower rice and cook, stirring occasionally, for 5-7 minutes or until nicely softened. Remove from the pan and set aside.

4. In the same pan heat the vegetable oil on a medium-high heat and add the marinated tofu. Cook for 10 minutes until the cubes become browned and crispy.

5. Serve tofu on a bed of cauliflower rice and garnish with chopped coriander leaves.

SERVES 2 | PREP + COOK TIME: 30 MINS + MARINATING | VEG | DAIRY FREE |

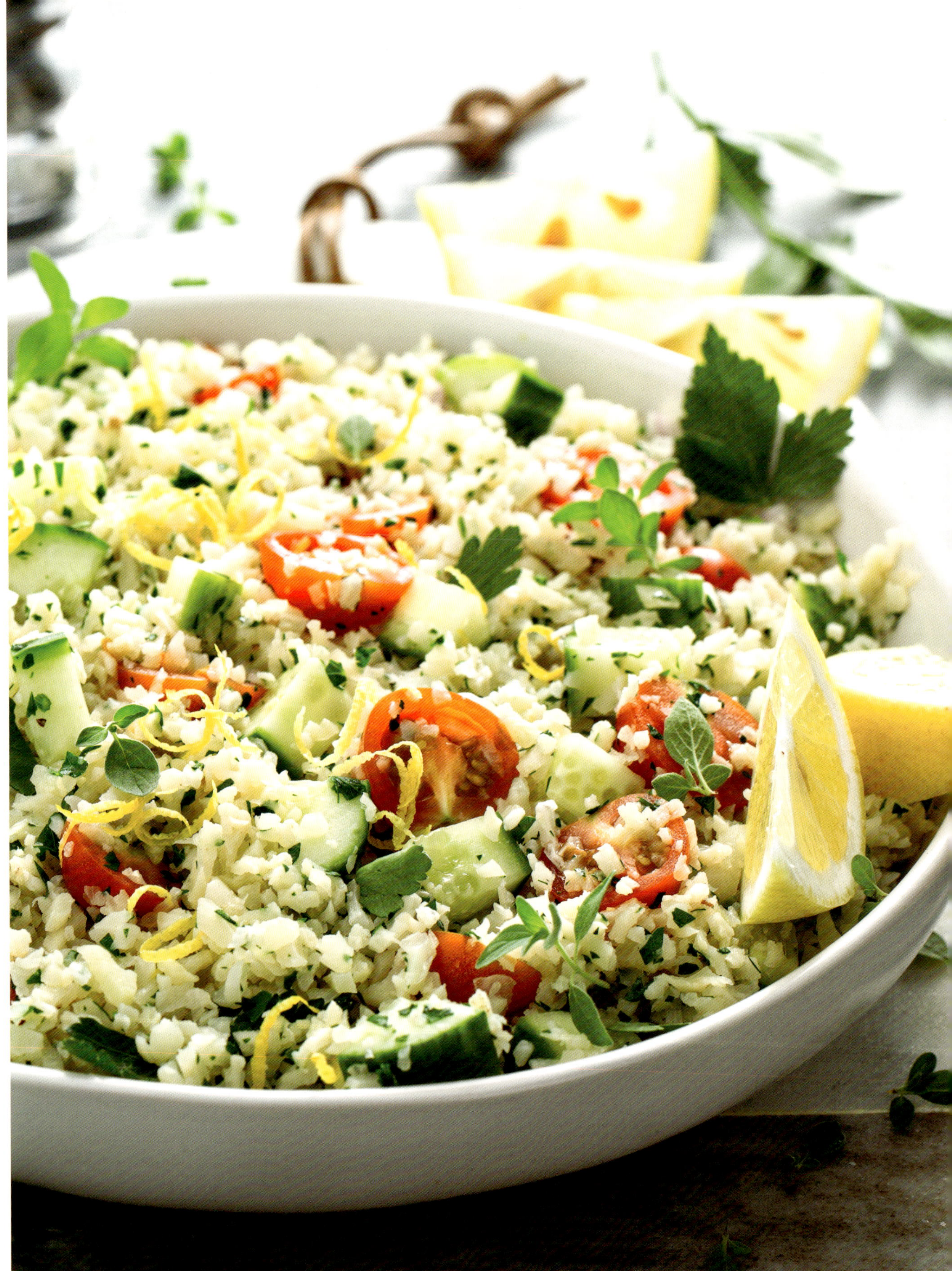

TABBOULEH CAULIFLOWER RICE

1 large head cauliflower (to make 3-4 cups cauliflower rice)

1 small cucumber, chopped

1 cup (225g) cherry tomatoes, halved

½ cup (20g) chopped fresh parsley

2 tbsps chopped fresh oregano

2 tbsps chopped fresh mint

Juice and zest of 1 large lemon

1 tbsp red wine vinegar

2 tbsps olive oil

Salt and pepper to taste

Lemon wedges to serve

STEPS

1. Divide cauliflower into florets and place in a food processor. Pulse for about 10-15 seconds until the cauliflower resembles rice. Alternatively use a box grater to grate the cauliflower into rice.
2. Place cauliflower rice in a large bowl. Add all vegetables and fresh herbs, and mix well.
3. Whisk together lemon juice, vinegar, oil, salt and pepper. Pour dressing over vegetable mixture and stir to coat.
4. Serve immediately with lemon wedges or refrigerate to let flavours meld.

SERVES 3-4 | PREP + COOK TIME: 30 MINS | VEG | GLUTEN FREE | DAIRY FREE |

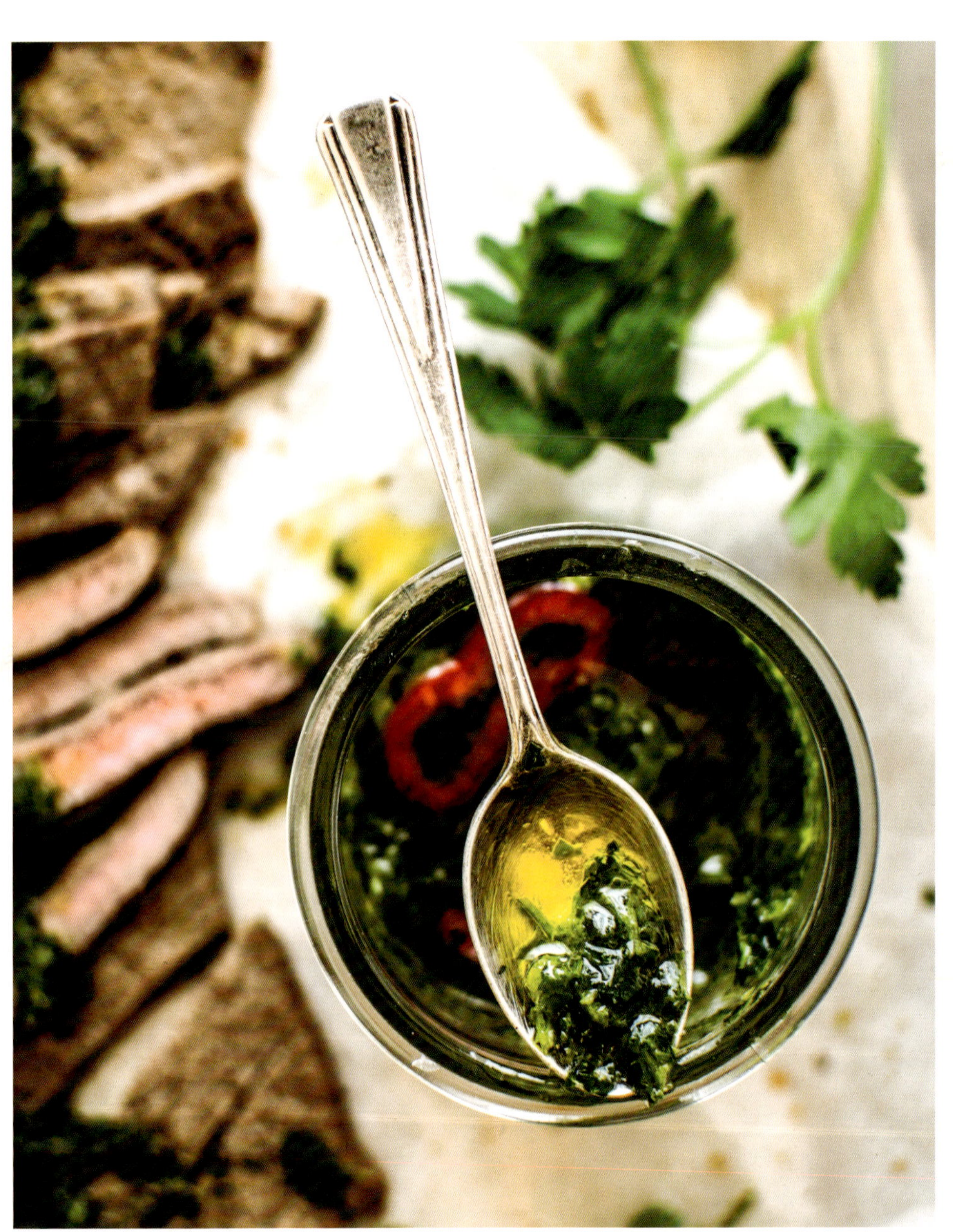

CHAPTER FOUR

(RED) MEAT MEALS

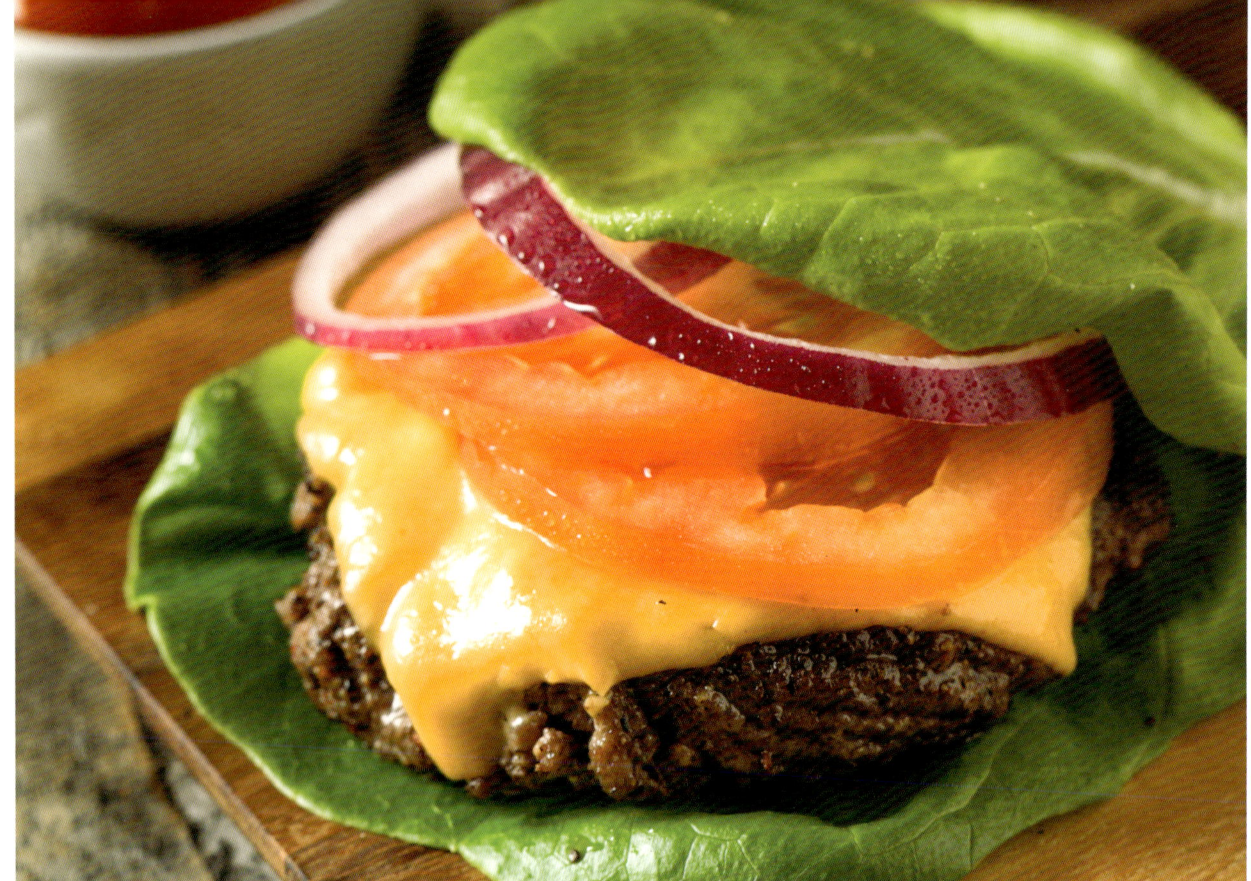

KETO CHEESEBURGERS

BURGERS

1.5kg beef mince

½ onion, very finely chopped

4 tsps garlic powder

4 tsps paprika

4 tbsps finely chopped fresh oregano

1 egg

4 cups (500g) grated cheese

Salt and pepper to taste

FILLINGS

4 large butter lettuce leaves

½ red onion, sliced into rings

1 medium tomato, sliced

¼ cup (60g) mayonnaise

STEPS

1. Place mince in a large bowl and add onion, garlic powder, paprika, oregano, egg and half the cheese. Season with salt and pepper. Use your hands to mix well.
2. Shape into eight patties.
3. Preheat the grill to medium. Line a baking tray with foil. Place the patties on the baking tray and place under the grill. Cook for 5 minutes then flip and top with the remaining grated cheese. Cook for 5 minutes more.
4. Assemble the burgers by placing one patty on top of a lettuce leaf. Top with sliced onions and tomatoes then a dollop of mayonnaise. Finish with a second lettuce leaf.

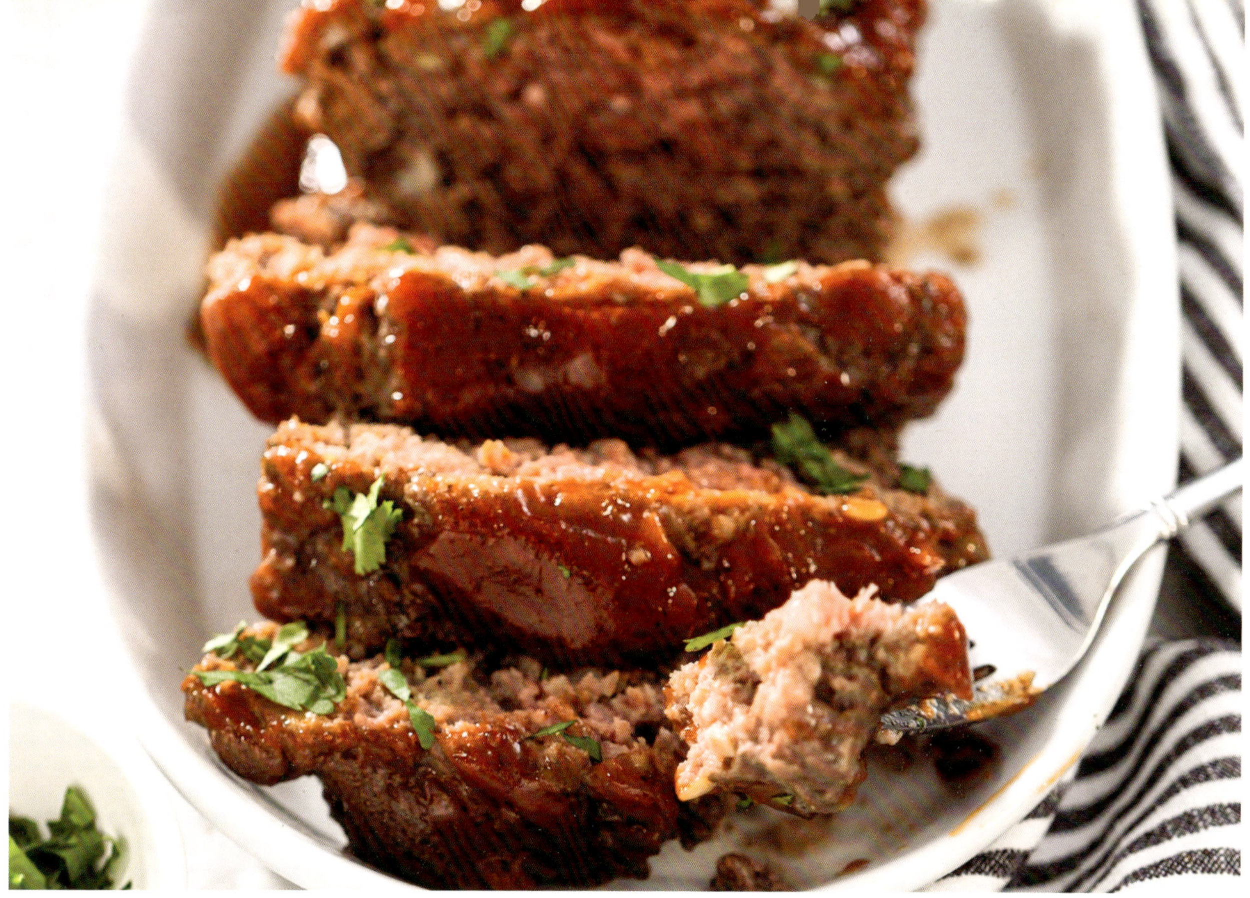

SERVES 8 | PREP + COOK TIME: 1 HOUR 25 MINS | GLUTEN FREE |

MEATLOAF WITH TOMATO GLAZE

1 large egg
1 tsp salt
½ tsp pepper
2 tsps garlic powder
2 tsps onion powder
½ tsp dried thyme
1kg beef mince
½ cup (60g) almond meal
½ cup (50g) grated Parmesan cheese
¼ cup (60ml) low-sugar ketchup
2 tbsps brown sugar
1 tbsp Dijon mustard
1 tbsp Worcestershire sauce
Fresh parsley to serve

STEPS

Preheat oven to 180°C.

1. In a large bowl, whisk together the egg, salt, pepper, garlic powder, onion powder and thyme. Add the beef mince, almond meal and Parmesan. Mix to combine.
2. In a small bowl, whisk together the ketchup, brown sugar, Dijon mustard and Worcestershire sauce to make the tomato glaze.
3. Press the mixture into a lined loaf tin and pour the tomato glaze over the top, reserving around 2 tablespoons for serving.
4. Bake the meatloaf for 60 minutes until cooked through in the centre. Remove from the oven and rest for 15 minutes.
5. Spoon the reserved tomato glaze on top and sprinkle with fresh parsley before slicing.

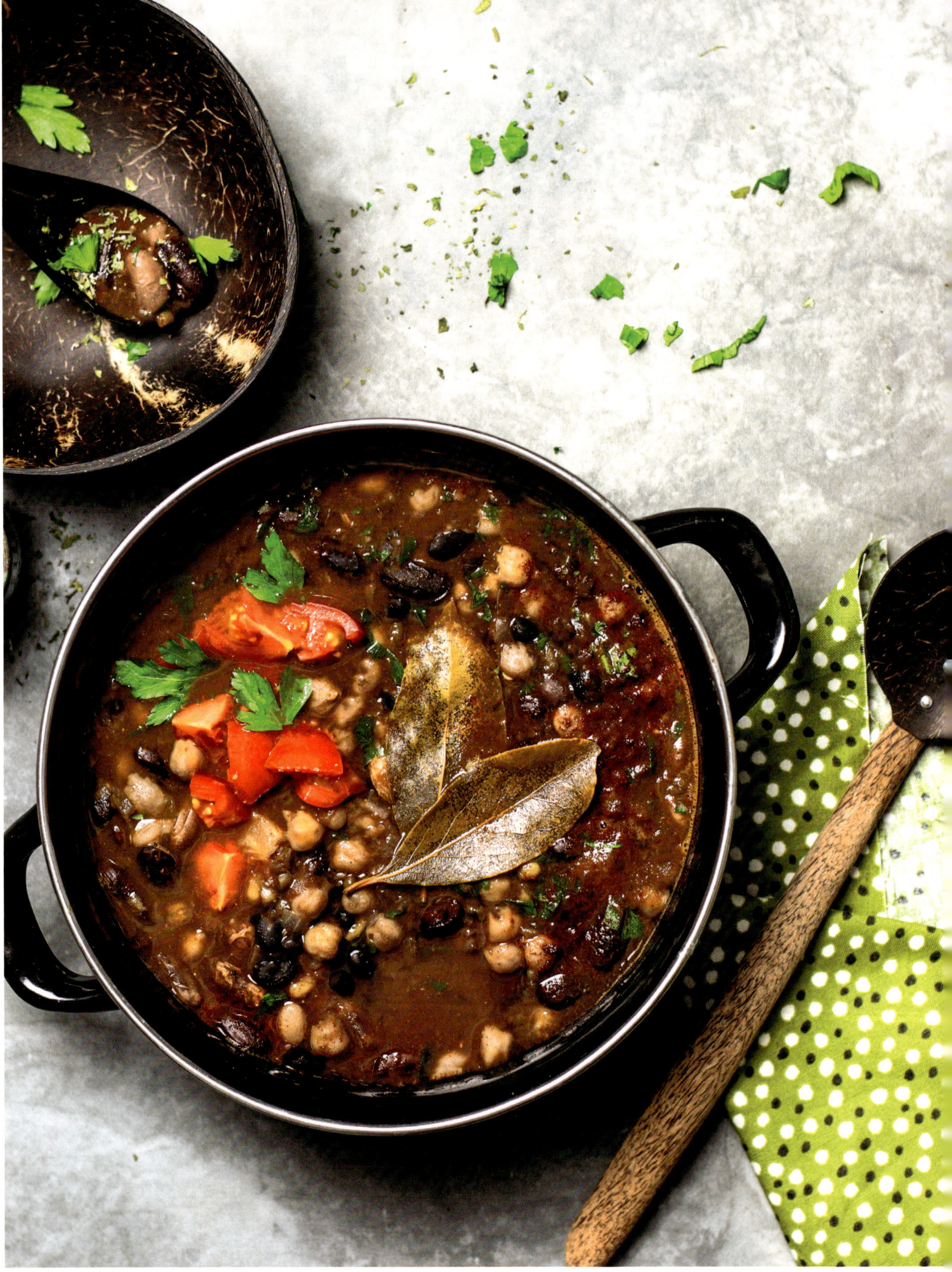

BEEF CHILLI

4 tbsps olive oil

1 small onion, diced

3 cloves garlic, minced

1 tsp chilli powder

1 tbsp paprika

1 tbsp ground cumin

1 tbsp ground coriander

1 tsp cinnamon

½ tsp pepper

1 tsp salt

1kg beef mince

2 tbsps tomato paste

1 x 400g cans diced tomatoes

2 bay leaves

1½ cups (375ml) beef stock

1 x 400g four bean mix (optional)

2 tbsps finely chopped fresh coriander + extra to garnish

1 large tomato, diced, to garnish

STEPS

1. Heat oil in a large saucepan over high heat. Add the onion and saute for 3-5 minutes until the onion is translucent. Add the garlic and spices and cook for 1 minute until fragrant. Add the beef mince and cook for 10 minutes, breaking apart with a spoon, until the beef is well browned.

2. Add the tomato paste, tinned tomatoes, bay leaves and beef stock and stir well. Reduce the heat to a low simmer and continue to cook, uncovered, for 30 minutes.

3. Add beans and chopped coriander. Adjust seasoning, adding more salt and pepper if desired.

4. Simmer for a further 10 minutes then remove bay leaves and serve with fresh tomato and extra coriander.

NOTE: Beans do contain some carbs, so do not exceed the amount stated in the recipe. A ½ cup of pinto beans contains 15g of carbs. This recipe contains less than ¼ cup per person but feel free to leave them out altogether if you wish.

SERVES 8 | PREP + COOK TIME: 1 HOUR | GLUTEN FREE | DAIRY FREE |

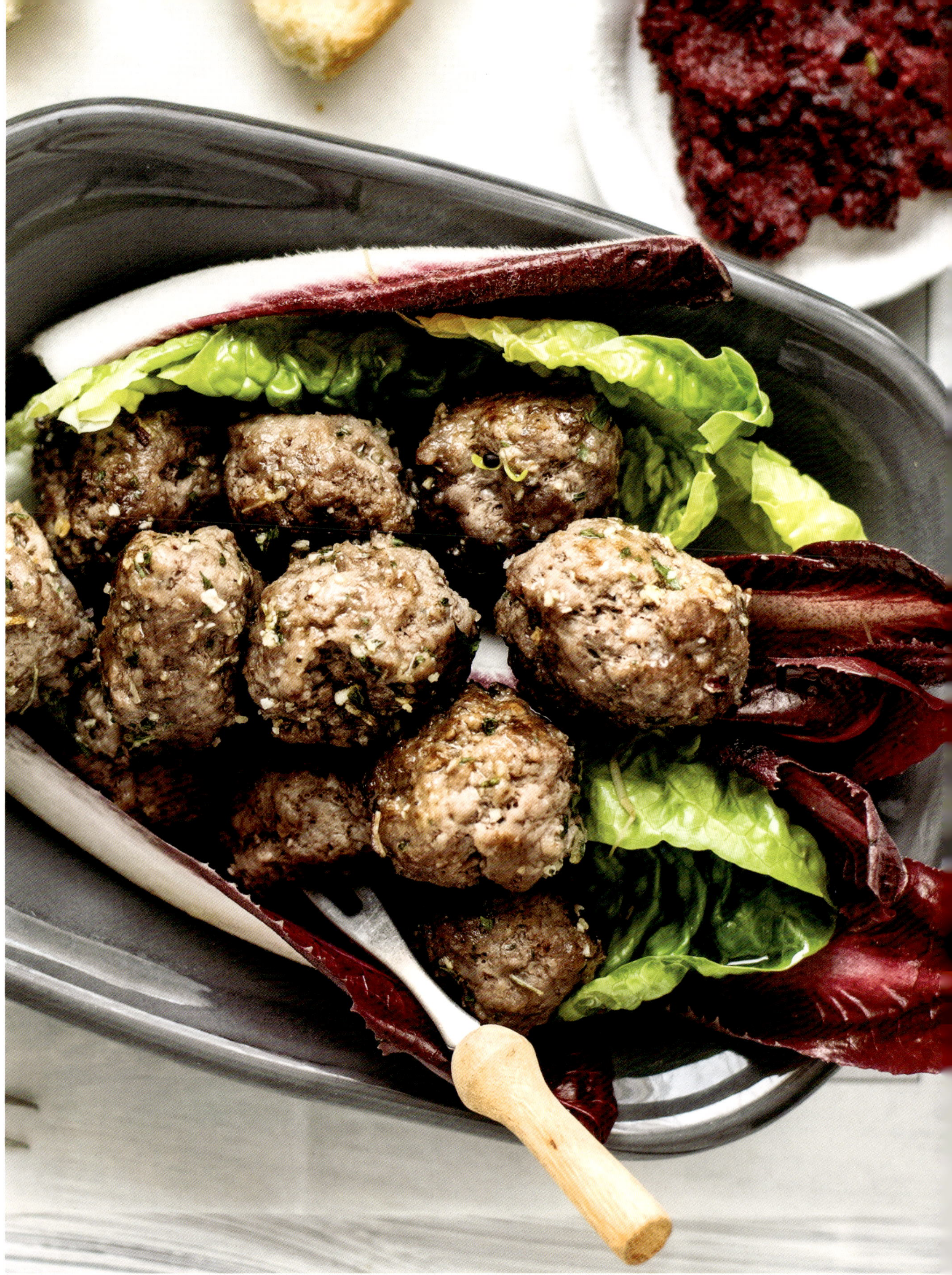

CHEESE & TARRAGON MEATBALLS

800g beef mince

½ cup (60g) grated mozzarella cheese

A few stems of fresh tarragon, leaves picked and roughly chopped

1 tbsp coconut flour

1 egg

1 small onion, finely chopped

2 cloves garlic, crushed

1 tsp dried dill

½ cup (125ml) water

Salt and pepper to taste

Olive oil for frying

Mixed lettuce leaves, to serve (optional)

STEPS

1. Place the beef, cheese, tarragon, coconut flour, egg, onion, garlic, dill, water and 1 teaspoon each of salt and pepper in a large bowl and mix thoroughly. Form tablespoons of mixture into small meatballs and place in the refrigerator to chill for 30-60 minutes.

2. Heat 2 tablespoons of oil in a large, deep-sided frying pan over medium heat. Fry the meatballs in batches for 10 minutes each, gently turning every 2 minutes to cook all over.

3. Season to taste and serve warm on a bed of mixed lettuce leaves.

SERVES 4 | PREP + COOK TIME: 1 HOUR + CHILLING | GLUTEN FREE |

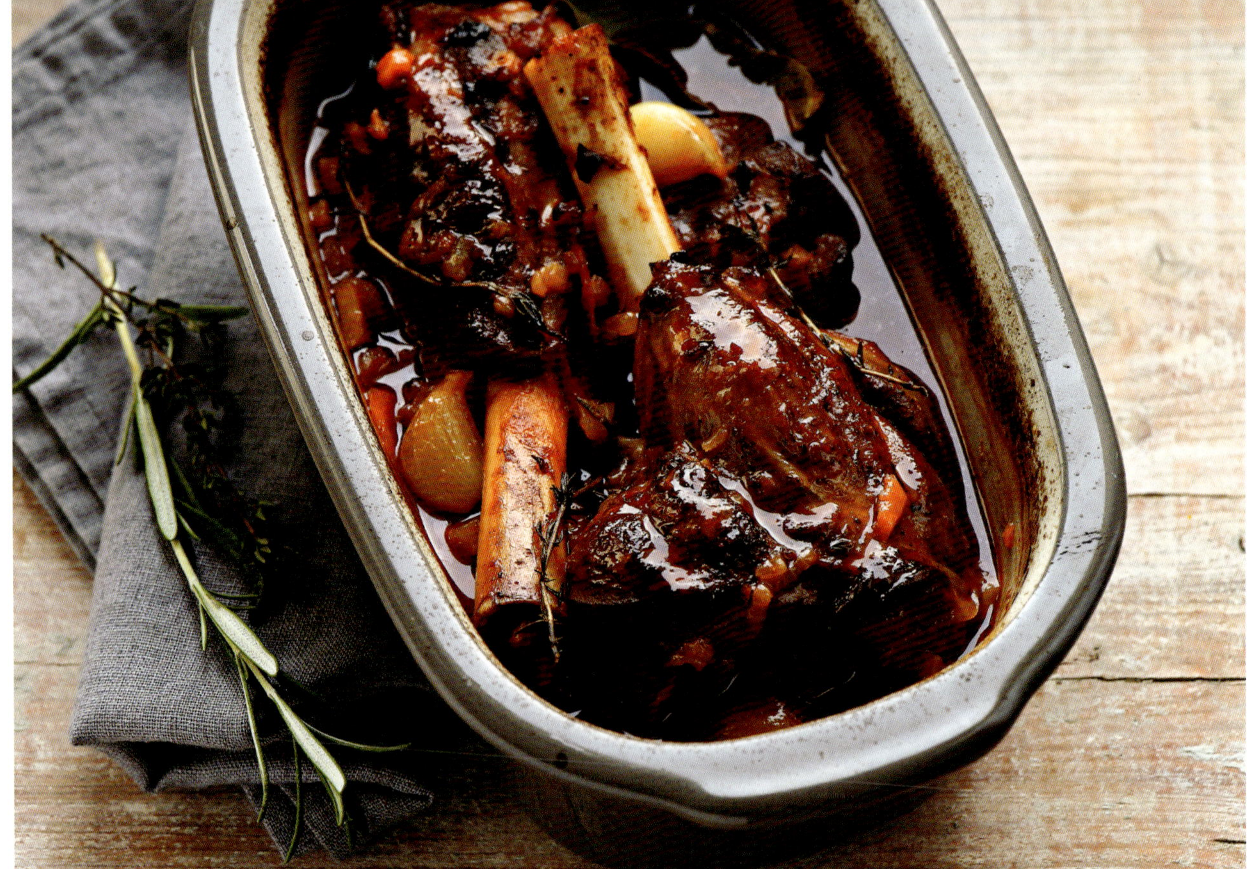

HERB LAMB SHANK

4 lamb shanks
1 tsp salt
½ tsp pepper
2 tbsps olive oil
1 onion, diced
1 carrot, diced
3 stalks celery, sliced
5 cloves garlic, peeled
2 cups (500ml) red wine
2 cups (500ml) lamb or chicken stock
4 sprigs thyme
2 bay leaves
4 sprigs rosemary

STEPS

Preheat the oven to 160°C.

1. Season the lamb shanks with salt and pepper.
2. Heat oil in a large casserole or Dutch oven over high heat. Add the lamb shanks and cook on all sides for 3-4 minutes until browned. Transfer the lamb to a plate and set aside.
3. Reduce the heat to medium-high. Add the onion, carrot and celery and cook for 3-5 minutes, stirring regularly, until the onion is soft and translucent. Add the garlic and cook for 1 minute until fragrant. Pour in the wine and stock. Add the thyme, bay leaves and rosemary.
4. Transfer to the oven and bake for 2½-3 hours until the lamb is very tender.

NOTE: This dish is great served with cauliflower mash.

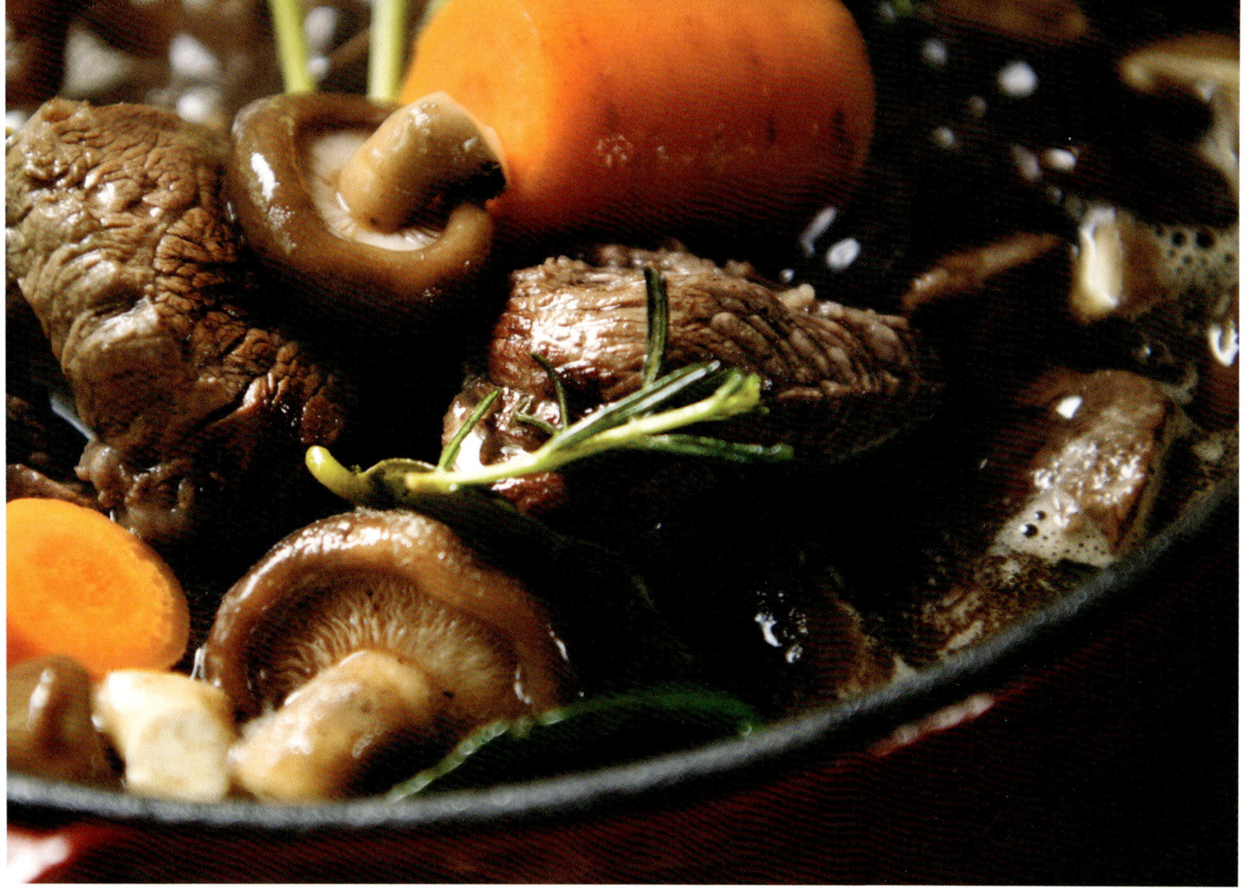

FARMHOUSE STEW

2 tbsps olive oil

800g stewing beef, fat trimmed and cubed

4 medium onions, peeled and quartered

3 cloves garlic, crushed

½ cup (125ml) red wine

2 tbsps tomato paste

1 tbsp fresh rosemary, chopped + 1 tbsp to serve

2 tbsps red wine vinegar

300g fresh mushrooms

3 medium carrots, thickly sliced

500g butternut pumpkin, cut into 3cm chunks

2 cups (500ml) beef stock

2 bay leaves

Salt and pepper to taste

STEPS

Preheat the oven to 170°C.

1. Heat oil in a large ovenproof casserole dish over medium heat. Add the beef and brown in batches then remove the pan and set aside.
2. In the same pan fry the onion and garlic until onion is translucent and garlic becomes fragrant.
3. Pour the red wine into the pan and bring to a boil, then simmer for 2 minutes.
4. Add the tomato paste, rosemary and vinegar and fry for a further 2 minutes. Add the mushrooms, carrot and pumpkin and cook for 5 minutes.
5. Return the beef to the pot and pour over the stock and add the bay leaves. Bake in the oven for 2 hours until the beef is tender. Remove from oven, season to taste and serve.

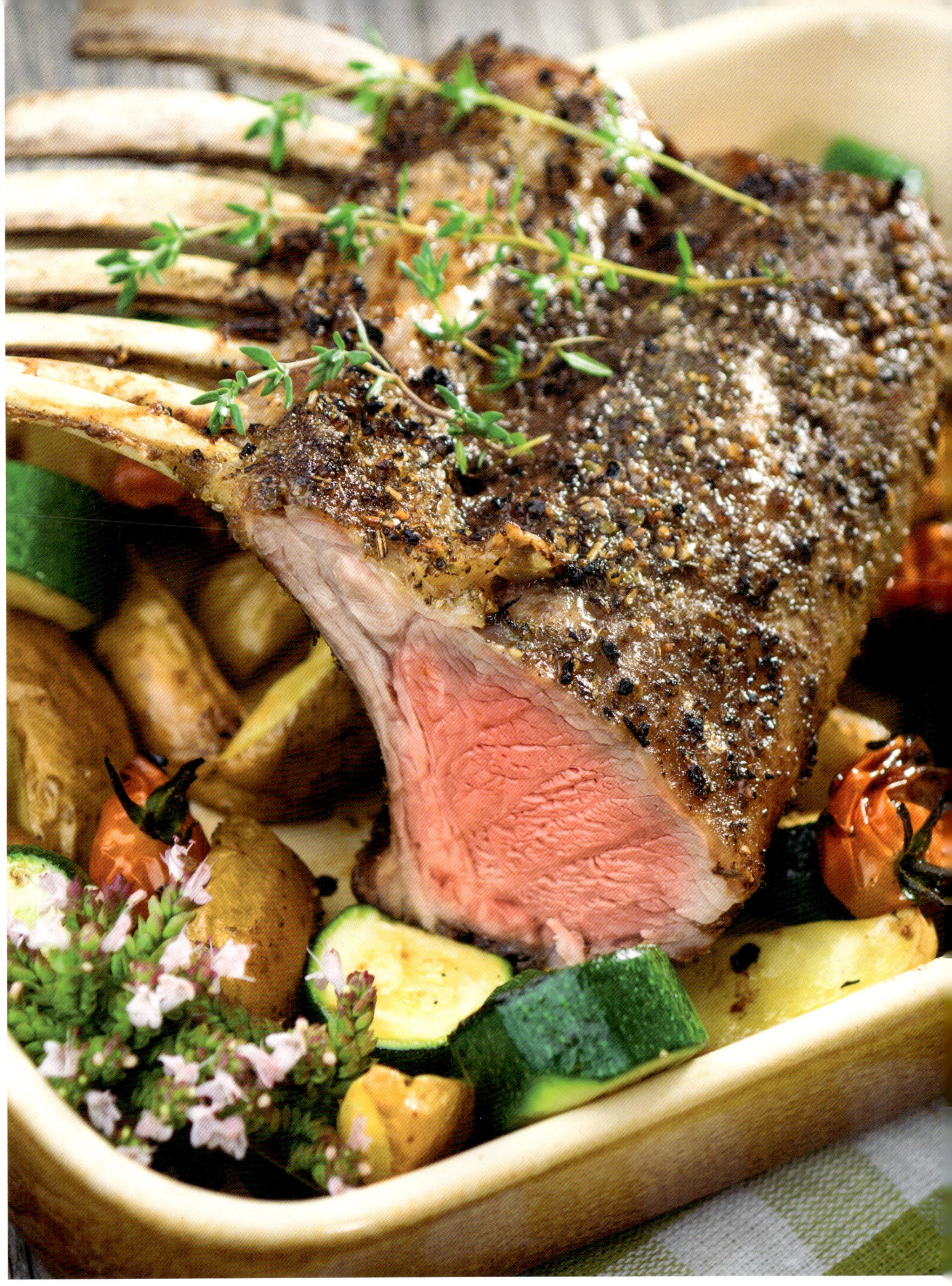

HERB-CRUSTED LAMB RACK WITH ROAST VEGETABLES

2 tbsps Dijon mustard

2 tbsps fresh rosemary, finely chopped

2 tbsps fresh thyme, finely chopped

2 cloves garlic, crushed

2 tbsps olive oil

Salt and pepper to taste

1 x 1kg lamb rack

3 medium potatoes, chopped (optional)

200g cherry tomatoes

3 zucchinis, thickly sliced

2 tbsps olive oil

1 tsp dried thyme

STEPS

Preheat oven to 220°C.

1. In a small bowl, mix together the Dijon mustard, rosemary, thyme, crushed garlic, olive oil, salt and pepper to create a herb crust mixture.
2. Season the lamb rack with salt and pepper, then brush the herb crust mixture all over the lamb, coating it evenly. Heat a heavy-based pan over medium-high heat. Place the lamb rack fat-side down in the pan and sear for about 3-4 minutes until browned. Flip the rack and sear the other side for an additional 3-4 minutes.
3. Transfer to a roasting pan and place in the oven. Roast for 20-25 minutes for medium-rare or longer if you prefer a well-cooked lamb.
4. While the lamb is roasting, prepare the roast vegetables. On a lined baking tray, toss the mixed vegetables with olive oil, dried thyme, salt and pepper until they are well coated. Place the tray in the oven alongside the lamb rack and roast for 20-25 minutes, or until the vegetables are tender and golden brown.
5. Remove the lamb rack from the oven and let it rest for 10 minutes before carving. Slice the lamb rack into individual chops and serve it alongside the roasted vegetables.

SERVES 4 | PREP + COOK TIME: 1 HOUR | GLUTEN FREE | DAIRY FREE |

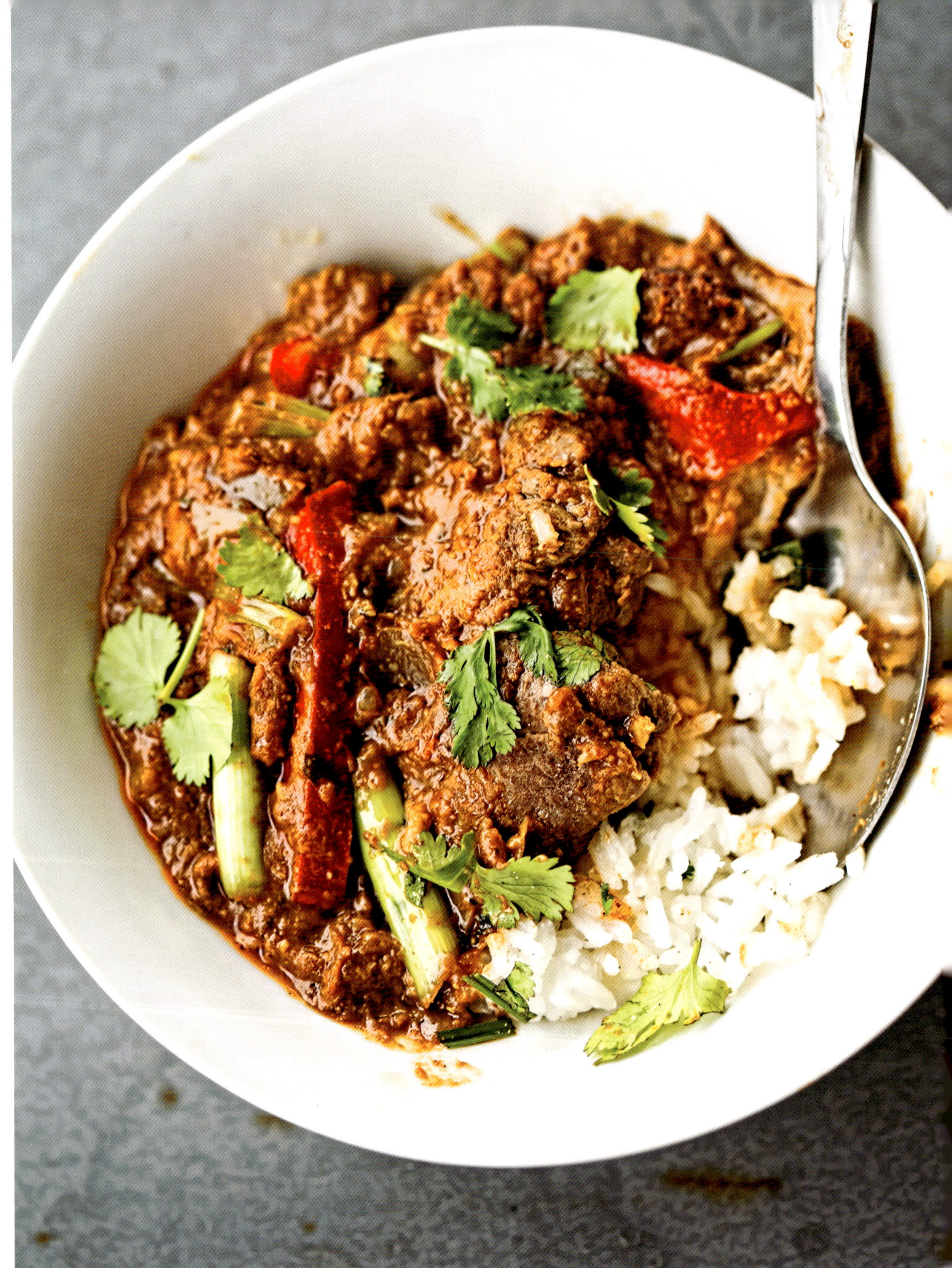

MALAYSIAN BEEF CURRY

SPICE PASTE

2 shallots, chopped

2 cloves garlic, crushed

2 dried chillies

1 stalk lemongrass, trimmed and chopped

2 tbsps finely grated ginger

½ tsp ground turmeric

1 tsp salt

CURRY

1½ tbsps vegetable oil

2 star anise

1 small cinnamon stick

2 cardamon pods, lightly crushed

1kg beef brisket, cut into 3cm cubes

Salt and pepper to taste

1 x 400ml can coconut milk

1 cup (250ml) hot water

Juice of 1 lime

3 mini red capsicums, chopped

STEPS

1. In a food processor add the shallots, garlic, dried chillies, lemongrass, ginger, turmeric and salt. Pulse until you have a smooth paste, adding a little water if it looks too dry. Transfer to a small bowl.

2. Heat the oil in a large, heavy-based saucepan over a medium heat. Fry the spice paste for 3-5 minutes, stirring occasionally, until it looks glossy and the oil starts to separate away from the spice mixture. Add the star anise, cinnamon and cardamon pods and stir well.

3. Add the beef and a little salt and cook for 4-5 minutes, stirring occasionally. Pour the coconut milk and hot water into the pan, stir well, and bring to a simmer. Cover the saucepan, reduce the heat to low and cook gently for 2 hours.

4. Remove from the heat after 2 hours and adjust the seasoning using salt, pepper and lime juice. Put back on a low heat and add the chopped capsicum and cook for a further 10 minutes or until capsicum softens.

NOTE: Serve with cauliflower rice for a low-carb alternative to white rice.

SERVES 4 | PREP + COOK TIME: 2 HOURS 30 MINS | GLUTEN FREE | DAIRY FREE |

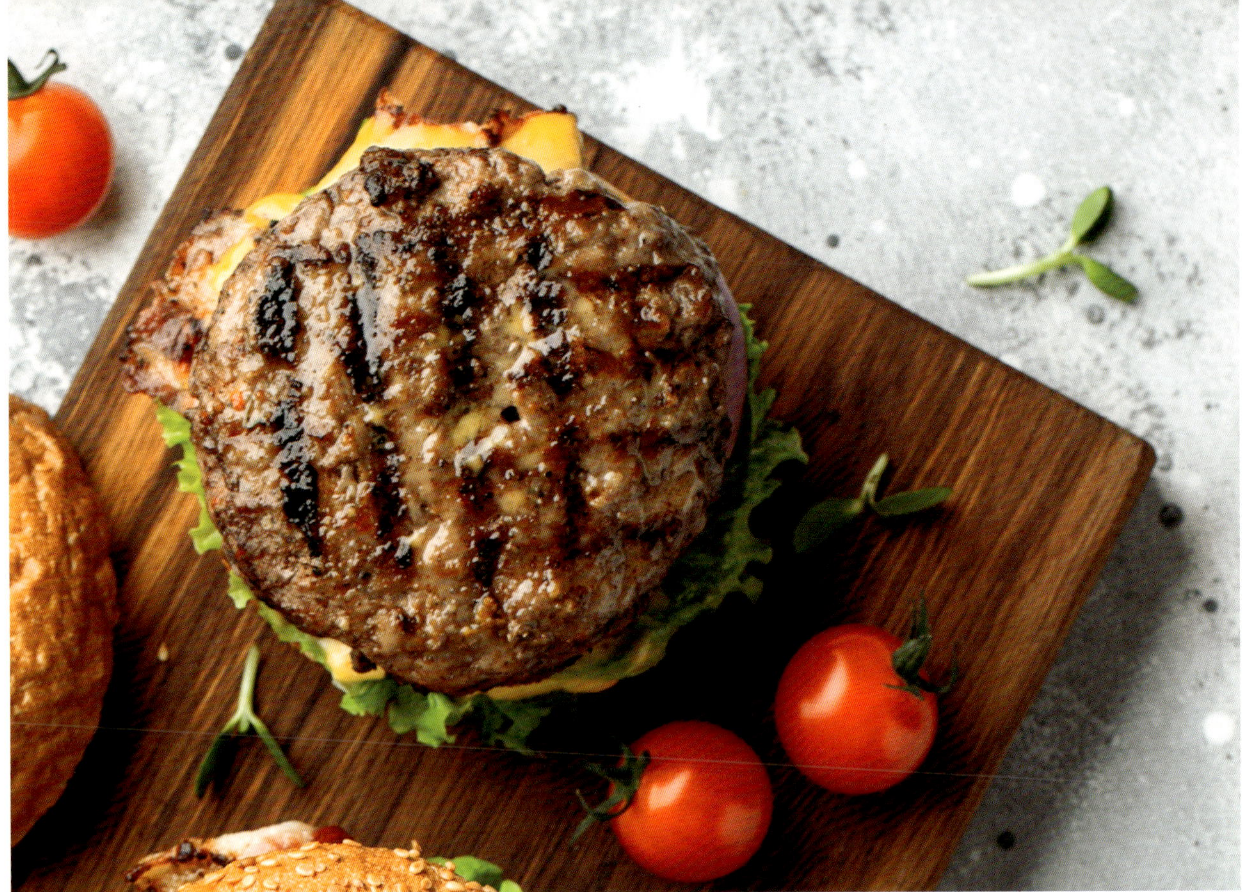

LAMB & BACON BURGERS

500g minced lean lamb

1 tbsp finely chopped fresh mint

1 tsp dried oregano

2 spring onions, finely chopped

Salt and pepper to taste

4 rashers bacon

1½ tbsps olive oil

1 large tomato, sliced

4 slices cheese

12 butter lettuce leaves

STEPS

1. In a large bowl, combine the lamb, mint, oregano, spring onion and a couple of good grinds of salt and pepper.
2. Shape the mixture into four patties.
3. Heat a large frying pan over medium-high heat and fry the bacon for 8 minutes until crispy. Remove from the pan and set aside.
4. Heat half the oil in the pan. Place the burgers on the pan and flatten slightly with a spatula. Cook the burgers 5 minutes on each side, taking care when turning them over so they stay together. Set aside.
5. Serve by layering equal portions of tomatoes and bacon and cheese on top of 2 lettuce leaves for each serving plate. Place a patty on top and then an additional lettuce leaf to complete the burger.

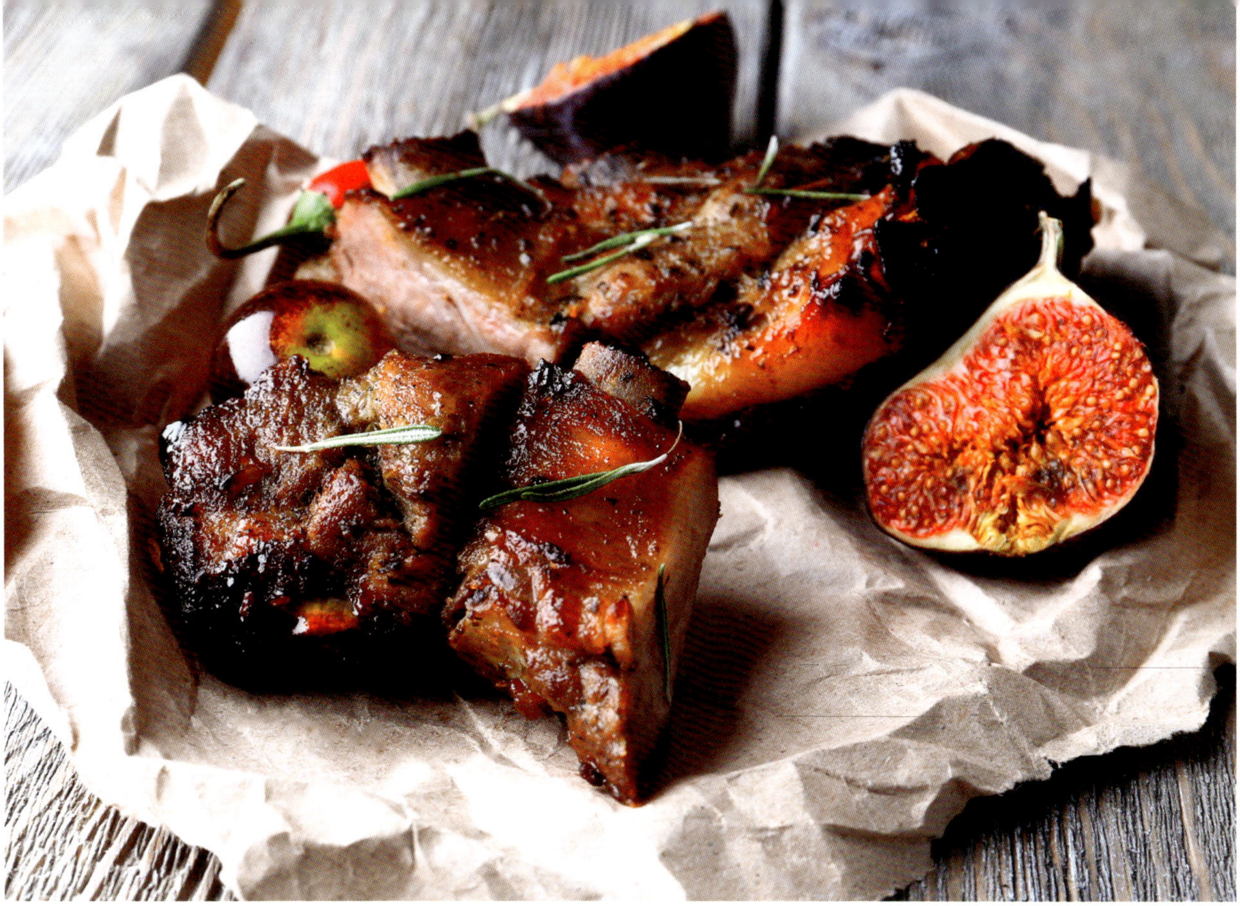

FIG & ROSEMARY LAMB BACKSTRAP

SERVES 2 | PREP + COOK TIME: 50 MINS | GLUTEN FREE | DAIRY FREE |

400g lamb backstrap fillets

6 purple figs, halved

1 tbsp olive oil

1 tbsp finely chopped rosemary + 1 tbsp rosemary leaves for garnish

Salt and pepper

½ cup (125ml) balsamic vinegar

1 tbsp maple syrup

STEPS

Preheat the oven to 180°C.

1. Season the lamb and figs with half the oil, the chopped rosemary and 1 teaspoon each of salt and pepper.
2. Heat a medium frying pan on medium-high heat. Sear the lamb for 1 minute on each side then place in a baking dish with the figs. Transfer to the oven to bake for 15 minutes.
3. Heat the rest of the olive oil, balsamic vinegar, maple syrup and a dash of salt in the frying pan until nearly bubbling. Reduce heat to low and cook for 5 minutes. Pour over the lamb and figs before the last 5 minutes of baking.
4. Once the lamb is out of the oven, let it sit for 5 minutes before slicing.

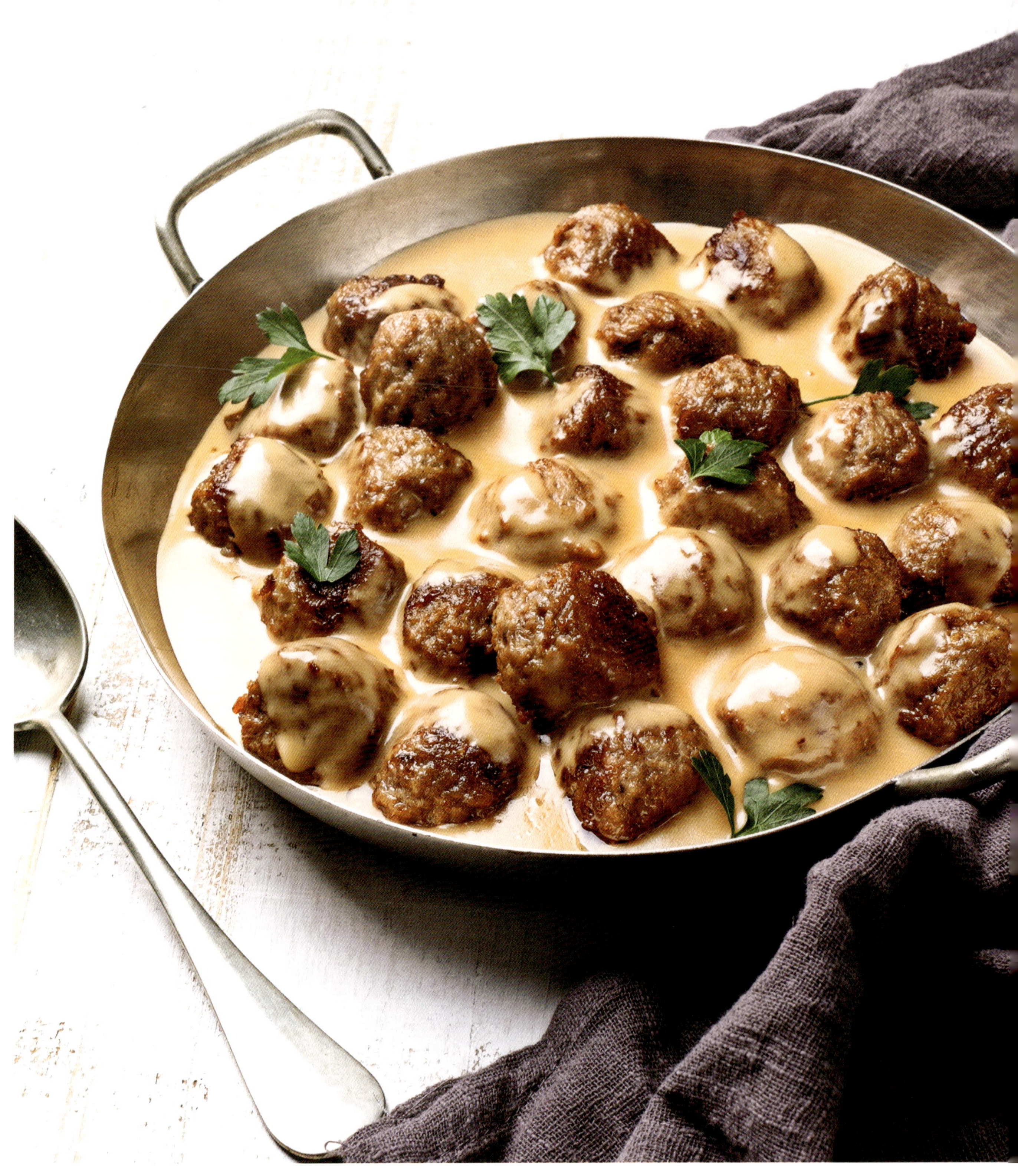

SWEDISH MEATBALLS IN GRAVY

MEATBALLS

500g beef mince

1 tbsp dried parsley

¼ tsp allspice

¼ tsp nutmeg

½ tsp garlic powder

½ tsp salt

½ tsp pepper

¼ onion, grated

1 tbsp olive oil

Parsley, chopped, to garnish

GRAVY

50g butter

1½ cups (375ml) beef stock

1 cup (125ml) thickened cream

2 tbsps Worcestershire sauce

½ tbsp Dijon mustard

Salt and pepper to taste

STEPS

1. In a mixing bowl, combine mince, parsley, spices, seasonings and grated onion. Combine with your hands, working the spices and onion through the meat. Roll into walnut-sized meatballs.
2. In a large frying pan heat olive oil on a medium heat and add the meatballs and cook for 5-6 minutes or until browned, turning gently. Remove from the pan and set aside.
3. Add the butter to the same pan. Use a spatula to scrape up any meat from the bottom of the pan. Add the beef stock, cream, Worcestershire sauce, Dijon mustard and salt and pepper. Stir to combine and taste for additional seasoning.
4. Return the meatballs to the pan. Simmer for 10-15 minutes until the meatballs are cooked through and sauce thickened to your liking. Sprinkle with chopped parsley and serve.

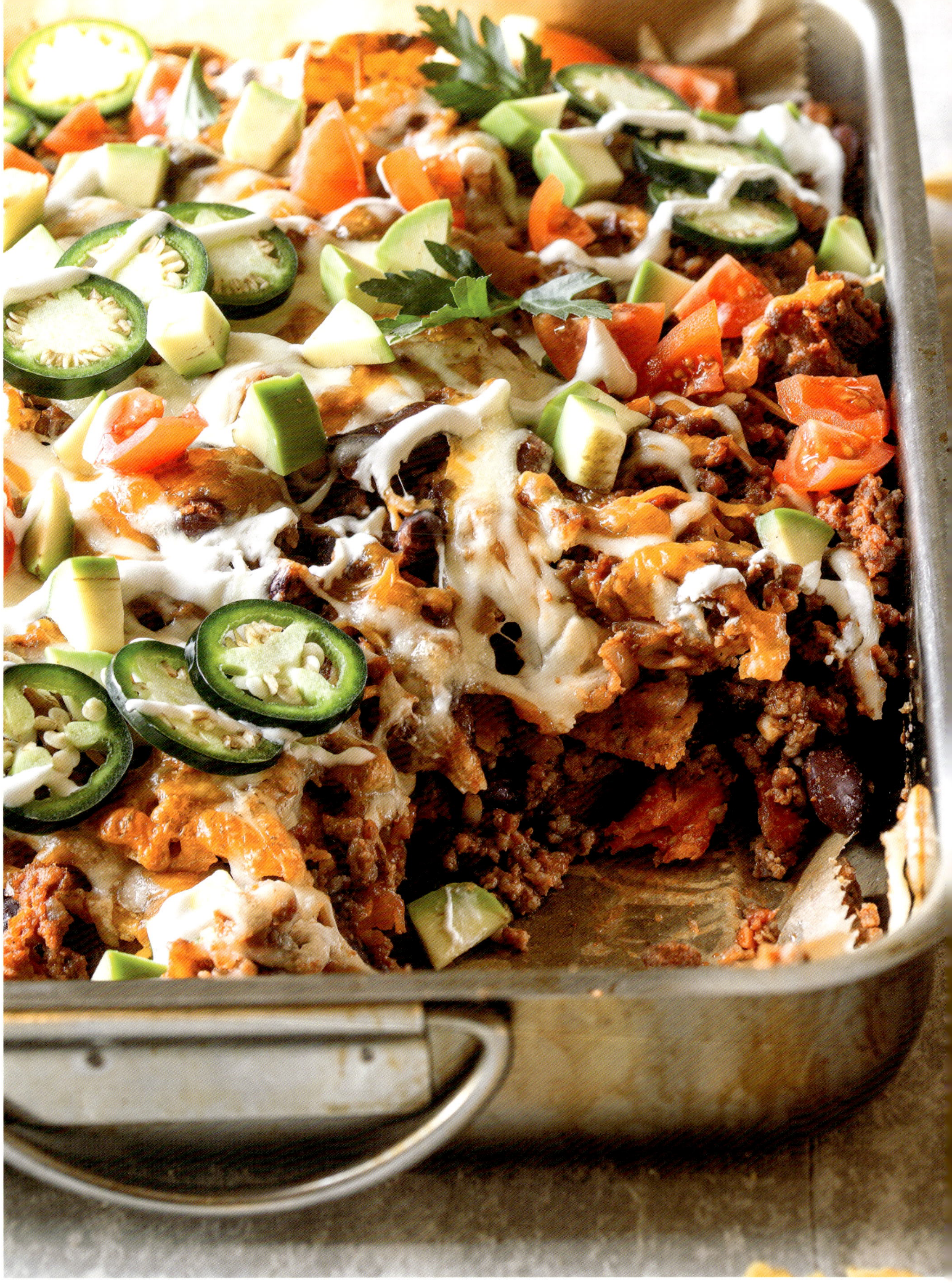

MEXICAN MINCE BAKE

500g beef mince
1 small onion, finely diced
2 cloves garlic, crushed
1 capsicum, diced
1 x 400g can diced tomatoes
1 x 400g can black beans, drained and rinsed
1 tbsp chilli powder
1 tsp ground cumin
1 tsp smoked paprika
Salt and pepper to taste
1 cup (125g) grated Cheddar or Mexican blend cheese
1 avocado, cubed
1 cup (225g) cherry tomatoes, quartered
1 jalapeno, finely sliced (optional)
¼ cup (60ml) sour cream
¼ cup (10g) chopped coriander

STEPS

Preheat oven to 190°C.

1. In a large pan, cook the mince on medium heat until browned. Drain any excess fat. Add the diced onion, garlic and diced capsicum to the pan and cook for 2-3 minutes until the vegetables have softened.
2. Stir in the diced tomatoes (including the juice), black beans, chilli powder, cumin, smoked paprika, salt and pepper. Mix well to combine all the ingredients. Simmer for 5-10 minutes to allow the flavours develop.
3. Transfer the mixture to a lined baking dish and spread it out evenly. Sprinkle the cheese over the top of the mince mixture then bake in the preheated oven for 20-25 minutes, or until the cheese is melted and bubbly.
4. Remove from the oven and let cool for a few minutes before sprinkling the avocado, tomatoes and jalapeno over the top. Dollop the sour cream evenly over the bake and garnish with coriander.

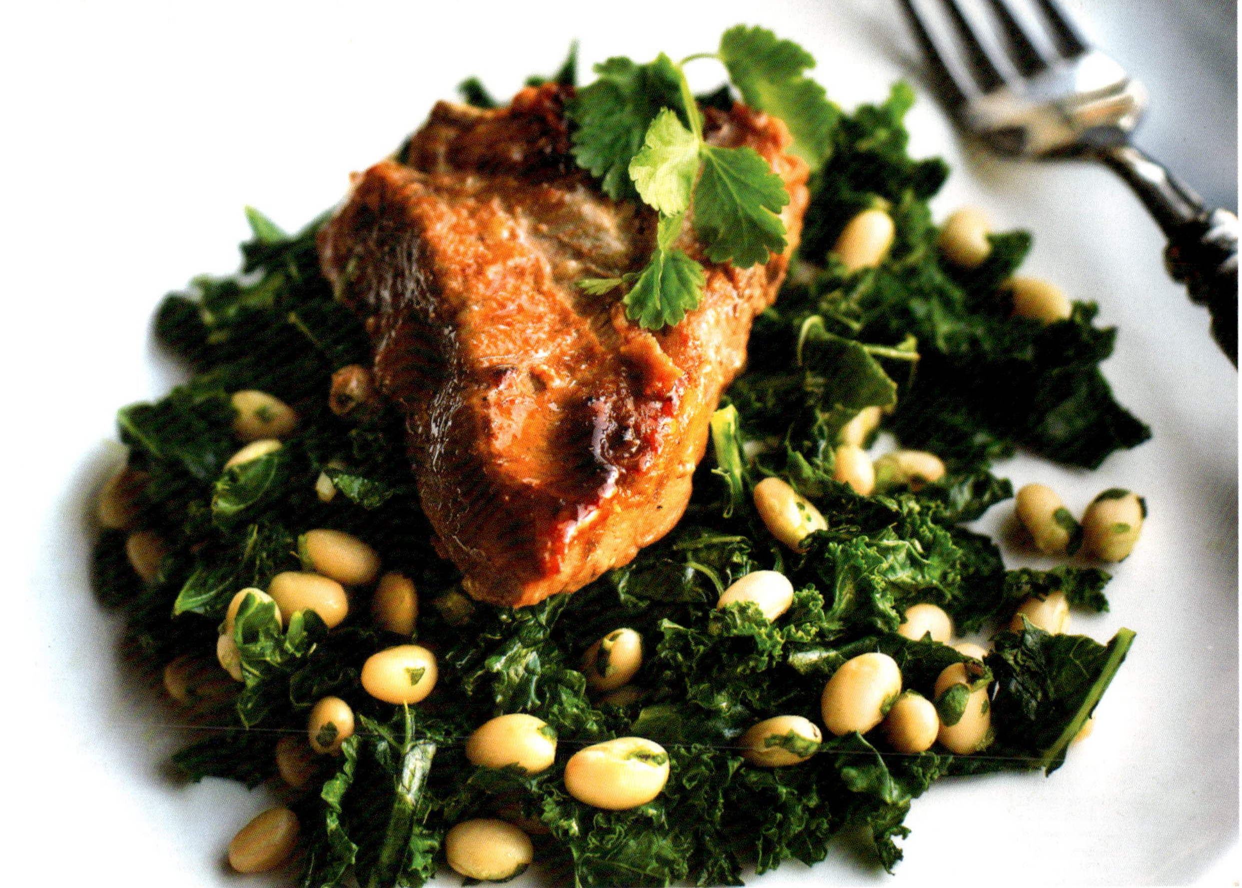

ROASTED LAMB CHOPS WITH KALE

2 tbsps coconut oil

2 cloves garlic, crushed

¼ tsp ground turmeric

½ tsp ground cumin

½ tsp ground oregano

Salt and pepper to taste

400g lamb chops

½ bunch kale, chopped

1 x 400g can cannellini beans, drained and rinsed

Pinch of nutmeg

½ tbsp lemon juice

¼ cup (60ml) vegetable stock

2 sprigs parsley, to garnish

STEPS

Preheat the oven to 200°C.

1. In a small bowl, mix together half the coconut oil, half the garlic, the turmeric, cumin, oregano, ½ teaspoon salt and a good grind of pepper. Rub into the lamb chops and set aside.
2. In a medium-sized saucepan, heat the rest of the oil over medium heat. Fry the rest of the garlic for 1 minute, then add the kale in batches. Once the kale is softened, stir through the beans, nutmeg, lemon juice and stock. Lower the heat, cover and cook for 10 minutes while you prepare the lamb.
3. Heat a large frying pan to medium-high heat. Fry the lamb chops for 5 minutes on each side or until browned nicely. Serve the lamb on top of the kale and beans and garnish with parsley.

SERVES 4 | PREP + COOK TIME: 30 MINS | GLUTEN FREE | DAIRY FREE |

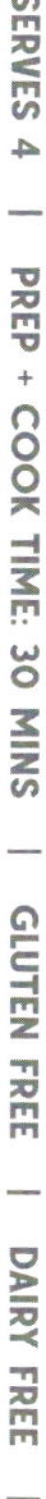

SPICY BEEF & MUSHROOM WRAPS

1 tsp sesame oil

500g beef mince

250g button mushrooms, halved

1 cup (110g) julienned or shredded carrots

4 tbsps tamari

3 cloves garlic, finely minced

Small piece ginger, grated

3 tbsps stevia brown sugar or other low-carb brown sugar substitute

½ tsp Sriracha

2 tsps cornflour

3 tsps water

12 medium cos lettuce leaves

Chopped coriander to serve

Asian dipping sauce (optional)

STEPS

1. Heat oil in a large frying pan over medium-high heat. Add the beef and cook, breaking up with a spoon, until browned. Add mushrooms and most of the carrots, leaving a handful for serving. Cook for a further 5-7 minutes until the carrots and mushrooms are tender.

2. Add the tamari, garlic, ginger, brown sugar substitute and Sriracha and stir well to combine.

3. Whisk together the cornflour and water in a small bowl. Add to the pan and stir well as the sauce thickens.

4. Remove the pan from the heat and serve the beef mixture in its sauce in lettuce wraps. Scatter with the remaining carrot and chopped coriander leaves. Serve with dipping sauce if desired.

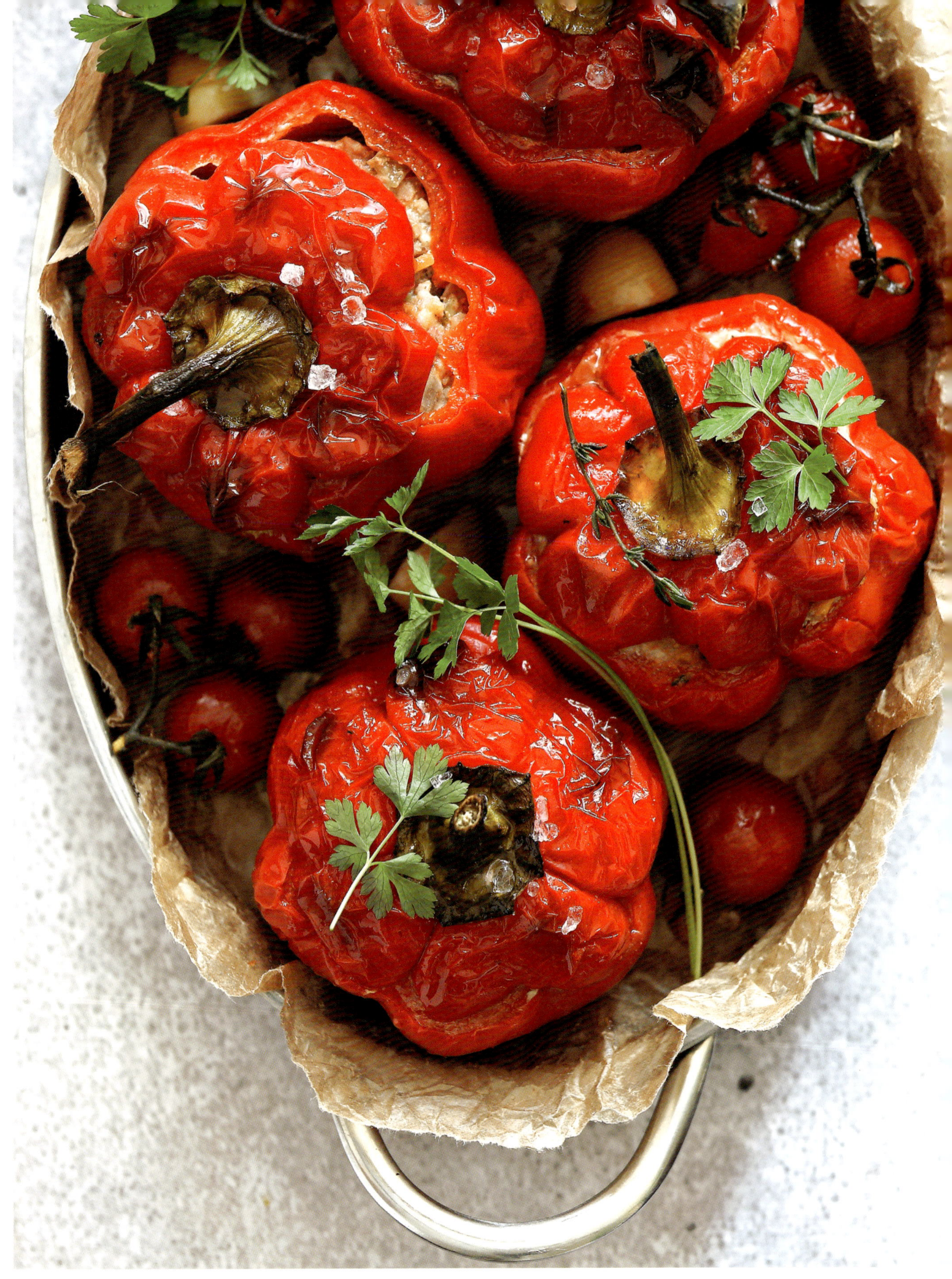

STUFFED ROASTED CAPSICUMS

4 large capsicums, any colour
8-10 vine-ripened tomatoes
1 tbsp olive oil
1 small onion, diced
2 cloves garlic, crushed
500g beef mince
1 cup (100g) cauliflower rice
½ cup (100g) diced tomatoes
1 tsp dried oregano
1 tsp dried basil
½ tsp smoked paprika
Salt and pepper to taste
1 cup (125g) grated mozzarella cheese
Fresh parsley, chopped, to garnish

STEPS

Preheat oven to 190°C.

1. Cut the tops off the capsicums and remove the seeds and membranes from the inside. Place the capsicums in a lined baking dish along with the tomatoes and set aside.
2. Heat olive oil in a large pan over medium heat. Add the diced onion and garlic to the pan and saute until they become fragrant and translucent. Add the mince to the pan and cook until browned.
3. Add the cauliflower rice, diced tomatoes, dried oregano, dried basil, paprika, salt and pepper to the pan. Stir well to combine all the ingredients. Cook for an additional 5 minutes, allowing the flavours to develop.
4. Spoon the filling mixture into the prepared capsicums, dividing it equally among them. Sprinkle mozzarella cheese on top of each stuffed capsicum and replace the tops.
5. Cover the baking dish with foil and bake in the preheated oven for 20-25 minutes, or until the capsicums are tender and the cheese is melted and bubbly. Remove from the oven and allow to cool slightly before serving.

SERVES 4 | PREP + COOK TIME: 45 MINS | GLUTEN FREE |

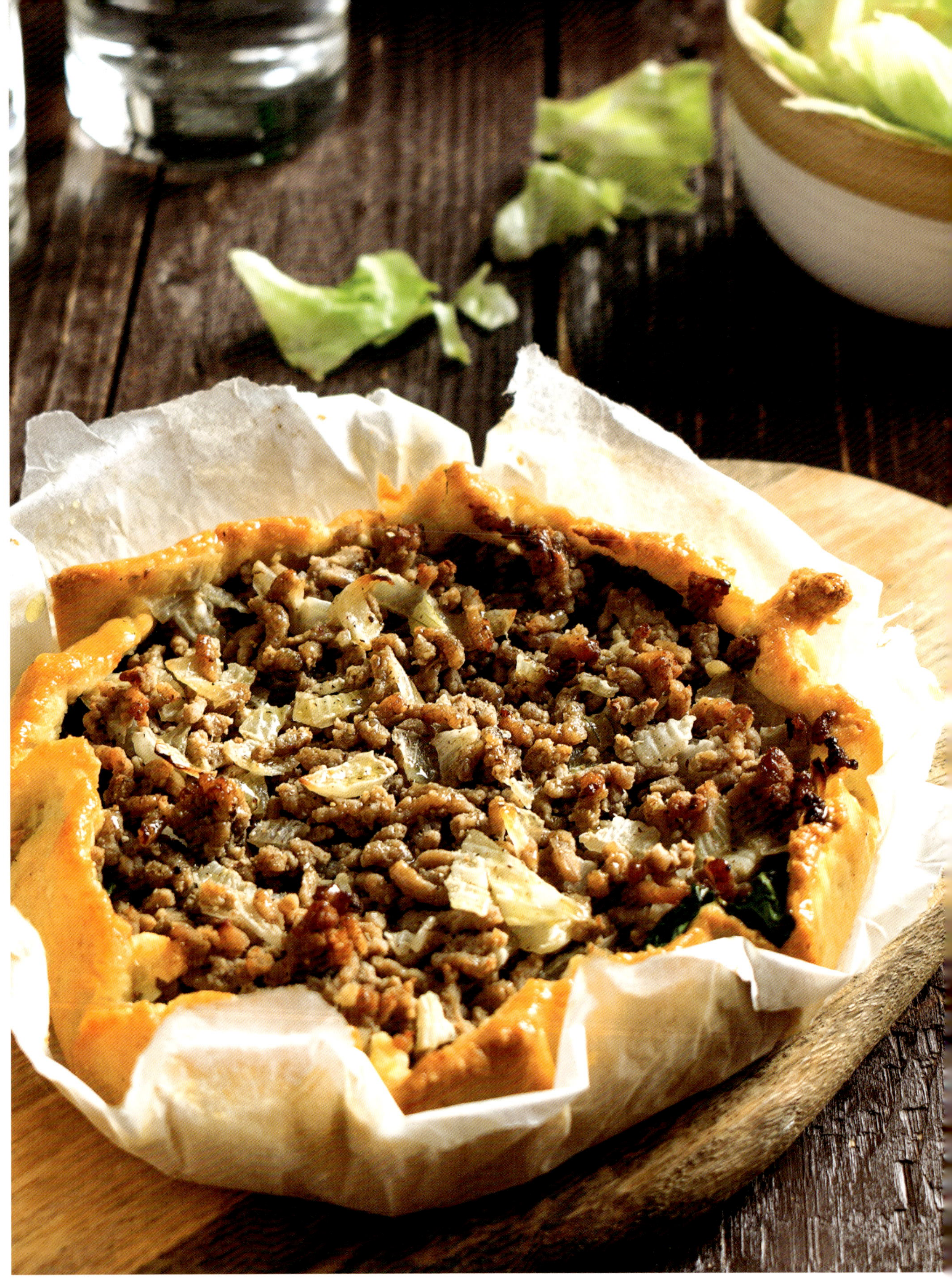

BEEF GALETTE

PASTRY (SEE NOTE)

1 cup (120g) almond meal

½ cup (50g) coconut flour

1 tsp xanthan gum

90g butter

60g cream cheese

2 eggs; 1 beaten for egg wash

½ tsp salt

FILLING

2 tbsps olive oil

1 small onion, sliced

350g beef mince

Salt and pepper to taste

1 tsp dried oregano

2 cups (60g) spinach leaves

STEPS

1. Place almond meal, coconut flour, xanthan gum, butter, cream cheese, one egg and salt in a food processor. Blend until the mixture forms a soft dough. Remove dough from the food processor and shape into a large disc. Wrap in greaseproof paper and chill in the fridge for 30 minutes.
2. Meanwhile, heat olive oil in a large frying pan over medium-high heat. Add onion and cook for 3-5 minutes until soft and translucent. Add beef and cook for 5 minutes until browned. Season with salt, pepper and oregano. Add spinach and stir until wilted. Drain off excess liquid. Set aside to cool.
3. Preheat the oven to 200°C. Line a baking tray with greaseproof paper.
4. Roll out the dough between two layers of greaseproof paper into a circle about ½ cm thick. Transfer to baking tray. Spoon the filling over the dough, leaving a 3cm border around the edges. Gently fold up the edges of the pastry to form a rough crust. Brush with egg wash.
5. Bake for 25-30 minutes until golden.

NOTE: Low-carb pastry mix is available to purchase from most supermarkets, and can be used in place of the pastry recipe in this book if preferred.

SERVES 4 | PREP + COOK TIME: 1 HOUR 15 MINS | GLUTEN FREE |

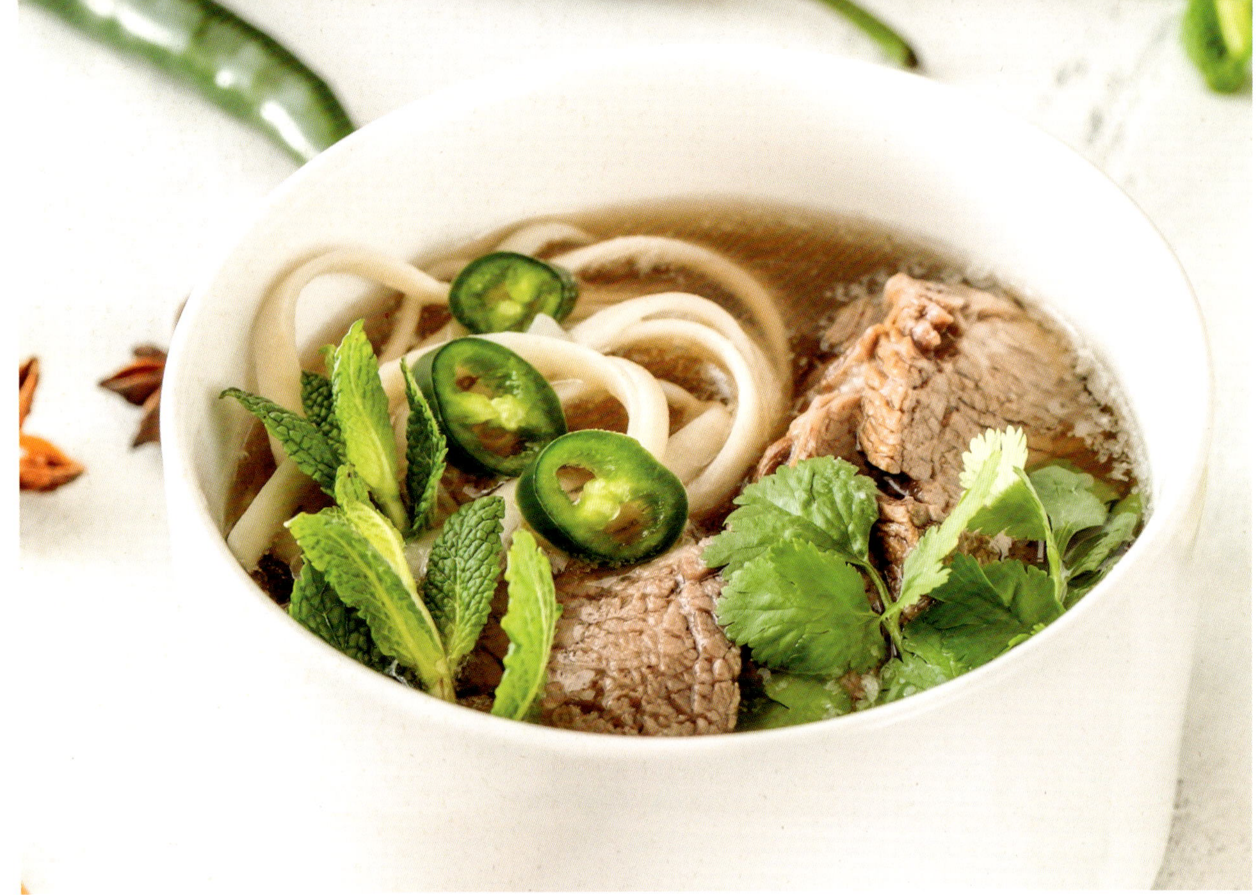

BEEF PHO

150g noodles (omit if following a strict low-carb diet)

1 tsp sesame oil

3 cups (750ml) beef stock

1 tsp finely chopped ginger

1 clove garlic, crushed

1 star anise

300g sirloin steak, sliced as thinly as possible

2 spring onions, cut into 4cm lengths

1 tsp fish sauce

1 tbsp fresh lime juice

Salt and pepper to taste

2 sprigs fresh mint, to garnish

Coriander leaves, to garnish

1 small green chilli, sliced

STEPS

1. If using noodles, prepare these first. Boil the noodles for 3 minutes, then drain and stir through sesame oil. Place into serving bowls and set aside.
2. Simmer the stock with the ginger, garlic and star anise for at least 30 minutes.
3. Add the beef, spring onions, fish sauce and lime juice and simmer for a further 5 minutes, until the beef is cooked.
4. Season to taste with salt and pepper.
5. Serve the hot soup poured over the noodles, and garnish with mint leaves, coriander leaves and the sliced chilli.

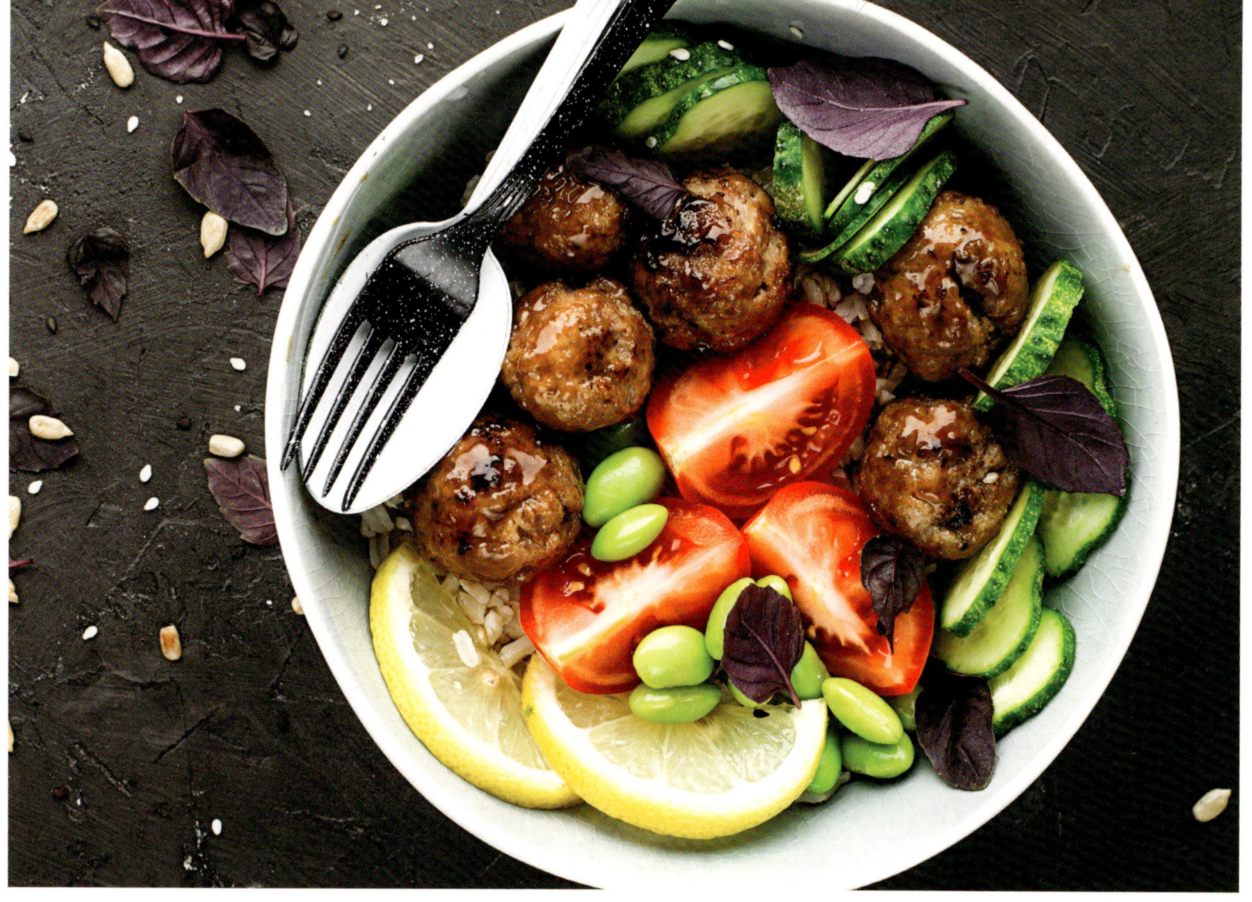

SERVES 4 | PREP + COOK TIME: 40 MINS | DAIRY FREE |

ASIAN MEATBALL BOWLS

MEATBALLS

500g beef mince
2 spring onions, finely sliced
2 cloves garlic, crushed
1 tbsp soy sauce
1 tbsp sesame oil
1 tbsp grated ginger
Salt and pepper to taste
1 tbsp vegetable oil

SALAD

2 cups (330g) cooked brown rice (optional)
4 Roma tomatoes, quartered
1 cucumber, sliced
¼ cup (45g) edamame
Honey soy dressing (see page 153)
Lemon slices to serve

STEPS

1. Place mince in a large bowl and add spring onions, garlic, soy, sesame oil and ginger. Season with salt and pepper and use your hands to mix well.
2. Shape into round meatball shapes, about 3cm in diameter.
3. Heat vegetable oil in a frying pan and cook meatballs in batches until nicely browned. Remove from heat and set aside.
4. To assemble the salad, divide brown rice (if using) evenly among four bowls and then layer with tomatoes, 3-5 meatballs each, sliced cucumber and edamame beans. Drizzle dressing over the top and garnish with lemon slices.

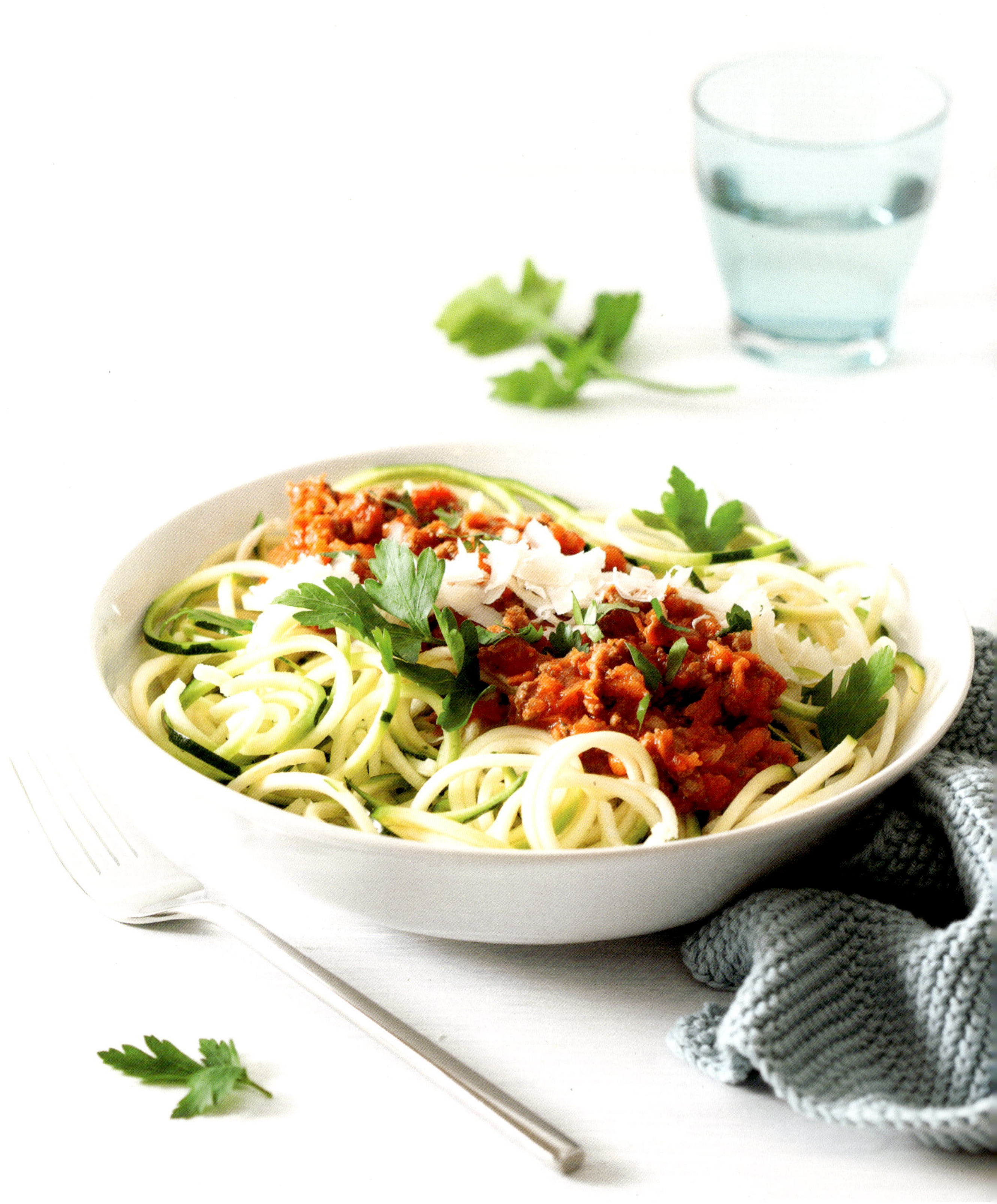

SIMPLE BOLOGNESE WITH ZOODLES

1 tbsp olive oil

1 onion, diced

2 cloves garlic, crushed

1 carrot, grated

1 tsp mixed Italian dried herbs

500g beef mince

2 x 400g cans crushed tomatoes

1 cup (250ml) beef or chicken stock

Salt and pepper to taste

3-4 medium zucchinis, spiralised into noodles

Parsley leaves to serve

Shaved Parmesan cheese to serve

STEPS

1. In a medium saucepan heat olive oil over a medium-high heat, add onion and garlic and saute until translucent. Add in grated carrot and dried herbs and saute for a further 2 minutes. Add in mince and cook until the meat is well browned, making sure to break apart any lumps. Add in the crushed tomatoes and half the stock and season with salt and pepper, then bring to a boil and reduce heat to simmer for around 20 minutes.
2. Meanwhile in a frying pan add the rest of the stock, bring to a simmer then add the zucchini and stir for 3 minutes until the zucchini is cooked through. Drain off any excess liquid and set aside for serving.
3. Remove mince mixture from the heat and set aside for serving.
4. Divide drained zucchini among bowls and ladle a generous amount of mince on top. Serve with parsley leaves, Parmesan and freshly cracked pepper.

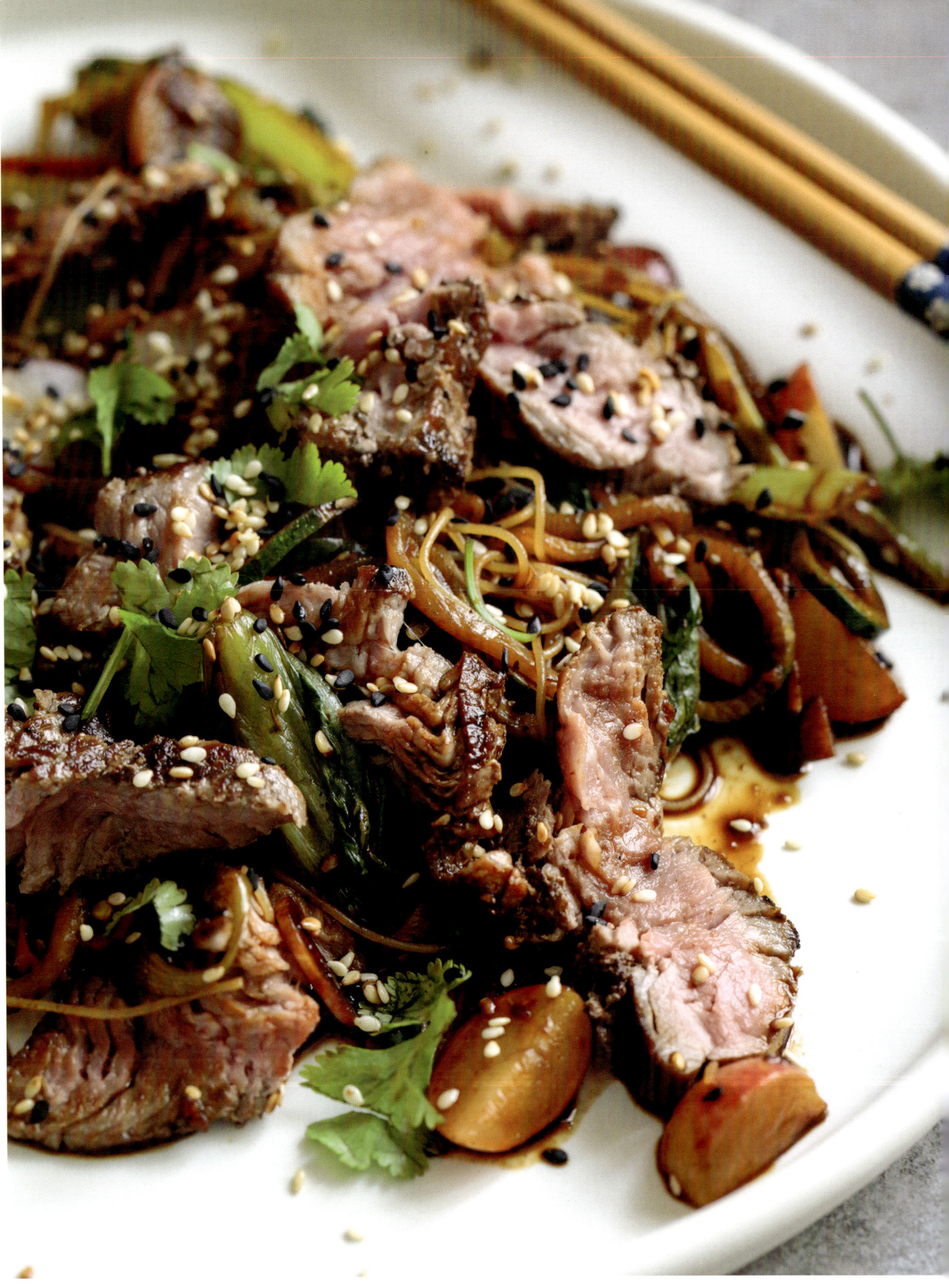

MONGOLIAN BEEF

½ cup (125ml) soy sauce

½ cup (125ml) water

2 tbsps brown sugar

200g brown rice noodles

2 tbsps vegetable oil

3 cloves garlic, minced

1 tsp grated ginger

500g flank steak, thinly sliced against the grain

1 bunch bok choy, chopped

4-6 radishes, quartered + 1 thinly sliced

TO GARNISH

2 spring onions, sliced diagonally

Sesame seeds

Coriander leaves

STEPS

1. In a small bowl, whisk together soy sauce, water and brown sugar. Mix until sugar has dissolved and set aside.
2. Cook the brown rice noodles according to the package instructions. Drain and set aside.
3. Heat vegetable oil in a large frying pan or wok over medium-high heat and add the minced garlic and grated ginger; saute for about 1 minute until fragrant. Add the flank steak to the pan and cook until it is browned on all sides.
4. Add bok choy and radishes and stir-fry for about 1 minute. Then add the soy sauce mixture and cooked noodles and fry for a further 2 minutes, making sure everything is well coated.
5. Remove from heat and serve immediately with spring onions, sesame seeds and coriander leaves.

SERVES 4 | PREP + COOK TIME: 30 MINS | DAIRY FREE |

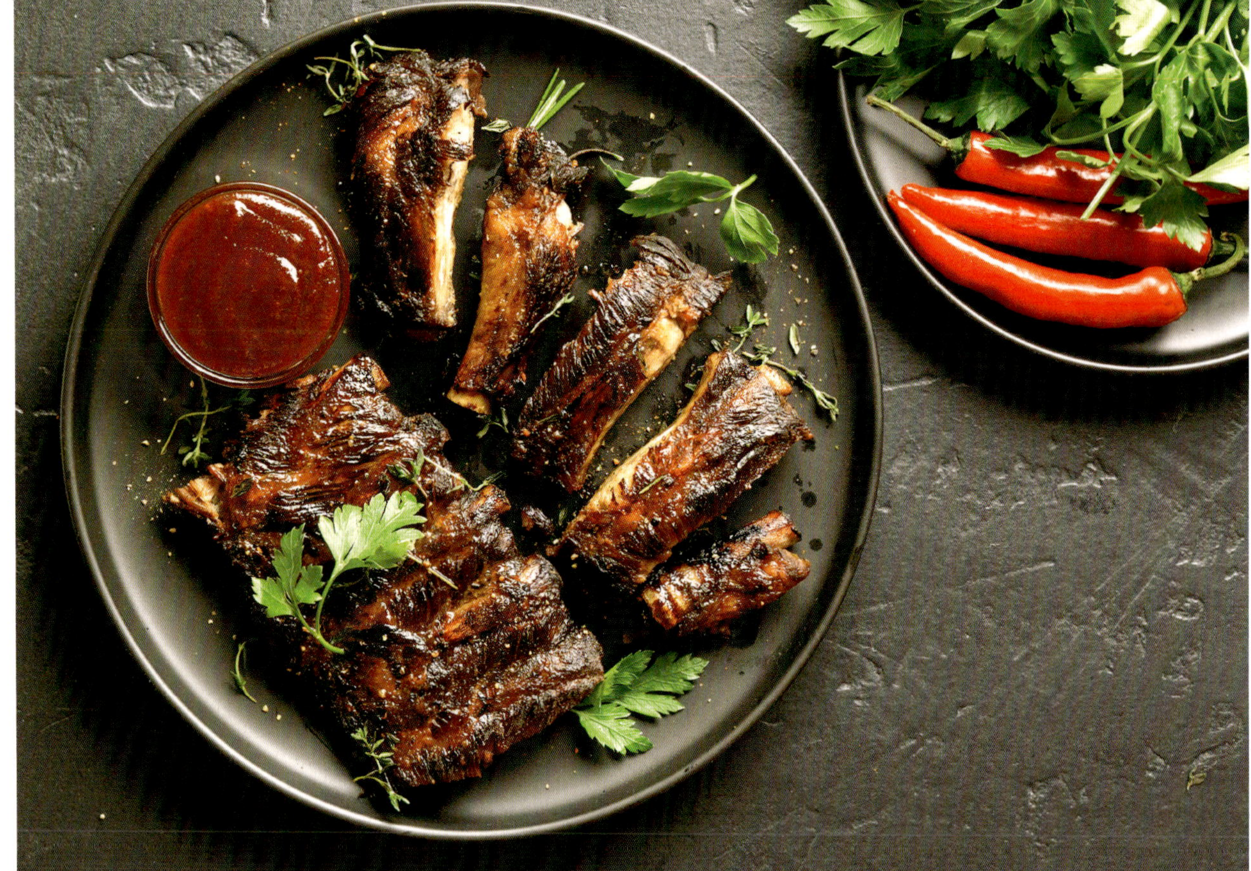

SPICY SPARE RIBS

1 tbsp brown sugar
1 tbsp paprika
1 tbsp chilli powder
1 tsp garlic powder
1 tsp onion powder
1 tsp cayenne pepper
½ tsp salt
½ tsp pepper
2 racks of spare ribs (1.5kg)
½ cup (125ml) Sriracha
Fresh coriander to garnish

STEPS

Preheat oven to 220°C.

1. In a small bowl, combine the brown sugar, paprika, chilli powder, garlic powder, onion powder, cayenne pepper, salt and pepper to make the spice rub.
2. Rub the spice mixture all over the spare ribs, ensuring they are well coated on both sides.
3. Place the seasoned spare ribs in a lined baking dish and bake for around 40-50 minutes or until the meat is tender and cooked through. During the last 15 minutes of grilling, baste the spare ribs with the Sriracha sauce, flipping and basting them every few minutes to create a sticky glaze.
4. Remove the spare ribs from the oven and let them rest for a few minutes before serving. Garnish with fresh coriander and extra Sriracha sauce.

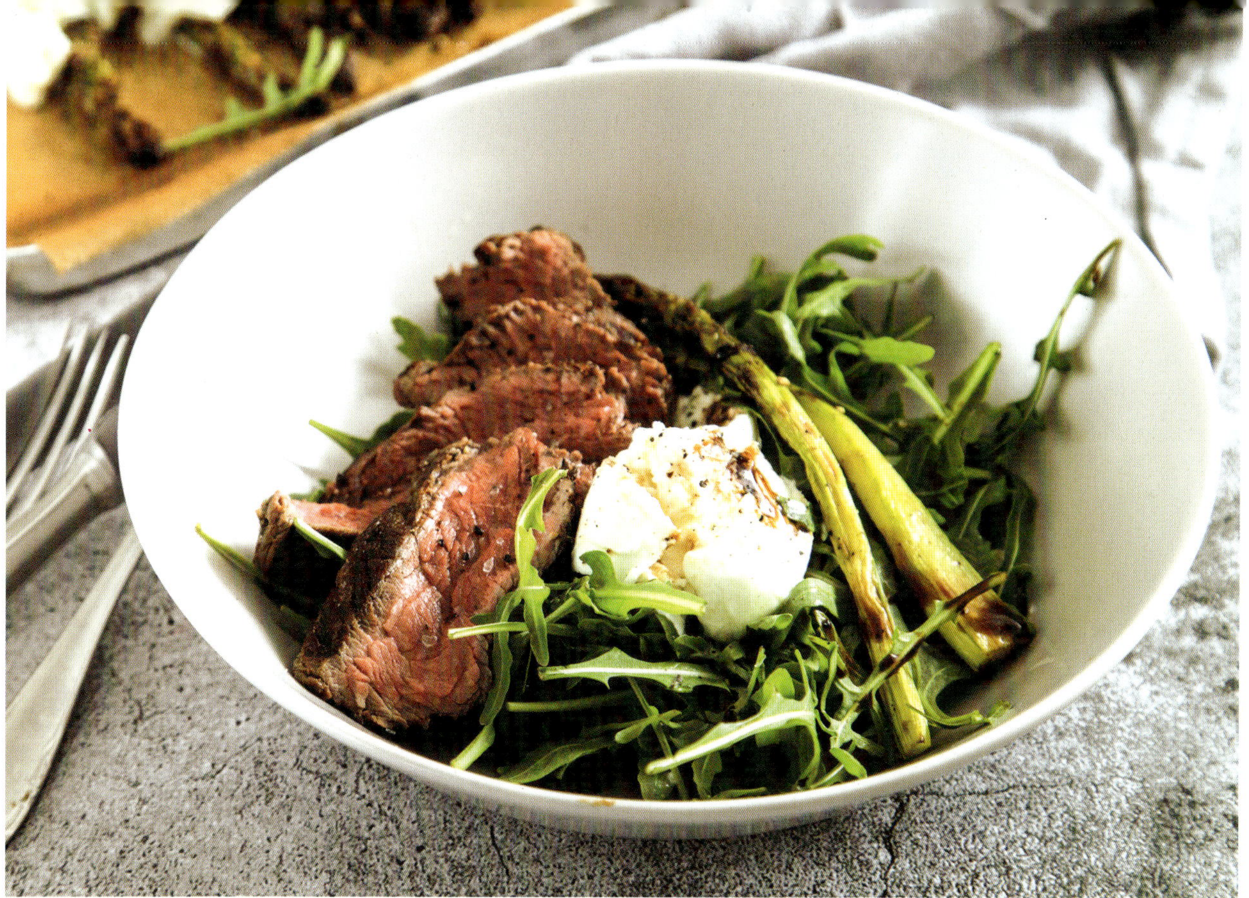

STEAK, ROASTED ASPARAGUS & BURRATA

500g asparagus spears, woody ends trimmed

2 tbsps olive oil + more for drizzling

1 tsp garlic powder

1 tbsp grated Parmesan cheese

Salt and pepper to taste

2 tbsps butter

2 rib-eye steaks (about 4cm thickness each)

2 cups (60g) rocket leaves

150g burrata

2 tsps balsamic vinegar

STEPS

Preheat oven to 200°C.

1. Toss the asparagus with olive oil, garlic powder, Parmesan cheese, salt and pepper and place asparagus on one half of a lined baking tray. Set aside.
2. Heat butter in a grill pan on high. Season both sides of the steaks with salt and pepper. Place steaks onto the grill pan and cook for 3 minutes on each side. Transfer to the baking tray with the asparagus and place in the oven. Roast for 10 minutes or until asparagus is tender.
3. Divide the rocket and burrata between two bowls.
4. Slice the steak and place on top of the rocket, along with the asparagus. Season with salt and pepper and drizzle with balsamic vinegar and a little more olive oil to serve.

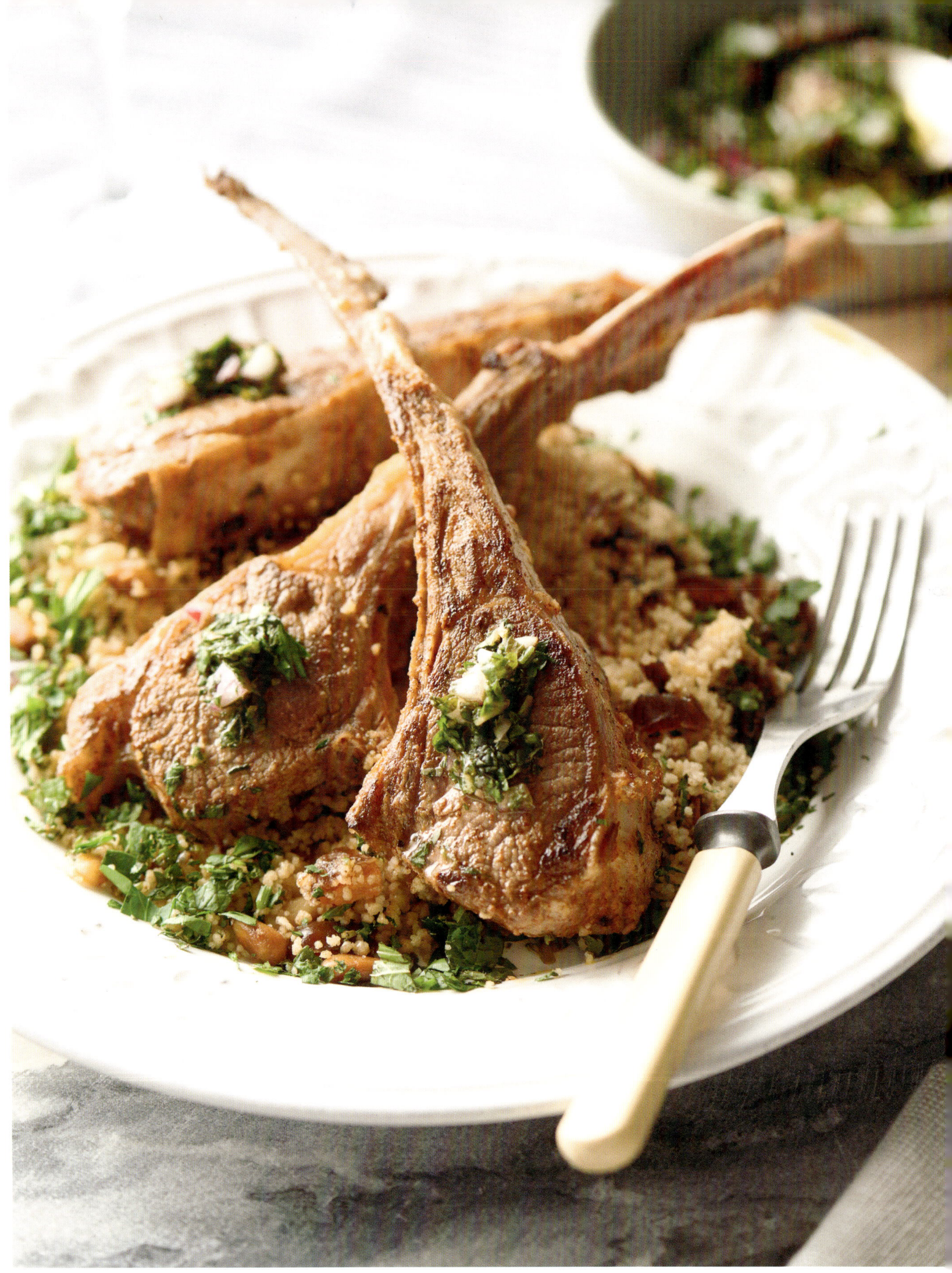

SPICED LAMB CUTLETS WITH COUSCOUS

½ cup (125ml) plain yoghurt

1 tbsp ground cumin

2 cloves garlic, crushed

Zest of 1 lemon

Salt and pepper to taste

8-10 lamb cutlets

2 tbsps olive oil

1 tbsp lemon juice

COUSCOUS SALAD

2 cups (330g) cooked couscous

½ cup (80g) mixed dried fruit (sultanas, apricots and cranberries)

½ cup (20g) chopped fresh parsley + extra to garnish

¼ cup (20g) chopped fresh mint

2 tbsps lemon juice

2 tbsps olive oil

2 tbsps pine nuts

Salt and pepper to taste

STEPS

1. Combine yoghurt, cumin, garlic, grated lemon zest, salt and pepper in a medium-sized bowl. Then add lamb cutlets, toss to coat and set aside to marinate for 30 minutes to 1 hour.

2. For the salad combine cooked couscous, dried fruit, parsley, mint, lemon juice, olive oil, pine nuts, salt and pepper and toss well to combine. Set aside for serving.

3. Preheat a barbecue, pan or grill to hot.

4. Add olive oil and cook cutlets on one side until the first sign of moisture appears on top, about 3-4 minutes. Turn over, brush with the lemon juice and cook for a further 3 minutes for medium-rare, or longer to your preference. Turn once only. Remove cutlets from heat.

5. Divide salad onto serving plates and top with warm cutlets, sprinkled with extra parsley.

SERVES 4 | PREP + COOK TIME: 15 MINS + MARINATING |

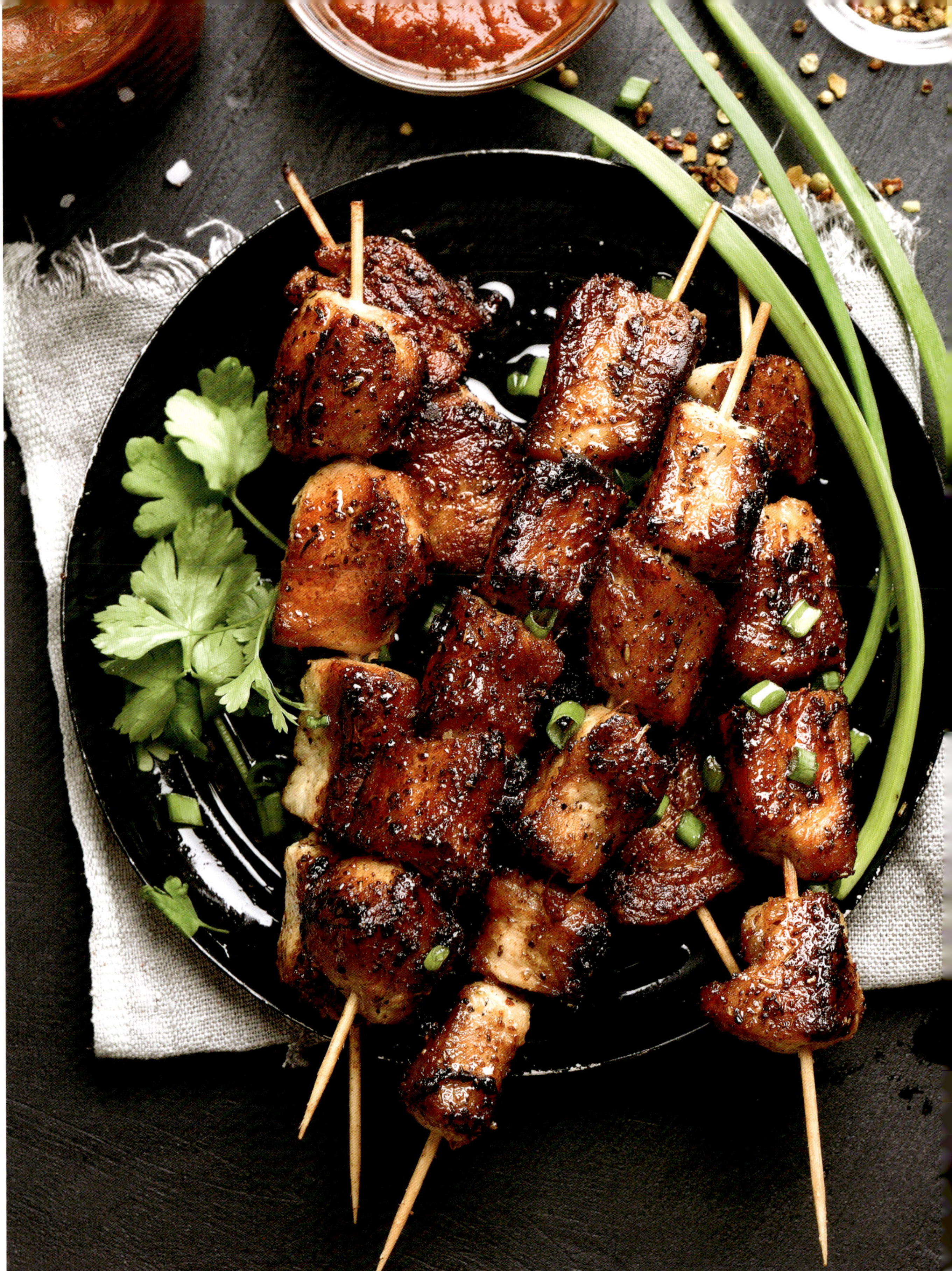

ASIAN-STYLE PORK KEBABS

¼ cup (60ml) soy sauce or tamari
2 tbsps hoisin sauce
2 tbsps honey
2 tbsps rice wine vinegar
2 cloves garlic, crushed
1 tsp grated ginger
1 tsp sesame oil
1 tsp vegetable oil
600g pork fillet, cut into 2cm cubes

TO GARNISH

Sliced spring onions
Coriander leaves
Sesame seeds

STEPS

1. In a bowl, whisk together the soy sauce, hoisin sauce, honey, rice wine vinegar, garlic, grated ginger, sesame oil and vegetable oil to make the marinade.
2. Place the pork cubes in a separate bowl and pour the marinade over the pork. Toss to coat the pork evenly. Marinate in the fridge for at least 30 minutes.
3. Preheat your grill to medium-high heat.
4. Thread the marinated pork cubes onto metal or soaked wooden skewers, leaving a small space between each piece.
5. Place the kebabs on the preheated grill and cook for about 10-12 minutes, turning occasionally, until the pork is cooked through and slightly charred on the outside. Remove the kebabs from the grill and let them rest for a few minutes before serving. Garnish with sliced spring onions, coriander leaves and sesame seeds.

SERVES 4 | PREP + COOK TIME: 25 MINS + MARINATING | DAIRY FREE |

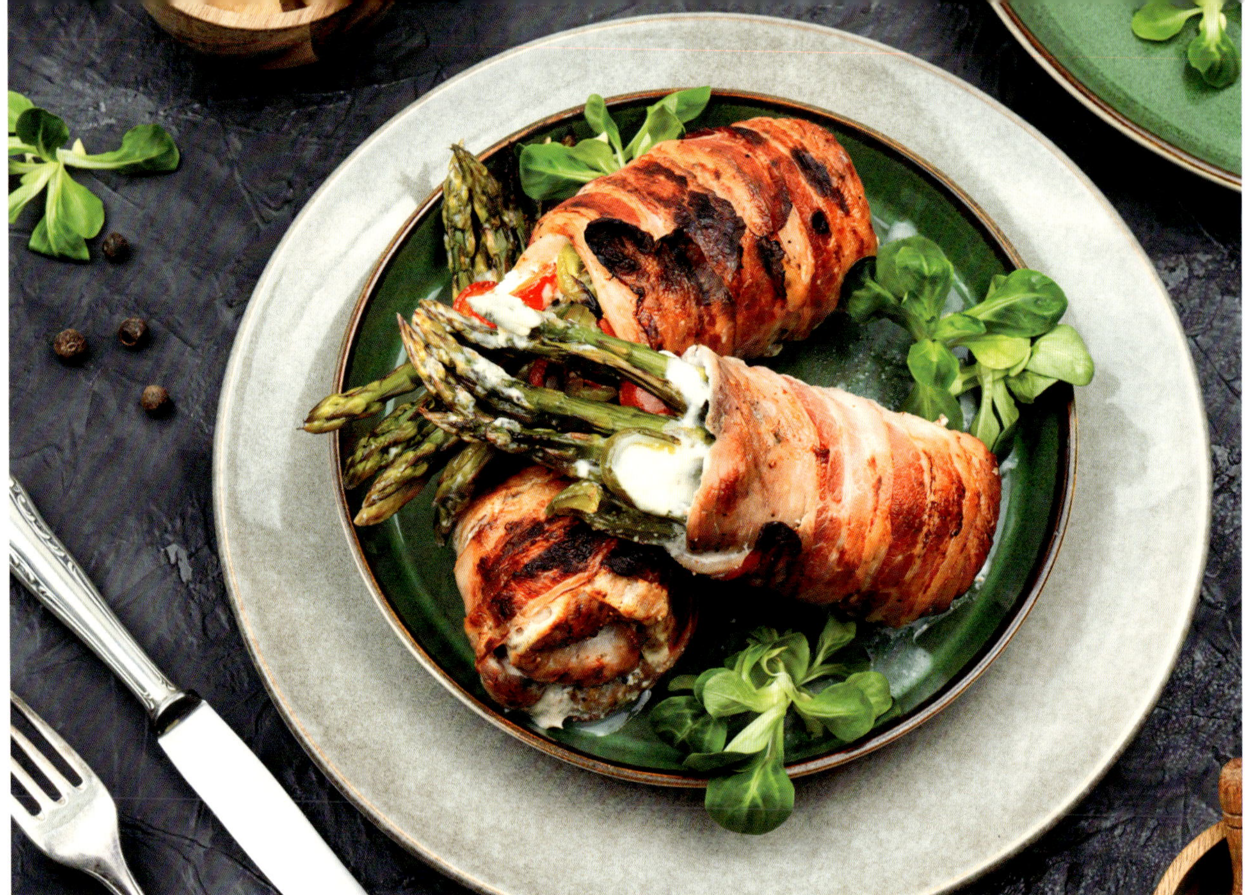

CHEESY BACON-WRAPPED ASPARAGUS

2 bunches of asparagus spears (about 20-24 spears)

10-12 rashers streaky bacon

1 cup (125g) grated Cheddar cheese

1 cup (225g) cherry tomatoes, halved

Salt and pepper to taste

STEPS

Preheat oven 200°C.

1. Trim the tough ends of the asparagus spears. Divide the asparagus into bundles of 4-6 spears, depending on their size.
2. Take two slices of bacon, lay them flat and place the asparagus bundle on top then add some cheese and chopped cherry tomatoes. Wrap the bundles up tightly with the bacon, making sure you enclose the filling. Repeat with the remaining asparagus bundles.
3. Place the wrapped bundles evenly on a lined baking tray. Bake in the preheated oven for 20-25 minutes or until the bacon is crispy and the asparagus is tender.
4. Remove from the oven and let cool slightly before serving.

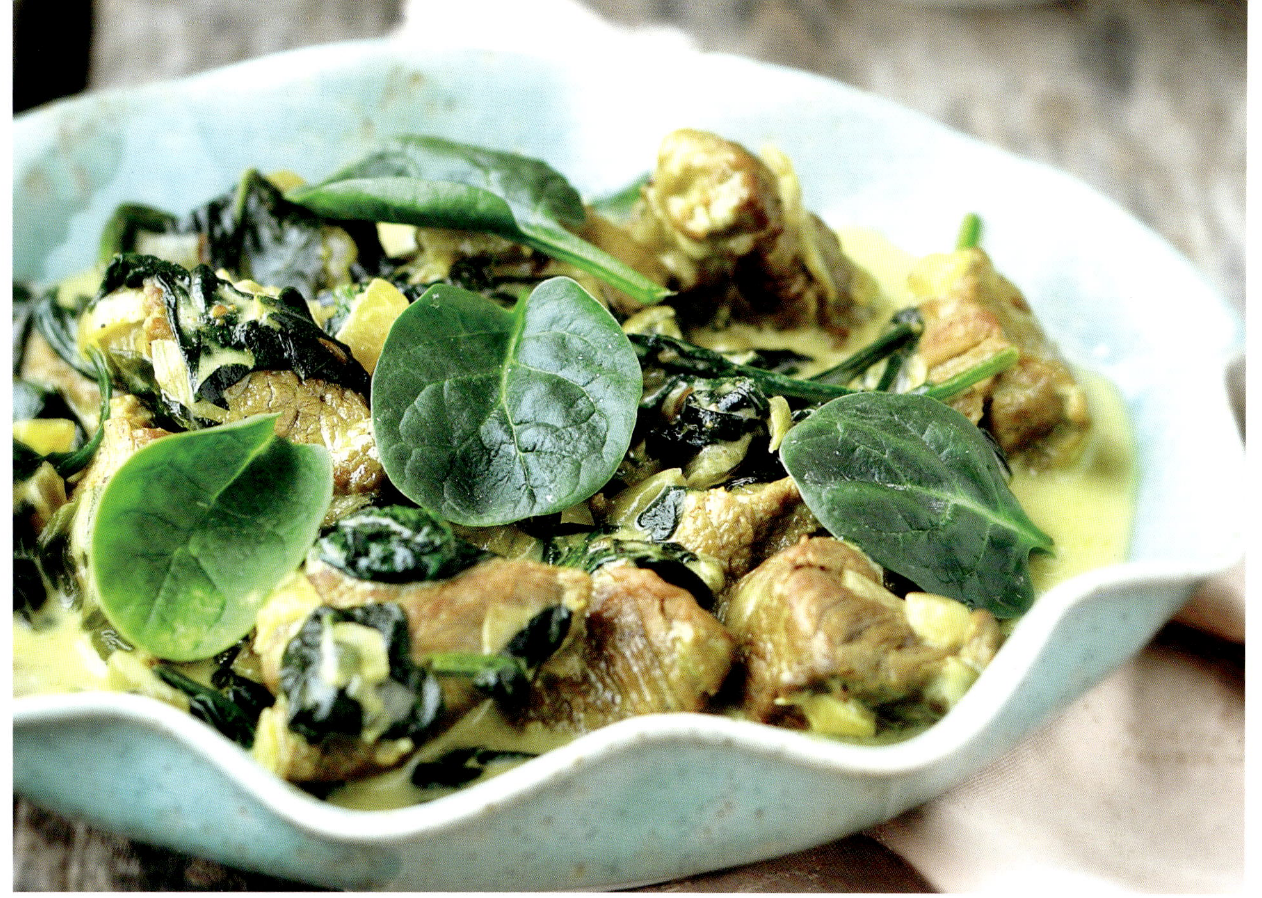

BRAISED BEEF IN CREAMY SPINACH SAUCE

2 tbsps olive oil

1 large onion, diced

6 cloves garlic, minced

750g sirloin steak, sliced across the grain

Salt and pepper to taste

300g baby spinach (reserve some leaves for garnish)

1 cup (250ml) thickened cream

¼ tsp nutmeg

STEPS

1. Heat olive oil in a large, deep frying pan over medium heat. Add onions and cook for 3-5 minutes until soft and translucent. Add garlic and cook for 30 seconds until fragrant.
2. Add beef, season with salt and pepper and stir-fry for 2-3 minutes until browned.
3. Add the spinach in batches. Cook each batch for a couple of minutes until it wilts before adding the next batch.
4. When all the spinach is wilted cook for a couple of minutes more until the liquid from the spinach starts to evaporate.
5. Stir in cream and nutmeg. Simmer for 3-4 minutes until the sauce thickens. Garnish with extra baby spinach leaves.

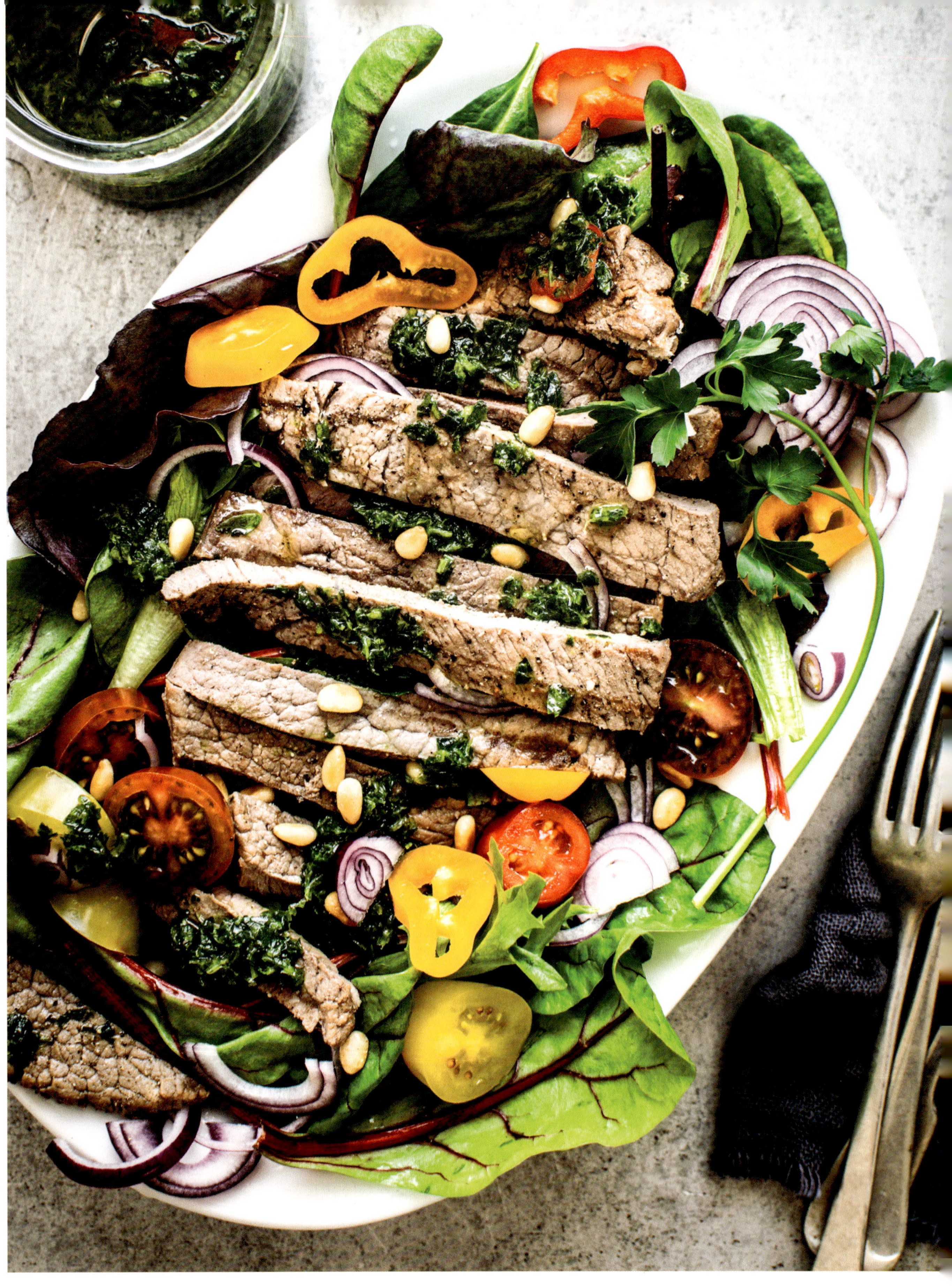

SALT & PEPPER SKIRT STEAK SALAD

500g skirt steak

Salt and pepper to taste

2 tbsps olive oil

SALAD

150g mixed lettuce leaves

⅔ cup (150g) cherry tomatoes, halved

½ red onion, halved and thinly sliced

1 cup (150g) mini capsicums, sliced

¼ cup (60ml) olive oil

1 tbsp lemon juice

Salt and pepper to taste

TO SERVE

¼ cup (60g) pesto (store-bought or see recipe page 69)

¼ cup (35g) toasted pine nuts (optional)

STEPS

1. Cut the steaks into 12-18cm-long pieces, small enough to fit on a grill pan. Thoroughly pat the pieces dry with paper towels on each side. Generously season each side of the steaks with salt and pepper.

2. Heat a large grill pan or cast-iron frying pan over high heat for 3 minutes. Once hot, add the olive oil.

3. Place the steak in the pan, then use tongs to press down firmly on the surface a few times. Sear the first side for about 2-4 minutes, depending on the thickness of the steak, until browned. Flip and cook for another 2-4 minutes. Work in two batches if needed. Transfer steak to a cutting board, loosely cover with foil and allow to rest for 10 minutes.

4. While the steak is resting layer the lettuce leaves, cherry tomatoes, onion and capsicum on a large serving plate and drizzle with olive oil and lemon juice. Season with salt and pepper.

5. Hold the carving knife at a 45-degree angle and slice the steak across the grain into 1cm-thick slices. Transfer to the plate and serve with dollops of pesto and toasted pine nuts.

SERVES 4 | PREP + COOK TIME: 25 MINS | GLUTEN FREE | DAIRY FREE |

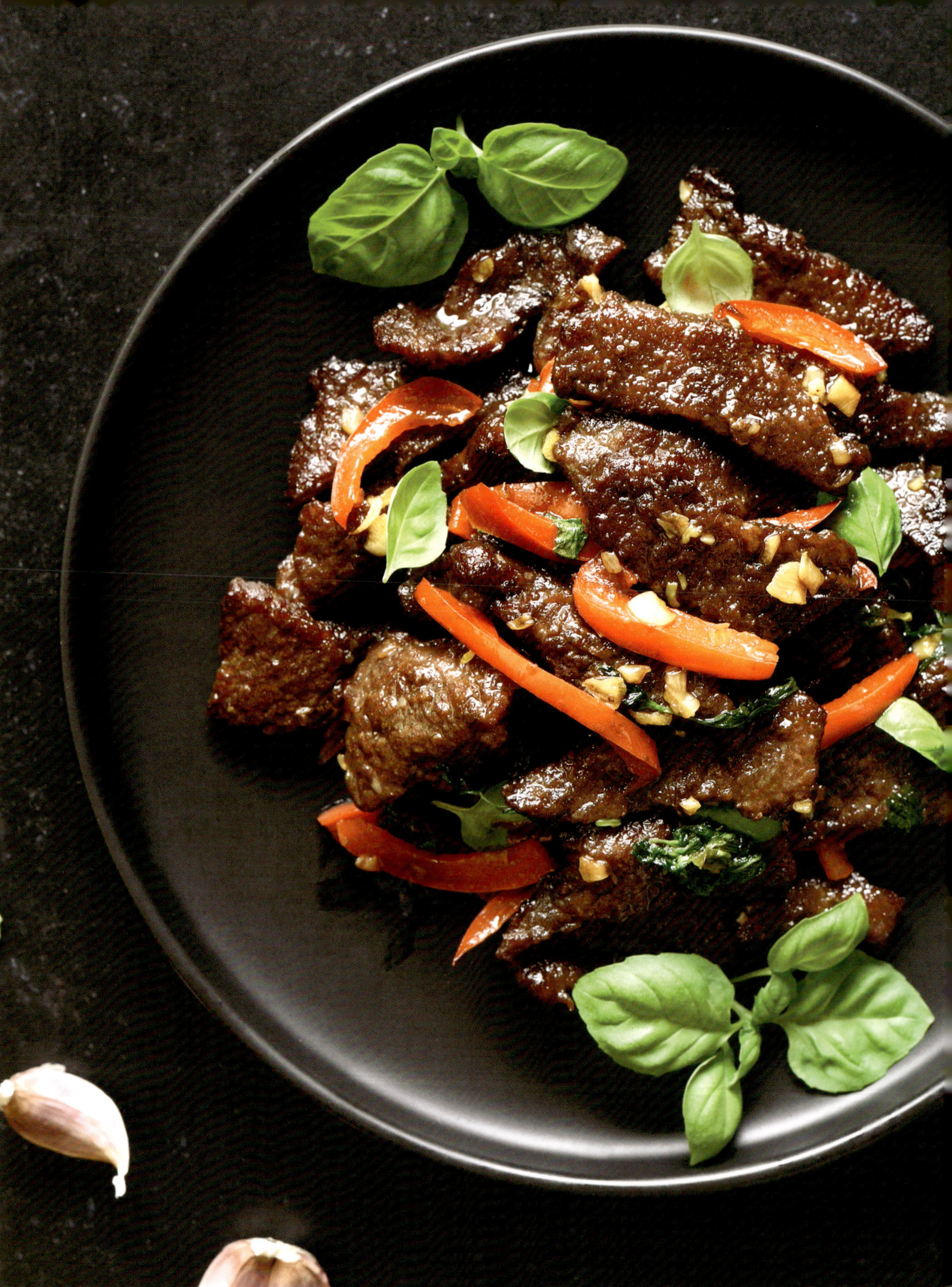

THAI STYLE BEEF STIR-FRY

2 tbsps soy sauce or tamari

1 tbsp oyster sauce

1 tbsp fish sauce

1 tbsp brown sugar

500g beef sirloin or flank steak, thinly sliced

2 tbsps vegetable oil

3 cloves garlic, crushed

1 small onion, thinly sliced

2 capsicums, thinly sliced

¼ cup (5g) Thai basil leaves + extra leaves to garnish

Crushed peanuts to garnish

STEPS

1. In a bowl, combine the soy sauce, oyster sauce, fish sauce, and brown sugar. Stir well to dissolve the sugar and set stir-fry sauce aside.
2. Place the sliced beef in a separate bowl and pour half of the stir-fry sauce over it. Toss to coat the beef and let it marinate for at least 15 minutes.
3. Heat the vegetable oil in a wok or large pan over high heat. Add the garlic, onion, capsicum and Thai basil to the hot oil and stir-fry for about 30 seconds until fragrant. Add beef to the wok and stir-fry for 2-3 minutes or until browned.
4. Pour the remaining stir-fry sauce over the beef and vegetables and stir-fry for an additional 1-2 minutes until everything is coated in the sauce and heated through.
5. Remove from heat and garnish with extra Thai basil and crushed peanuts.

SERVES 4 | PREP + COOK TIME: 30 MINS | DAIRY FREE |

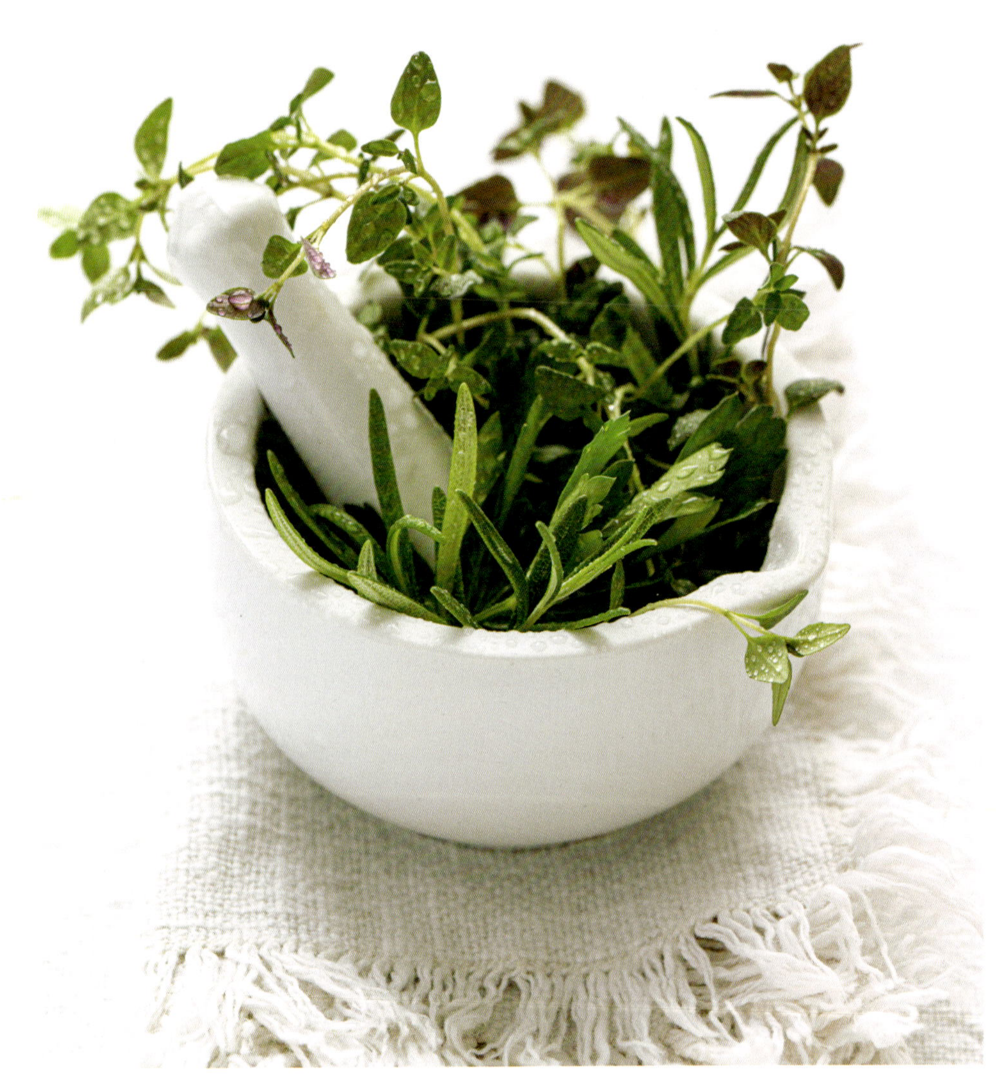

FISH & CHICKEN

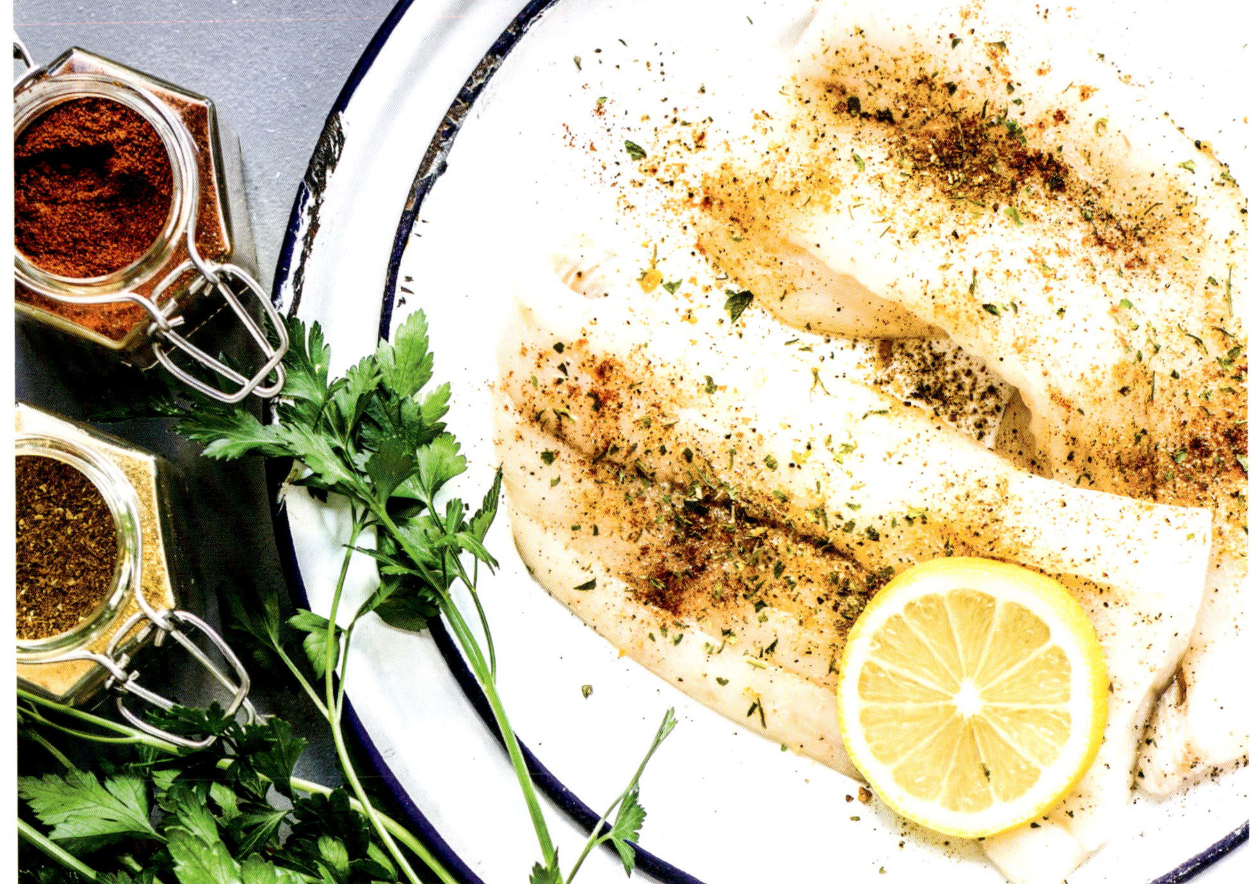

SIMPLE SPICED FISH

½ tbsp dried mixed herbs

½ tbsp smoked paprika

½ tbsp garlic powder

½ tbsp onion powder

1 tbsp salt

2 tbsps pepper

2 large firm white fish fillets

2 tbsps lemon juice

TO SERVE

Lemon wedges

Salad leaves

STEPS

1. Place the mixed herbs, smoked paprika, garlic and onion powders, salt and pepper in a small bowl and mix to combine.
2. Prepare the fillets by patting the fish dry and sprinkling the spice mix over the entire fillet.
3. Heat a pan to medium-high heat and cook the fish for 2-3 minutes on each side, or until the fish is cooked through. Turn the heat off and add lemon juice to the hot pan.
4. Serve with lemon wedges and salad leaves.

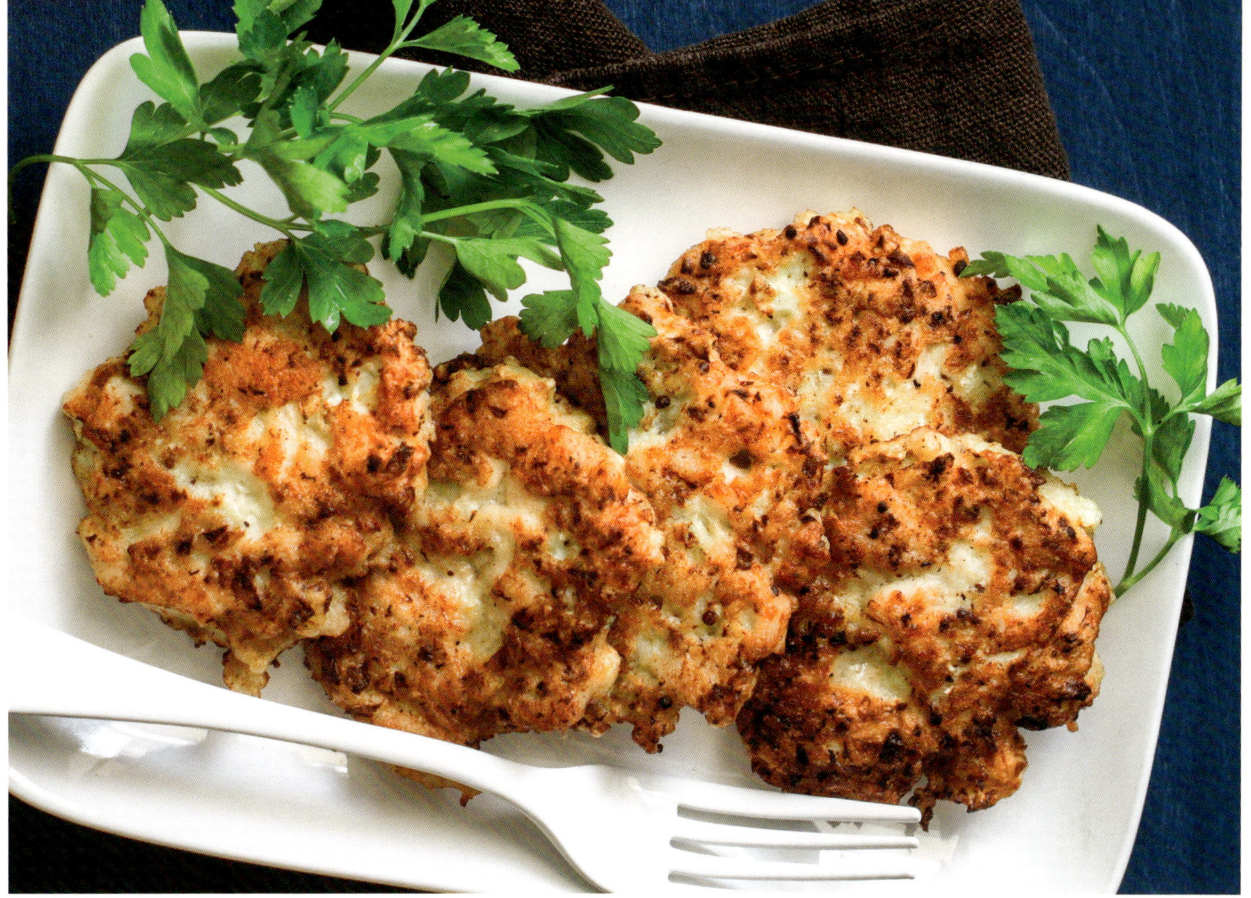

CAULIFLOWER & CHICKEN FRITTERS

1 medium head cauliflower, chopped
400g chicken mince
2 large cloves garlic, crushed
¾ cup (90g) grated Cheddar cheese
½ cup (60g) almond meal
1 tbsp seeded mustard
2 small eggs, lightly beaten
¼ cup (25g) coconut flour
Salt and pepper to taste
Olive oil for frying

STEPS

1. Place all the ingredients except the olive oil in a large bowl and combine thoroughly.
2. Shape ⅓ cup-sized portions into fritters and place in the refrigerator for at least 30 minutes to chill.
3. Heat 2 tablespoons of oil in a large nonstick frying pan over medium heat. Fry the fritters in batches for 5 minutes on each side until golden. Drain the fritters on paper towels. Add more oil as needed while frying.

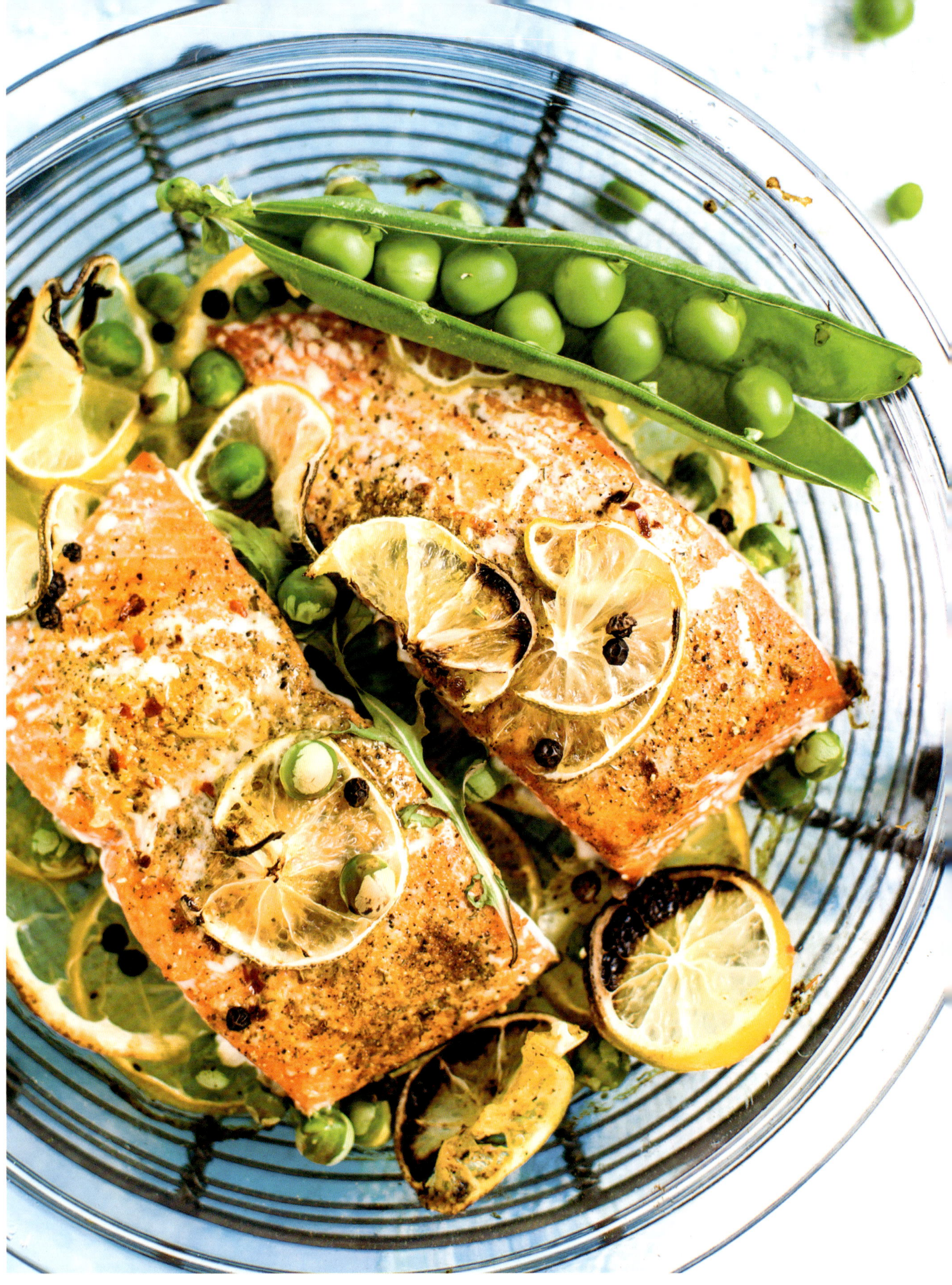

LEMON BAKED SALMON FILLETS

2 large salmon fillets, skin removed

1 tbsp olive oil

Salt and pepper to taste

½ tbsp paprika

1 clove garlic, minced

1 tbsp lemon zest

1 lemon, cut into slices

½ cup (125ml) dry white wine

SALAD

2 cups (230g) snow peas, trimmed

120g rocket leaves

2 tbsps olive oil

2 tbsps fresh lemon juice

Salt and pepper to taste

STEPS

Preheat the oven to 200°C.

1. Drizzle salmon with olive oil and rub evenly into the salmon fillets. Sprinkle with salt, pepper and paprika then top with the minced garlic and lemon zest and set aside.
2. To make the salad add the snow peas, rocket leaves, olive oil, lemon juice and salt and pepper into a bowl and toss to combine.
3. Arrange lemon slices on the bottom of a small baking dish then place the salmon on top.
4. Pour the wine into the baking dish, and then cover with aluminium foil. Bake the salmon until the fish flakes and white bubbles of protein appear on the surface, 12-15 minutes, depending on the thickness of the fillets. Check the salmon after 10 minutes to see its progress.
5. Divide salad between two serving plates and place warm salmon on top.

SERVES 2 | PREP + COOK TIME 35 MINS | GLUTEN FREE | DAIRY FREE |

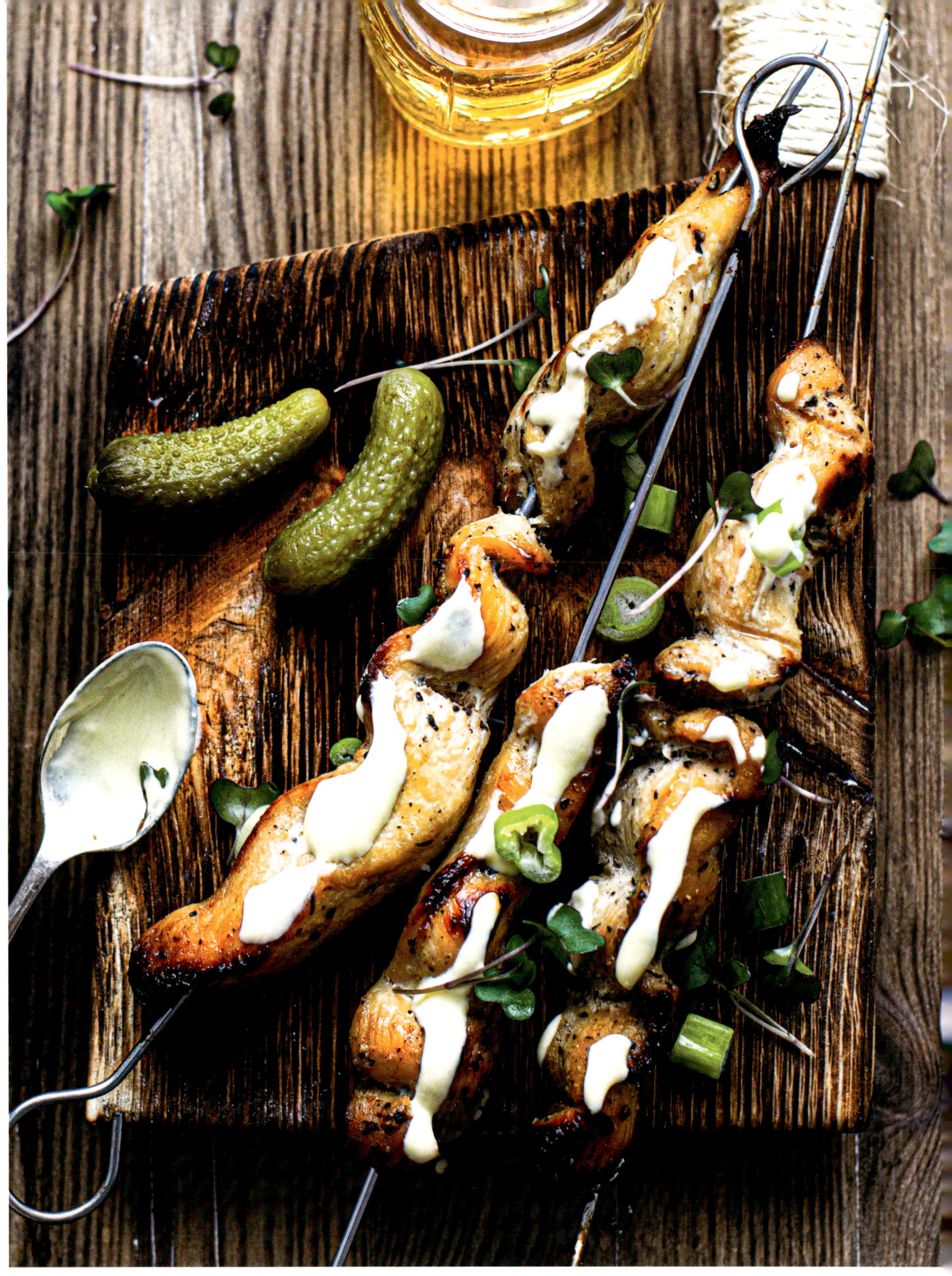

MUSTARD CHICKEN SKEWERS

1 tbsp apple cider vinegar

4 tbsps Dijon mustard

3 tbsps seeded mustard

300g chicken breast fillets, cut into 3cm cubes

½ cup (125ml) Greek yoghurt

2 tbsps honey

Salt and pepper to taste

2 tbsps olive oil

1 clove garlic, crushed

TO SERVE

Sliced spring onions

Micro herbs

Sliced cucumber pickles

STEPS

1. Combine the vinegar, 1 tablespoon of Dijon and 1 tablespoon of seeded mustard together and coat the chicken pieces with it. Cover the chicken and place in the refrigerator for at least 2 hours.

2. For the dipping sauce add Greek yoghurt, honey and 1 tablespoon of Dijon mustard to a small bowl and mix well to combine. Season with salt and pepper and set aside.

3. Mix together the oil, ¼ teaspoon each of salt and pepper, garlic and the rest of the mustards in a small bowl.

4. Thread the chicken pieces onto metal or soaked wooden skewers and heat a grill plate on high heat. Place the skewers on the grill and brush with the mustard oil. Grill for 2 minutes on all four sides, brushing each time with the oil.

5. Serve hot with dipping sauce and sliced spring onions, micro herbs and cucumber pickles.

SERVES 2 | PREP + COOK TIME: 20 MINS + MARINATING | GLUTEN FREE |

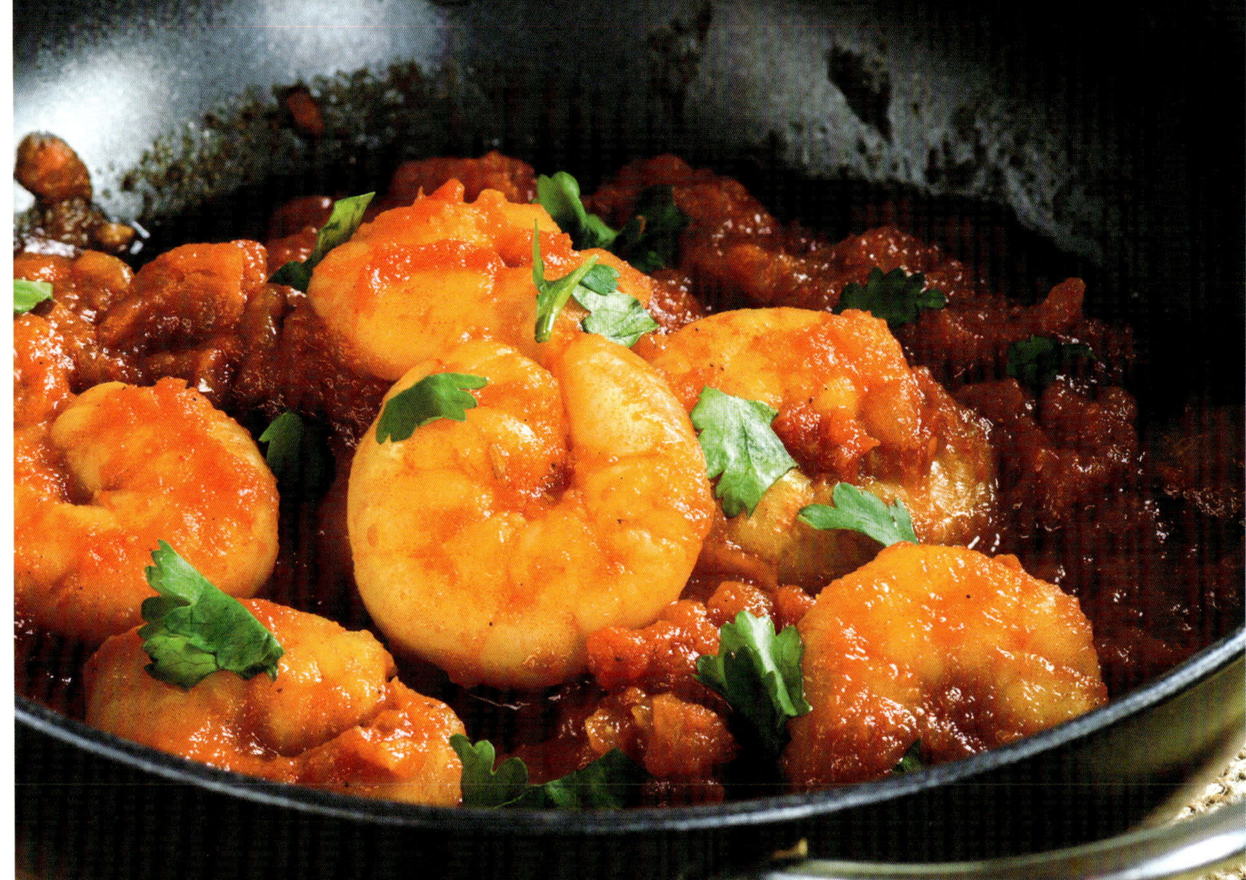

PRAWN MASALA

2 tbsps vegetable oil

450g prawns, peeled and deveined

1 large onion, finely chopped

Small piece of ginger, grated

2 cloves, crushed

1 tsp turmeric

1 tsp chilli powder

1 tsp ground cumin

1 tsp coriander

½ tsp garam masala

½ tsp ground fenugreek

Salt to taste

1 x 400g can diced tomatoes

Cauliflower rice to serve

Fresh coriander leaves, chopped, to garnish

STEPS

1. Heat half the vegetable oil in a pan over medium heat. Add the prawns to the pan and cook for 4-5 minutes, or until they turn pink and are cooked through. Remove from pan and set aside.

2. In the same pan, heat the rest of the oil and add the chopped onions and saute until they become translucent. Then add the ginger and garlic and cook for another minute until fragrant.

3. Add the turmeric, chilli, cumin, coriander, garam masala, fenugreek and salt. Mix well and cook for 2-3 minutes to allow the spices to release their flavours. Then add the diced tomatoes and mix until combined.

4. Add the prawns back to the pan and simmer for 2-3 minutes to allow the flavours to meld together. Serve with cauliflower rice and fresh coriander.

SERVES 4 | PREP + COOK TIME: 15 MINS | GLUTEN FREE | DAIRY FREE |

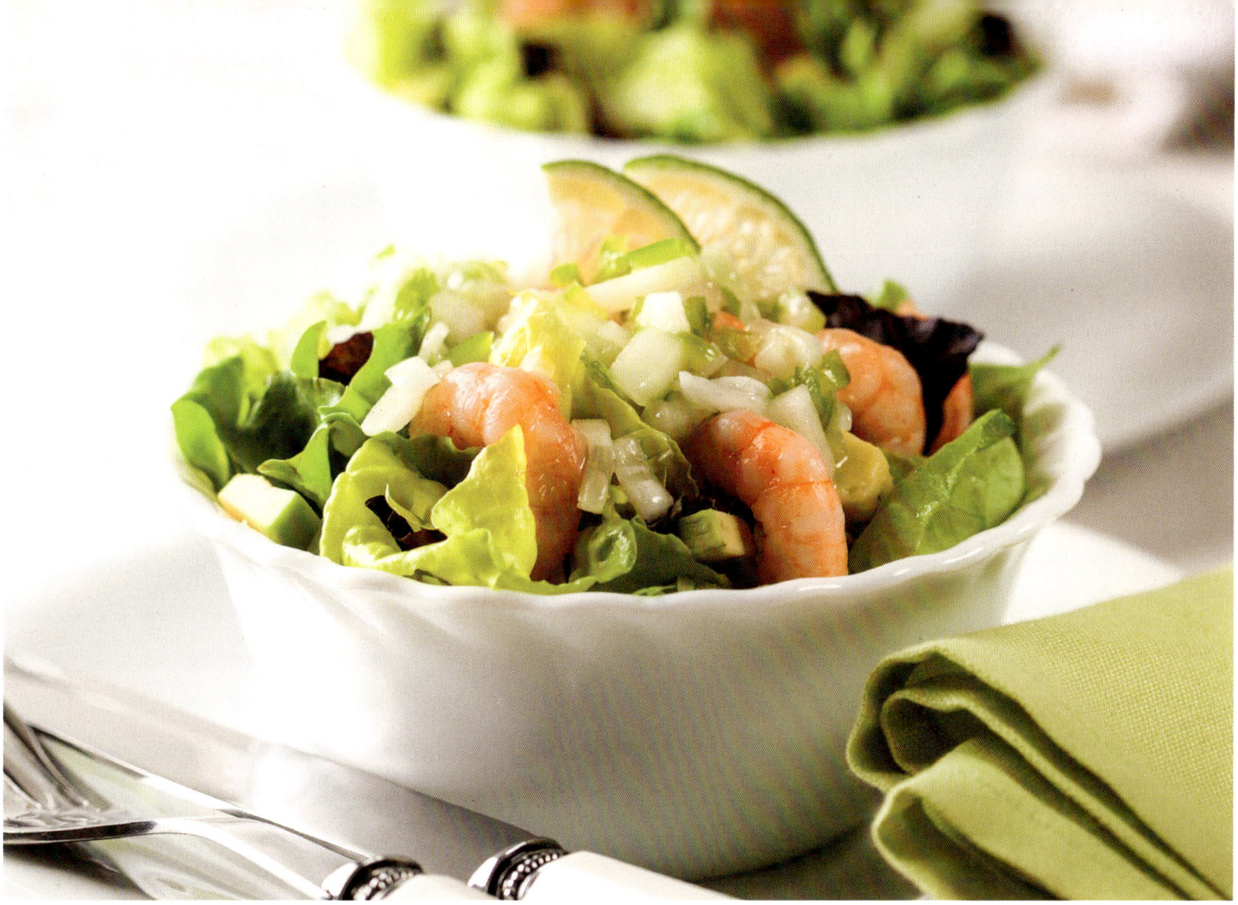

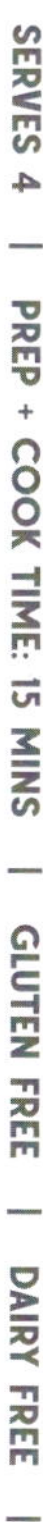

PRAWN, AVOCADO & CUCUMBER SALAD

1 large lime, juiced
2½ tbsps olive oil
2 tbsps apple cider vinegar
½ small white onion, finely chopped
4 cups butter or cos lettuce leaves
2 large avocados, diced
2 small Lebanese cucumbers, diced
600g cooked, peeled, deveined prawns
Salt and pepper to taste

STEPS

1. In a small bowl add lime juice, olive oil and cider vinegar and whisk to combine, then add the onion and let it sit for 10-15 minutes to slightly pickle.

2. In a large serving bowl add the salad leaves, avocado, cucumbers and cooked prawns, gently tossing to combine.

3. To serve pour the onion dressing over the salad and season with salt and pepper to taste.

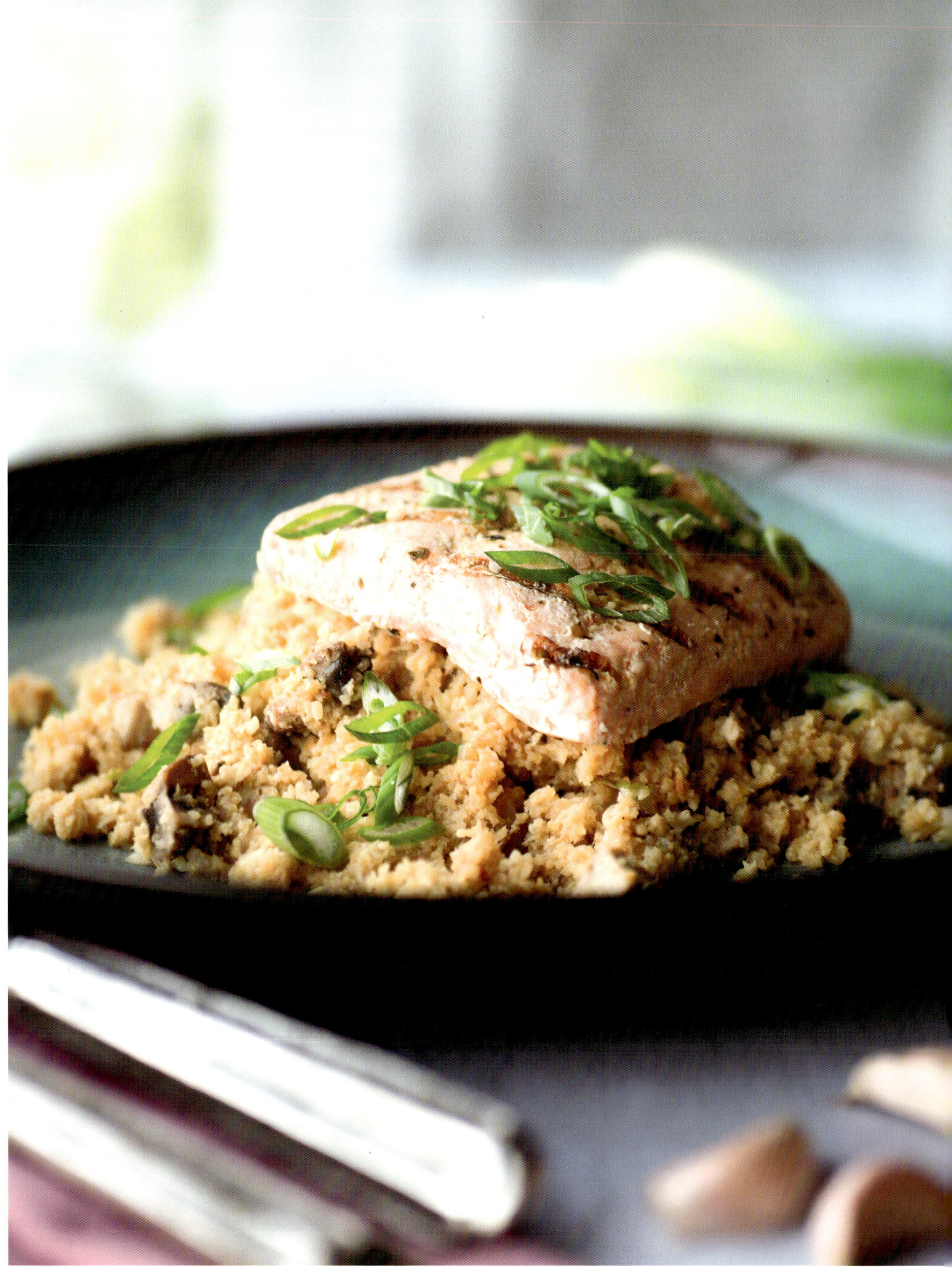

BAKED SALMON ON CAULIFLOWER RICE

¼ cup (60ml) soy sauce
1 tbsp rice wine vinegar
2 tbsps grated fresh ginger
2 tbsps lime juice
½ tbsp chilli sauce
2 cloves garlic, crushed
2 x 150g skin-on salmon steaks
1 small head cauliflower
1 tbsp sesame oil
200g button mushrooms, chopped
2 spring onions, sliced

STEPS

Preheat oven to 220°C.

1. In a small bowl, mix together the soy sauce, vinegar, ginger, lime juice, chilli sauce and garlic. Place the salmon steaks in a baking dish and pour the sauce over the top. Bake for 15 minutes or until the salmon is cooked through. Cover and set aside.

2. Meanwhile break the cauliflower into pieces then place them in a food processor. Pulse until the cauliflower begins to resemble rice.

3. Heat the oil in a large frying pan over medium heat. Add the mushrooms and cook for 5 minutes. Add the cauliflower, cover and cook for 5 minutes.

4. Pour 1½ tablespoons of the sauce from the baking dish over the top of the rice and gently stir through. Heat for a further minute.

5. Serve the salmon steaks on top of the cauliflower, garnished with spring onion.

SERVES 2 | PREP + COOK TIME: 40 MINS | DAIRY FREE |

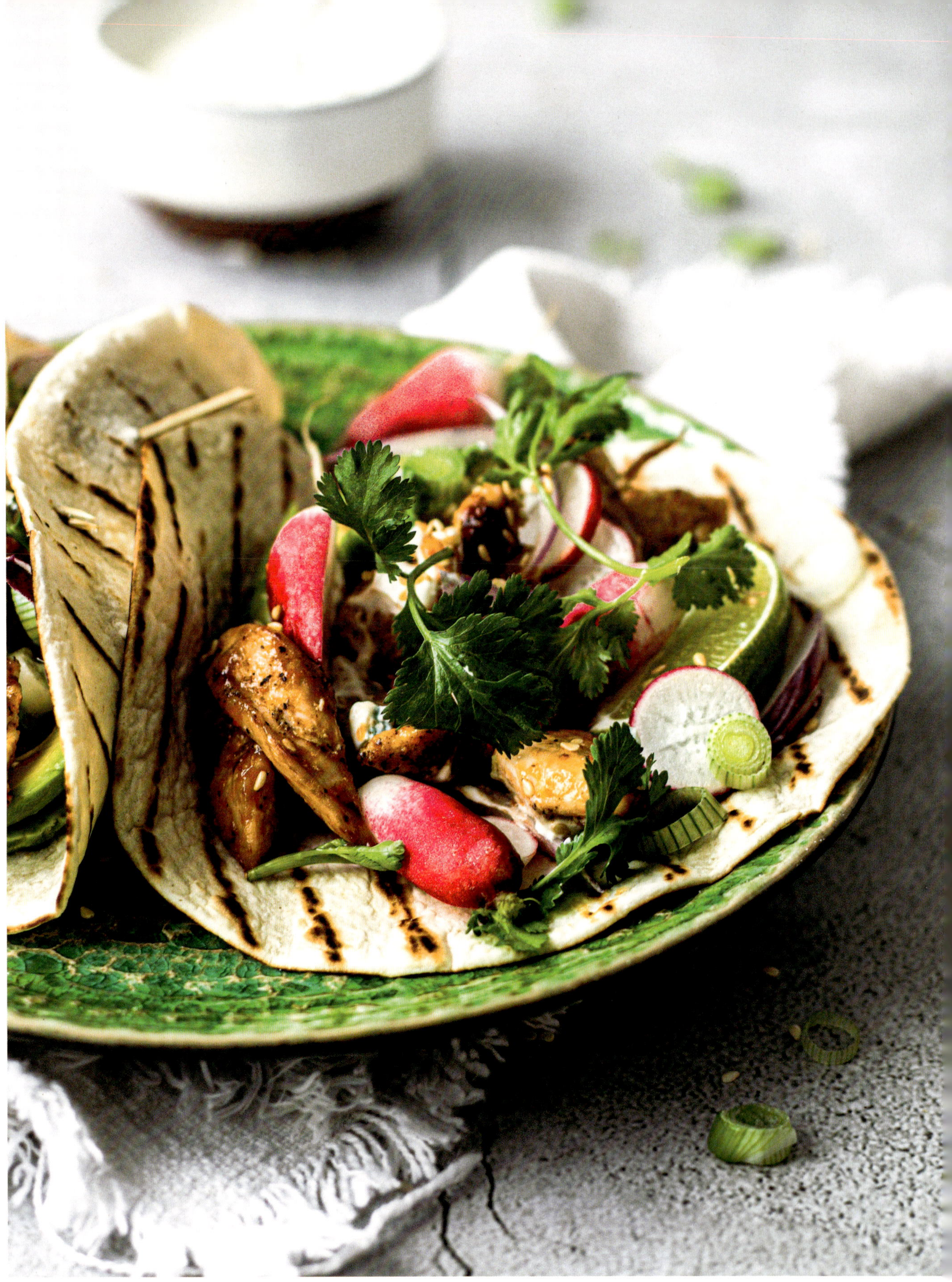

CHICKEN TACOS

CHICKEN

2 cloves garlic, minced

1 tsp chilli powder

½ tsp ground cumin

½ tsp paprika

1 tsp sesame seeds

½ tsp salt

¼ tsp pepper

2 tbsps olive oil

450g boneless, skinless chicken breasts

TACOS

8 small corn tortillas

½ cup (120g) store-bought mayonnaise

4-6 radishes, sliced and quartered

½ avocado, diced

½ cup (75g) sliced onion

½ cup (20g) chopped fresh coriander

Green onions, sliced (optional)

Lime wedges to serve

STEPS

1. In a bowl, combine the garlic, chilli powder, cumin, paprika, sesame seeds, salt, pepper and olive oil to make a marinade. Add the chicken to the mixture and toss until the chicken is well coated. Let it marinate for at least 30 minutes.

2. Heat a frying pan over medium-high heat. Cook the chicken for about 6-8 minutes per side, or until cooked through. Cooking time may vary depending on the thickness of the chicken. Remove the chicken from the pan and let it rest for a few minutes before slicing into 1-2cm pieces.

3. For the corn tortillas heat a grill pan or dry frying pan and warm each one individually until slightly browned and set aside until serving.

4. To assemble the tacos dollop some mayonnaise on a tortilla and place a few slices of grilled chicken on top. Then layer with radishes, diced avocado, onion and fresh coriander and green onions. Serve with lime wedges.

SERVES 4 | PREP + COOK TIME: 30 MINS + MARINATING | GLUTEN FREE | DAIRY FREE |

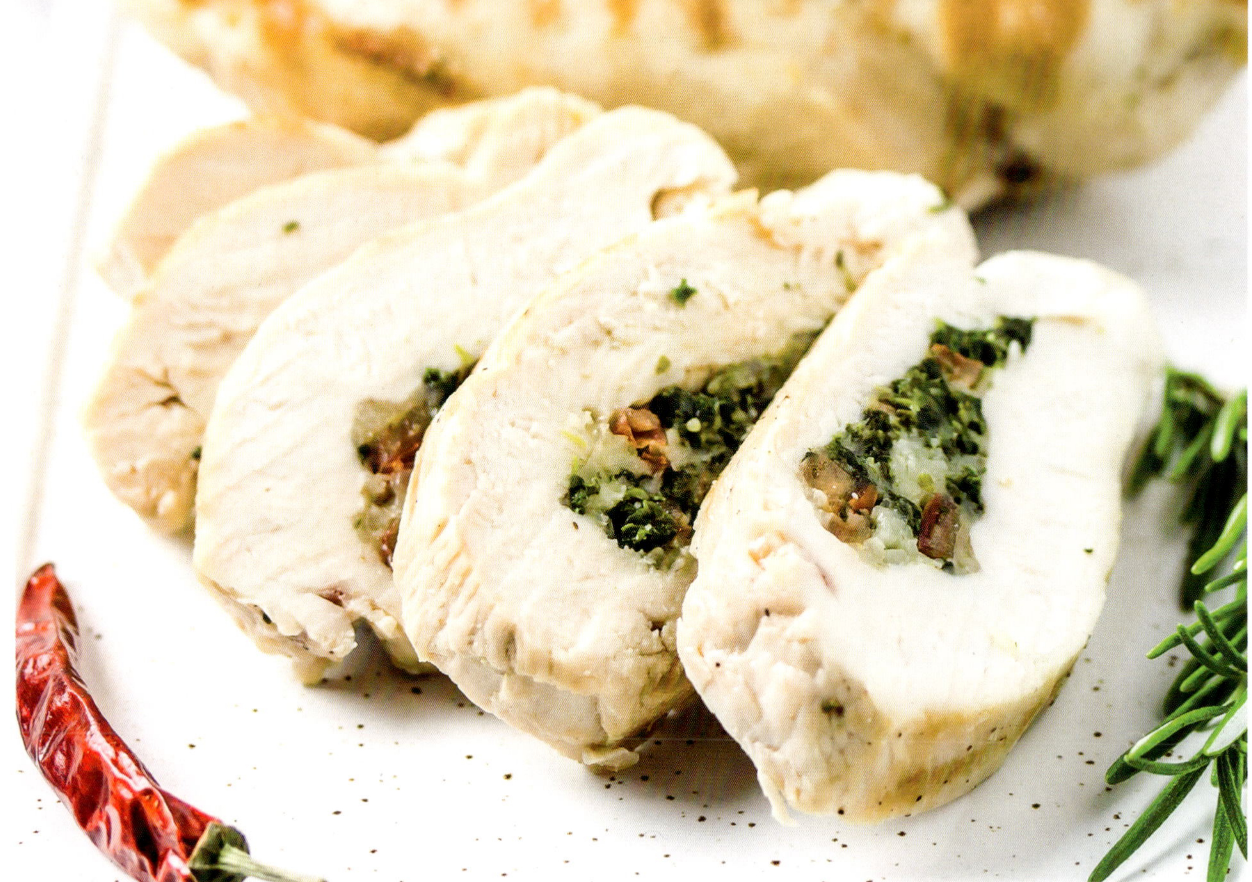

STUFFED CHICKEN BREAST

4 large, skinless chicken breasts

300g frozen chopped spinach, thawed and drained well

4 slices of prosciutto, finely diced

½ cup (125g) ricotta cheese

¼ cup (25g) finely grated Parmesan cheese

Salt and pepper to taste

½ cup (125ml) dry white wine

2 tbsps olive oil

STEPS

Preheat oven to 180°C.

1. Place backing paper down on a chopping board and arrange chicken pieces in a single layer. Pound each chicken breast down to 2cm thick and set aside.
2. In a medium-sized bowl, combine spinach, prosciutto, ricotta, Parmesan, salt, and pepper.
3. Divide spinach mixture between each of the four chicken breasts and roll up each breast, then place seam down in a small, shallow baking dish.
4. Pour wine over chicken then season with salt and pepper and drizzle with olive oil. Cover and bake for 35-45 min. Remove chicken from pan and let rest for 10 minutes. Slice the chicken and serve with salad greens.

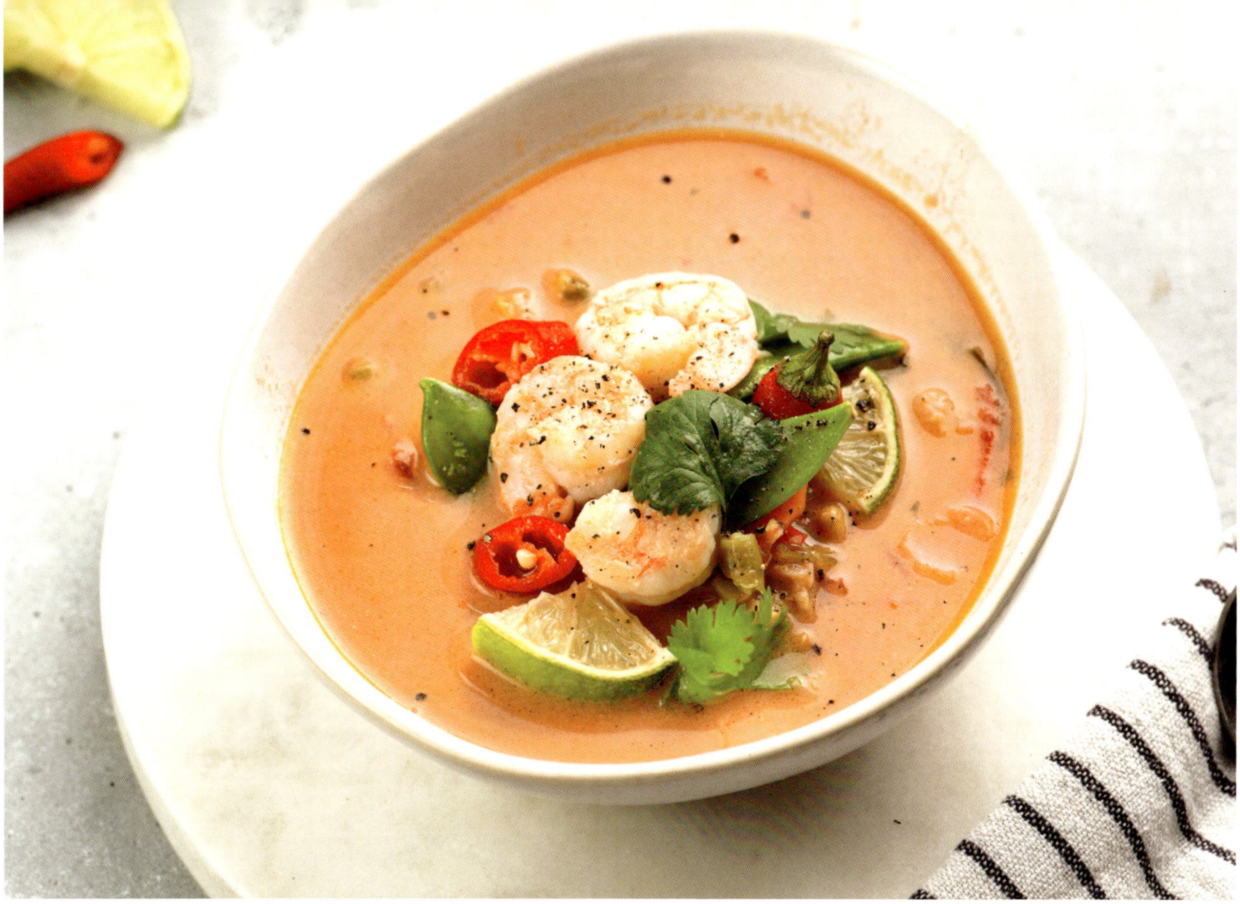

SERVES 4 | PREP + COOK TIME: 30 MINS | GLUTEN FREE | DAIRY FREE |

COCONUT PRAWN CURRY SOUP

1 tbsp vegetable oil
1 onion, finely chopped
2 cloves garlic, crushed
1 tbsp grated ginger
1 tbsp red curry paste
1 x 400ml can coconut milk
2 cups (500ml) vegetable stock
500g prawns, peeled and deveined
1 cup (40g) snow peas, trimmed
1 tbsp fish sauce (optional)
Juice of 1 lime
Salt and pepper to taste
Fresh coriander leaves, chopped, to garnish

STEPS

1. Heat vegetable oil in a large pot or saucepan over medium heat. Add the chopped onion and saute until it becomes translucent then add the garlic and grated ginger. Cook for another minute until fragrant.
2. Stir in the red curry paste and cook for 1-2 minutes, stirring constantly.
3. Add the coconut milk and stock to the saucepan and stir well to combine.
4. Bring the broth to a simmer and let it cook for 5 minutes to allow the flavours to develop.
5. Add the prawns and snow peas to the pan and simmer for about 5-7 minutes, or until the prawns are cooked through. Stir in the fish sauce (if using) and lime juice. Season with salt and pepper to taste and garnish with coriander.

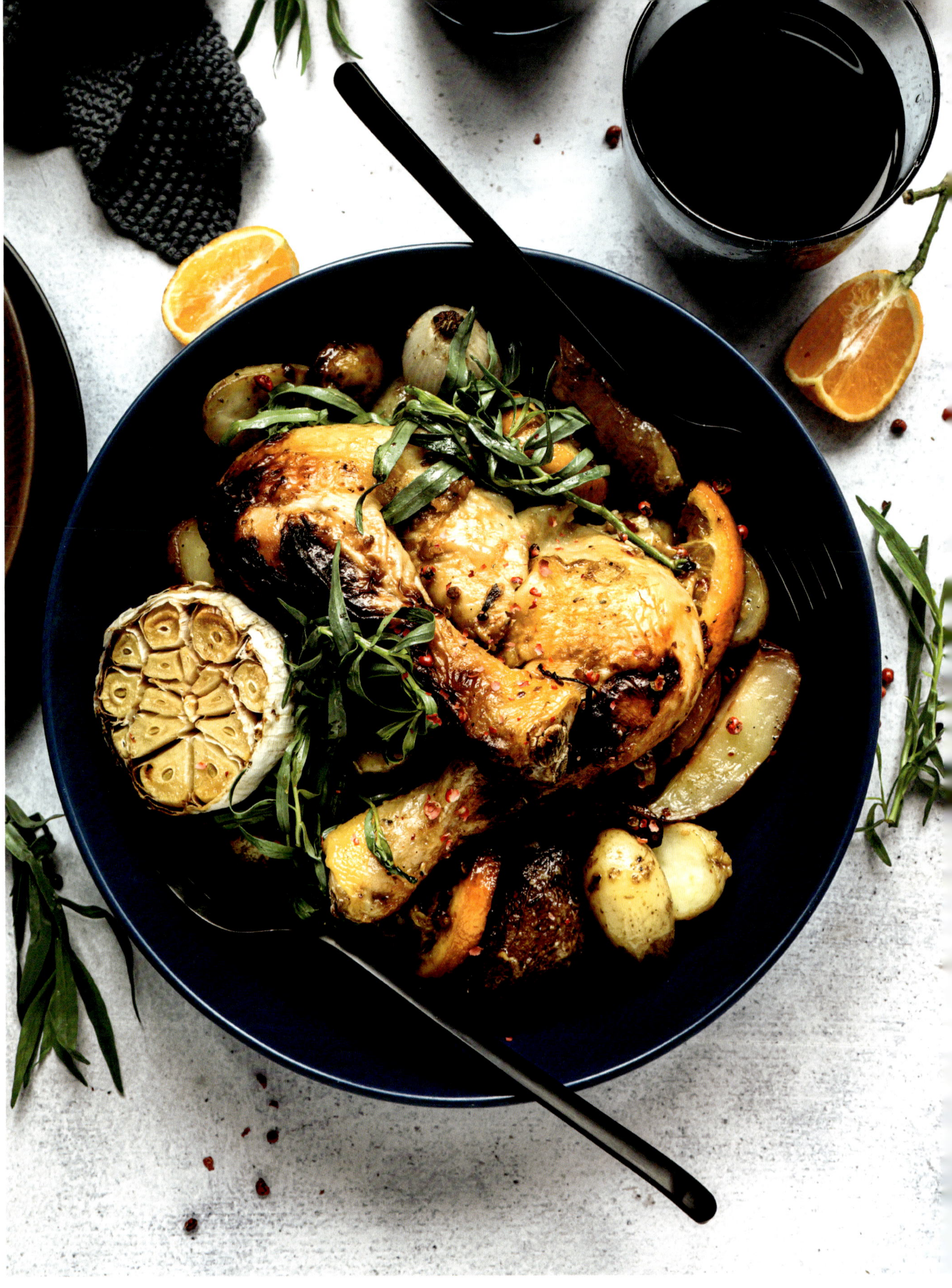

CHILLI GARLIC ROAST CHICKEN

3 cloves garlic, crushed
¼ cup (60ml) lemon juice
¼ cup (60ml) olive oil
1 tsp dried chilli flakes
2 tbsps finely chopped rosemary
2 tbsps finely chopped oregano
2 tsps salt + more to taste
1 tsp pepper + more to taste
1 small brown onion, cut into wedges
300g baby potatoes, halved (see note)
1 head garlic, cut in half crossways
½ orange, sliced
4 chicken Marylands, skin on

STEPS

Preheat the oven to 200°C.

1. In a large bowl whisk together crushed garlic, lemon juice, olive oil, chilli flakes, half the rosemary, half the oregano and the salt and pepper. Then add in onion, potatoes, the head of garlic and sliced orange; toss to combine.
2. Add the chicken to the bowl with the vegetables and toss everything together until chicken is well coated.
3. Arrange the chicken pieces and all the vegetables in a large baking dish. Then place in the oven and bake for 35-40 minutes.
4. Serve each Maryland with an equal portion of baked vegetables.

NOTE: Omit the potatoes if following a strict low-carb diet.

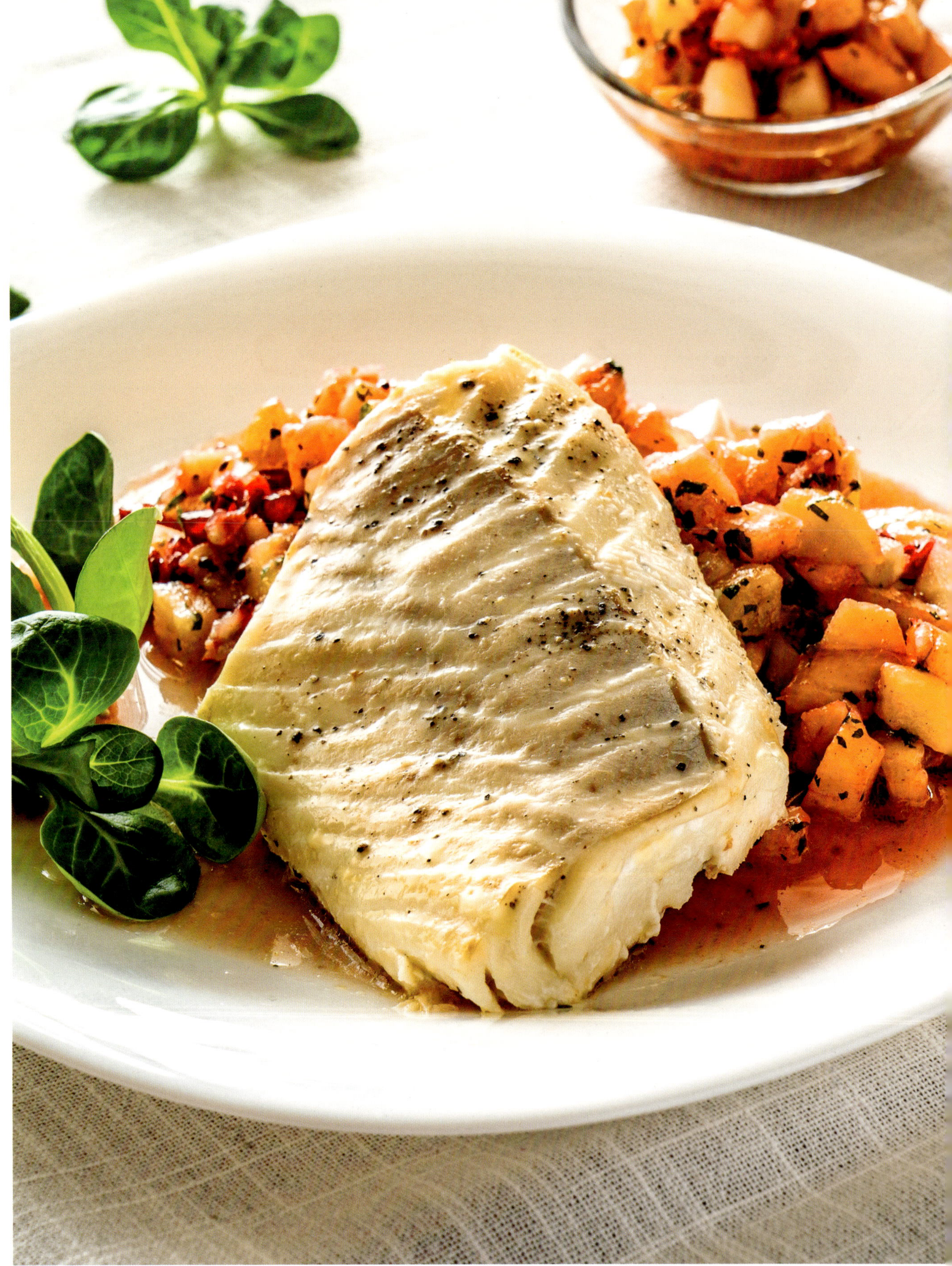

GRILLED FISH WITH PINEAPPLE SALSA

FISH

2 tbsps olive oil

½ tsp garlic powder

½ tsp salt

¼ tsp pepper

4 firm white fish fillets (such as snapper)

Lemon wedges to serve

SALSA

1 cup (200g) diced pineapple

1 yellow capsicum, diced

½ small red onion, diced

1 jalapeno pepper, deseeded and chopped

2 tbsps finely chopped coriander

1 tbsp lime juice

Salt and pepper to taste

STEPS

Preheat the grill to medium-high heat.

1. In a small bowl, combine the olive oil, garlic powder, salt and pepper to make a marinade. Brush both sides of the fish fillets with the marinade.
2. Place the fish fillets on a lined oven tray and cook for about 4-5 minutes per side, or until the fish is opaque and flakes easily with a fork. Cooking time may vary depending on the thickness of the fillets.
3. While the fish is grilling, prepare the pineapple salsa. In a medium bowl, combine the diced pineapple, diced capsicum, red onion, jalapeno, chopped coriander, lime juice, salt and pepper and stir well to combine.
4. Remove the fish from the grill and let it rest for a couple of minutes.
5. To serve, divide salsa evenly among four plates and place the grilled fish on top.

SERVES 4 | PREP + COOK TIME: 30 MINS | GLUTEN FREE | DAIRY FREE |

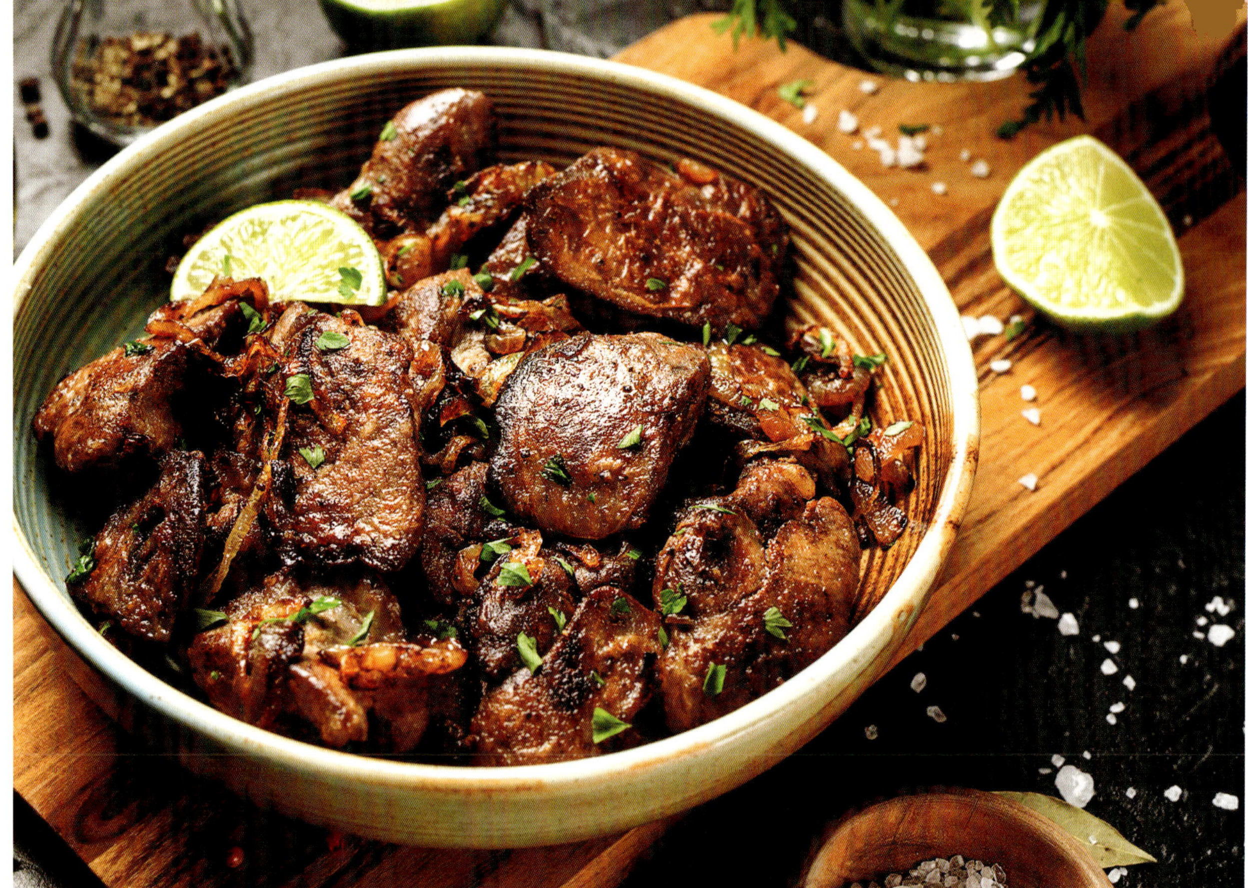

FRIED CHICKEN LIVER WITH ONIONS

2 tbsps ghee

2 medium onions, quartered and sliced

2 small cloves garlic, crushed

1 tsp smoked paprika

1 tbsp apple cider vinegar

600g chicken livers, trimmed and cleaned

¼ cup (10g) parsley, roughly chopped + parsley leaves to garnish

1 lime, quartered, to serve

Salt and pepper to taste

STEPS

1. Heat the ghee in a medium frying pan over low heat. Fry the onion and garlic for 15 minutes until the onion has softened. Add the paprika and vinegar and cook for another 2 minutes.

2. Increase the heat to medium-high and add the livers. Fry for 5 minutes, turning halfway, until slightly browned. Add the parsley and cook for 1 more minute.

3. Season to taste. Garnish with fresh parsley leaves and serve hot with lime wedges.

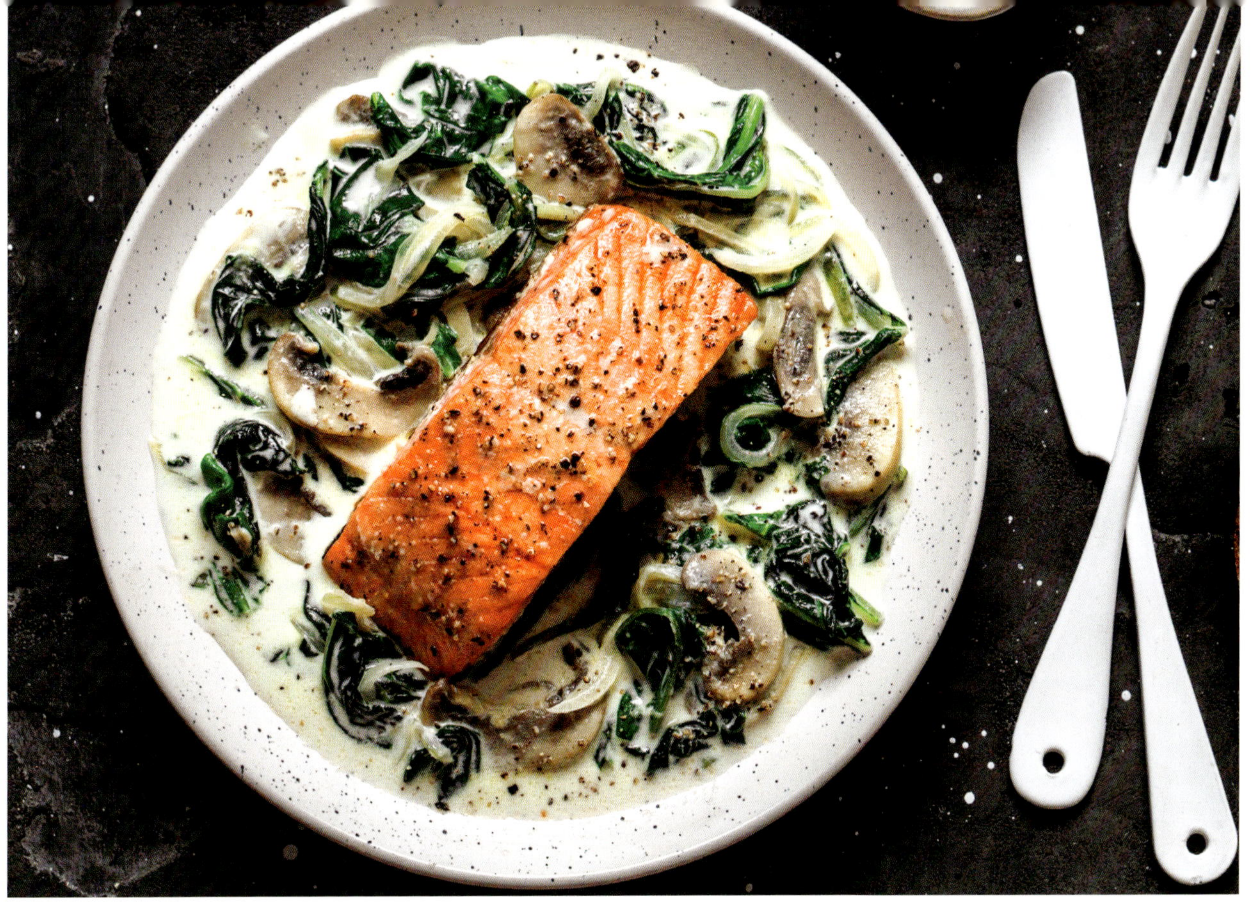

SERVES 4 | PREP + COOK TIME: 25 MINS | GLUTEN FREE |

SALMON WITH CREAMY SAUCE

4 salmon fillets, patted dry

Salt and pepper to taste

2 tbsps olive oil

3 cloves garlic, crushed

1 cup (75g) sliced mushrooms

¼ cup (60ml) vegetable or chicken stock

1 cup (250ml) cream

1 cup (30g) baby spinach, roughly chopped

STEPS

1. Season salmon with salt and pepper then heat half the oil in a large nonstick pan over medium heat. Add salmon and cook for 4-5 minutes or until golden. Gently flip the fillets onto the other side and continue to cook for 4-6 minutes, or until cooked through and skin is crispy. Remove salmon from the pan and set aside.
2. Heat remaining oil in the same pan over medium-high heat then add garlic and cook until fragrant. Add the mushrooms and cook until slightly browned. Add stock and cream and season with salt and pepper.
3. Reduce the heat to low and simmer until sauce is thickened, then stir in spinach and cook until wilted, about 1-2 minutes.
4. Return the salmon to the pan, and spoon the creamy spinach and mushrooms on top.

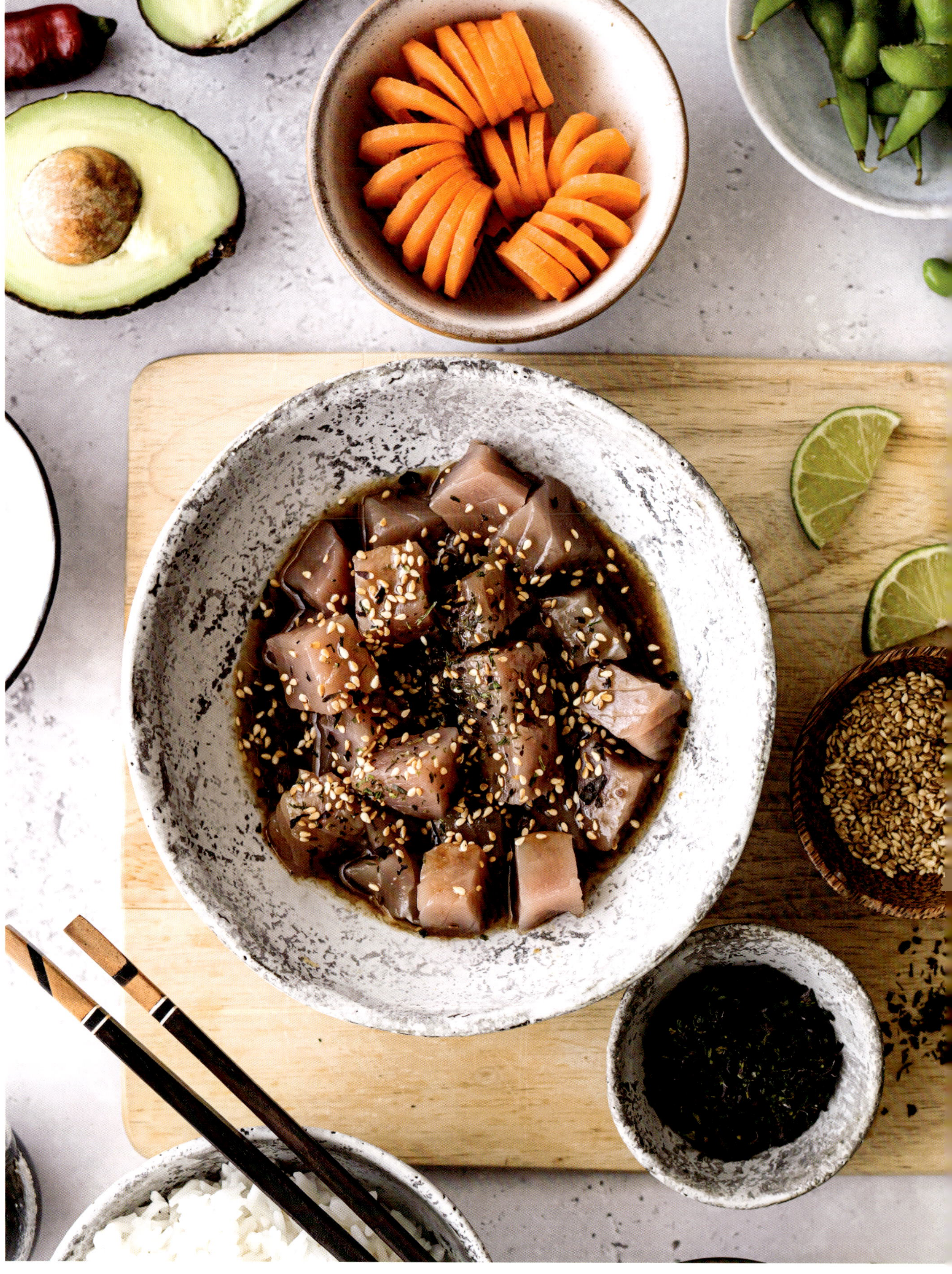

JAPANESE MARINATED TUNA

SERVES 4 | PREP + COOK TIME: 15 MINS | DAIRY FREE |

200g sashimi-grade tuna (see note)

2 tbsps soy sauce

1 tbsp sesame oil

1 tbsp sesame seeds

TO SERVE

Toasted sesame seeds

Seaweed flakes

STEPS

1. Rinse the tuna and pat dry with a paper towel to remove excess moisture. Cut the raw tuna into bite-sized cubes.
2. In a small bowl, whisk together soy sauce, sesame oil, and half of the sesame seeds.
3. Combine the tuna cubes and the sesame oil mixture and mix until each piece of the tuna is nicely coated. You can then put it in the fridge for at least 10-20 minutes to let the flavours meld, but it's not required.
4. Garnish with toasted sesame seeds and seaweed flakes.

NOTE: Check your local supermarket for vacuum-packed sashimi-grade fish, or ask your fishmonger.

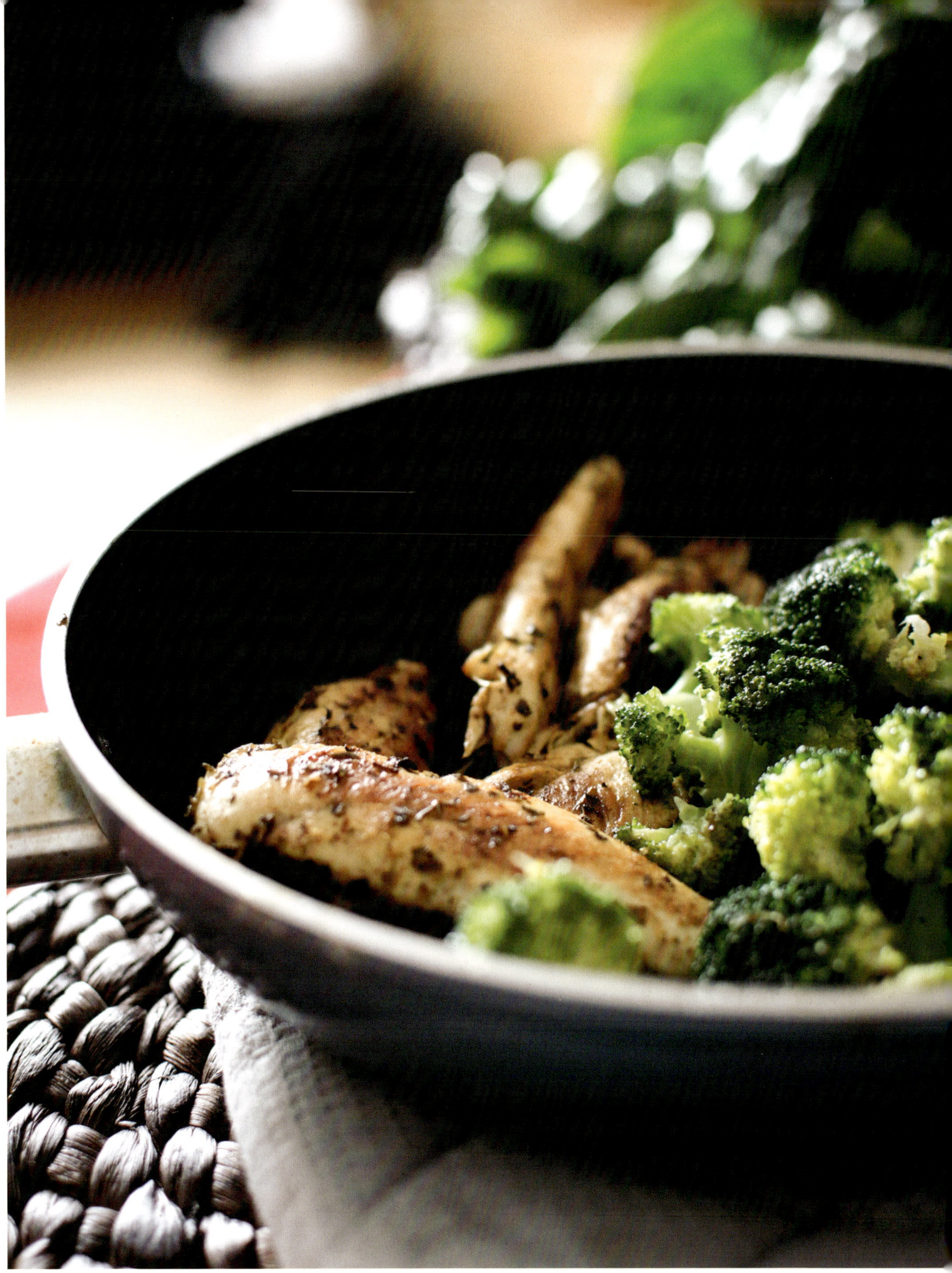

HERBY CHICKEN WITH BROCCOLI

CHICKEN

2 cloves garlic, crushed

1 tsp dried thyme

1 tsp dried rosemary

½ tsp dried oregano

Salt and pepper to taste

2 tbsps olive oil

500g chicken tenderloins

ROASTED BROCCOLI

4 cups (300g) broccoli florets

2 cloves garlic, crushed

2 tbsps olive oil

Salt and pepper to taste

Lemon wedges to serve

STEPS

Preheat the oven to 200°C.

1. In a small bowl, combine the garlic, dried thyme, dried rosemary, dried oregano, salt, pepper and olive oil to make a herb marinade.
2. Place the chicken in a baking dish and rub the herb marinade all over the chicken, making sure it's evenly coated. Bake the chicken in the preheated oven for about 20-25 minutes, or until cooked through. Remove the chicken from the oven and cover to keep warm.
3. Meanwhile, in a large bowl, combine the broccoli florets, garlic, olive oil, salt and pepper. Toss until the broccoli is evenly coated.
4. Spread the seasoned broccoli florets on a baking tray in a single layer. Bake in the oven for 15-20 minutes or until tender.
5. Serve the herby chicken alongside the roasted broccoli. Squeeze over fresh lemon juice.

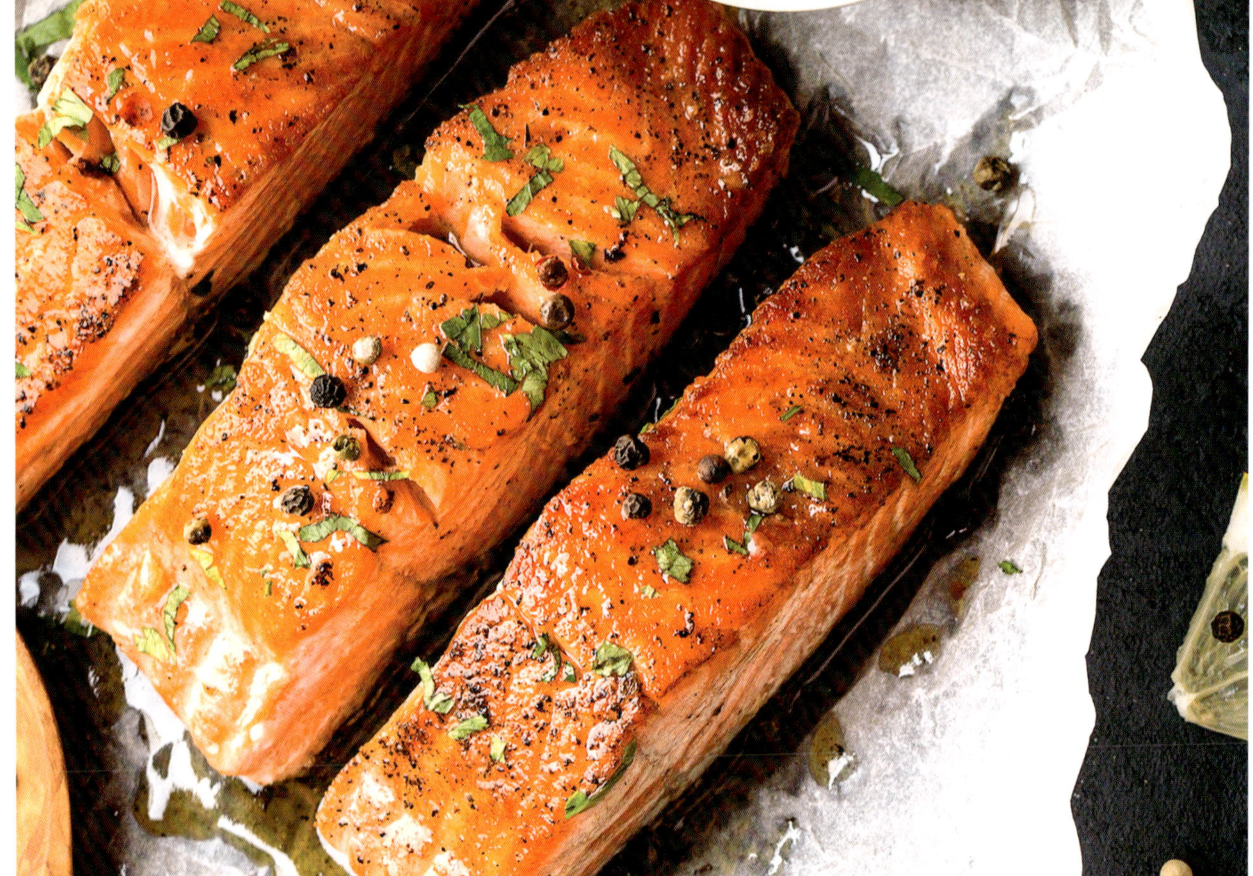

SWEET BAKED SALMON

4 skinless salmon fillets

3 tbsps fresh lemon juice

2 tbsps low-sugar or sugar-free honey substitute (e.g. stevia or erythritol-based honey substitute)

2 tbsps olive oil

2 cloves garlic, minced

½ tsp salt + more to serve

½ tsp pepper + more to serve

Parsley, finely chopped, to garnish

STEPS

Preheat oven to 200°C.

1. In a small bowl add lemon juice, honey substitute, olive oil, garlic and salt and pepper. Whisk well to combine.
2. Place the fillets in a casserole dish and drizzle the lemon mixture over the top.
3. Bake for 20 minutes until the salmon is cooked through.
4. Let the fillets sit for 5 minutes before serving. Garnish with fresh parsley and extra salt and pepper.

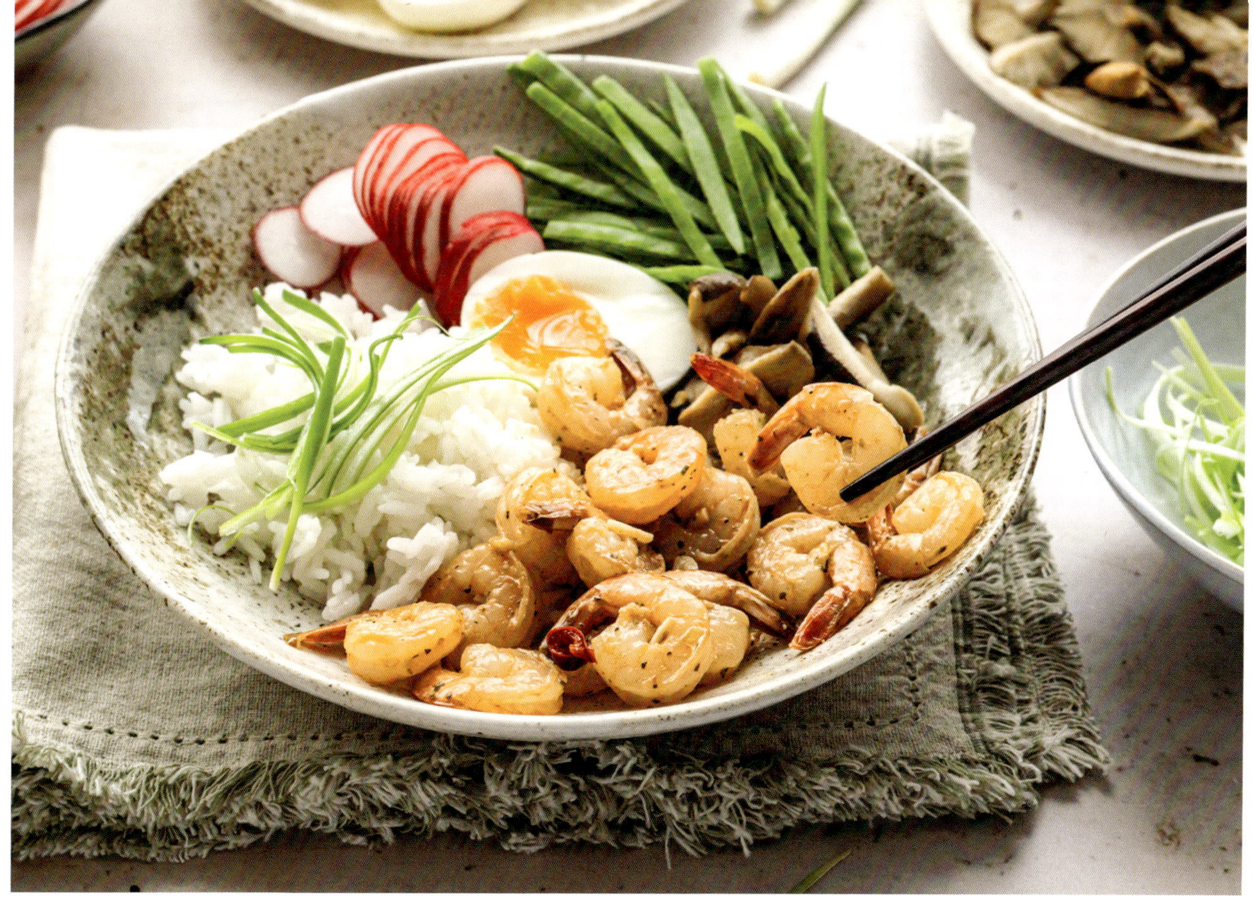

GARLIC PRAWNS & COCONUT RICE

2 cups (310g) rice (see note)
1 x 400ml can coconut milk
1½ cups (375ml) water
1 tsp salt
¼ cup (60ml) olive oil
4 tbsps butter
6 cloves garlic, finely chopped
Small piece ginger, grated
500g prawns, peeled and deveined
Salt and pepper to taste

TO SERVE

1 cup (100g) snow peas, julienned
2-4 radishes, finely sliced
2 spring onions, julienned
Boiled eggs (optional)

STEPS

1. Place the rice, coconut milk, water and salt in a medium saucepan. Stir, then cover and cook on medium heat until boiling. Turn down heat as low as possible. Cook for 20 minutes, allowing rice to absorb the liquid. Turn heat off and leave, covered, for a further 10 minutes.

2. Heat the oil and butter in a frying pan until butter is just melted. Reduce heat to low. Add chopped garlic and ginger and saute until fragrant. Then add prawns and salt and pepper. Cook for 1 minute. Turn and cook for another minute or until prawns turn a deeper pink colour and are cooked through.

3. Fluff up the coconut rice and divide among bowls. Spoon prawns on top then layer the vegetables and eggs and garnish with spring onions.

NOTE: Replace rice with cauliflower rice if following a strict low-carb diet.

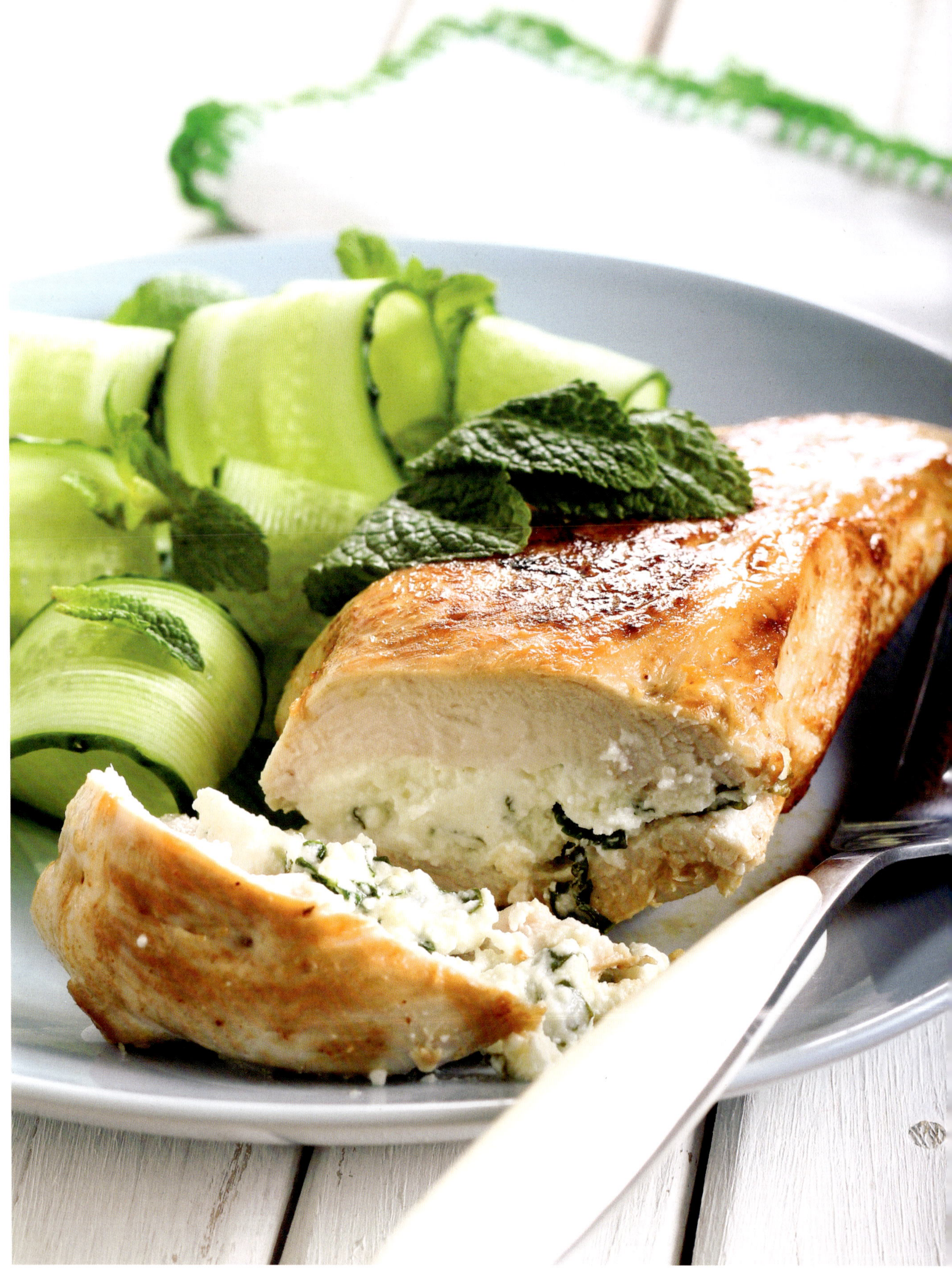

CHICKEN BREASTS STUFFED WITH FETA & MINT

SERVES 4 | PREP + COOK TIME: 35 MINS | GLUTEN FREE |

4 boneless, skinless chicken breasts

Salt and pepper to taste

½ cup (120g) crumbled feta cheese

2 tbsps finely chopped fresh mint leaves + mint leaves for garnish

2 cloves garlic, crushed

1 tbsp olive oil

1 cucumber, cut into ribbons, to serve

STEPS

Preheat oven to 200°C.

1. Season the chicken breasts on both sides with salt and pepper. Use a sharp knife to cut through the middle of each chicken breast but not all the way through.
2. In a small bowl, add crumbled feta, mint, garlic and salt and pepper, and mash the ingredients together.
3. Gently stuff each piece of chicken with the feta mix, then place the chicken breasts in a greased baking dish. Pour over olive oil and bake for 20-25 minutes or until chicken is cooked through and browned nicely.
4. Serve with cucumber ribbons and fresh mint.

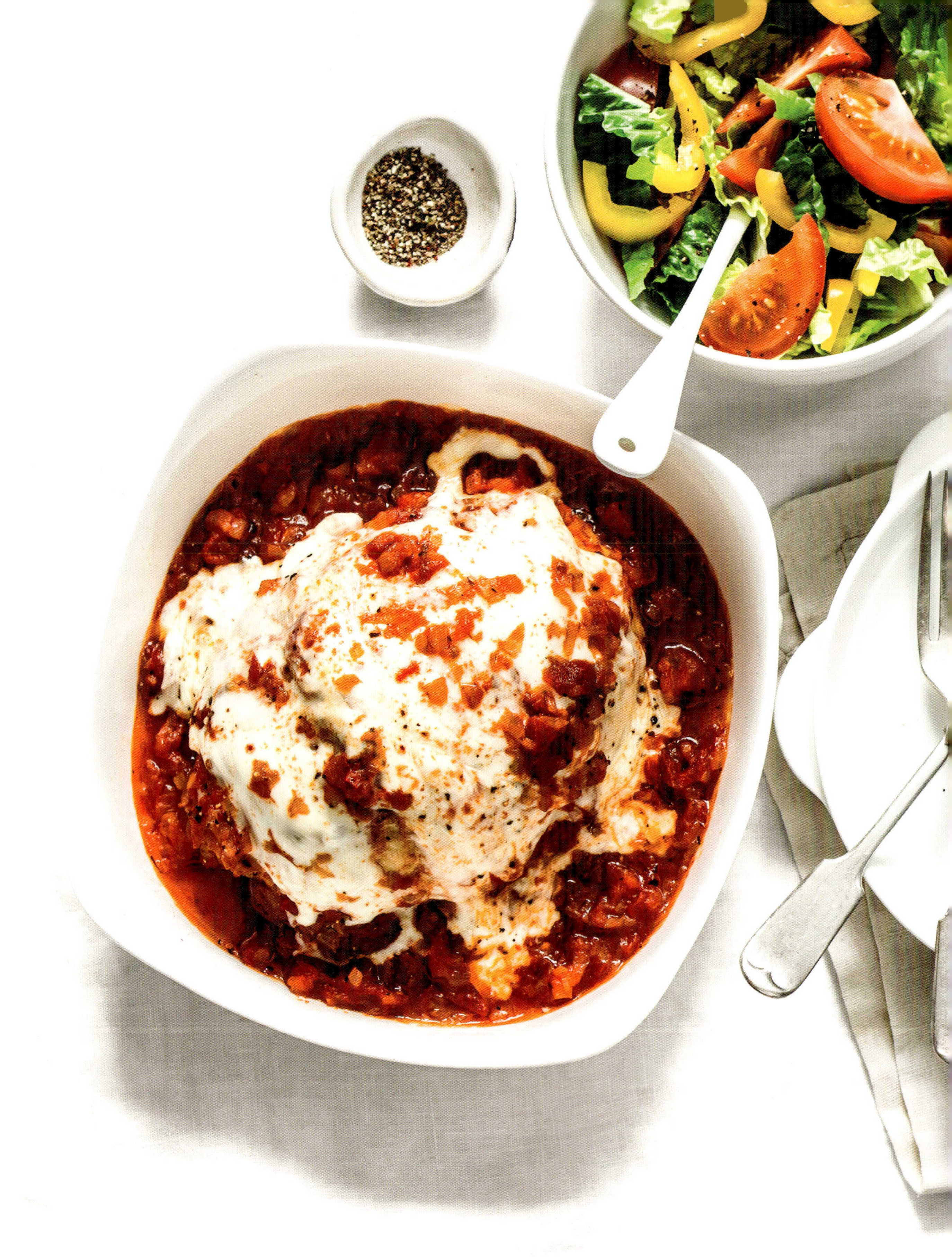

CHICKEN MEATLOAF IN TOMATO SAUCE

MEATLOAF

1kg chicken mince

1 small onion, finely chopped

2 cloves garlic, crushed

1 stalk celery, finely chopped

1 carrot, grated

1 cup (125g) breadcrumbs (you can use almond flour for a lower-carb option)

¼ cup (60ml) milk

¼ cup (25g) grated Parmesan cheese

2 tbsps chopped fresh parsley

1 tsp dried basil

1 tsp dried oregano

Salt and pepper to taste

1 egg, lightly beaten

TOMATO SAUCE

1 tsp olive oil

1 small onion, finely chopped

2 cloves garlic, crushed

¼ cup (60g) tomato paste

½ tsp sugar or sugar substitute (optional)

2 x 400g cans crushed tomatoes

Salt and pepper to taste

WHITE SAUCE

2 tbsps unsalted butter

2 tbsps plain flour

2 cups (500ml) milk

Salt and pepper to taste

STEPS

Preheat oven to 200°C.

1. In a large bowl, combine the chicken mince, onion, garlic, celery, carrot, breadcrumbs, milk, grated Parmesan cheese, parsley, basil, oregano, salt, pepper and the beaten egg. Mix well until all the ingredients are evenly combined.

2. Transfer chicken mixture to a greased loaf tin, shaping it into a loaf shape. Bake in the oven for 50-60 minutes or until loaf is cooked through. Set aside to rest after cooking.

3. To make the tomato sauce, heat olive oil in a saucepan over a medium heat. Add onion and garlic and saute until fragrant, then add tomato paste, sugar and crushed tomatoes, mixing well to combine. Simmer for 5-10 minutes to allow the flavours to develop. Season to taste and take off the heat and set aside.

4. In a separate saucepan, melt the butter over medium heat. Once butter has melted, add flour and whisk continuously for about 1-2 minutes, creating a smooth roux. Gradually pour in the milk while whisking constantly. Continue whisking the mixture until it thickens and comes to a gentle simmer. This usually takes about 5-7 minutes. Take off the heat add salt and pepper and set aside for serving.

5. To assemble, spoon half the tomato sauce into a large ceramic dish then remove the chicken loaf from the tin and place on top. Spoon the rest of the tomato sauce over the chicken loaf and then ladle the white sauce on top, making sure the loaf is well covered. Serve immediately.

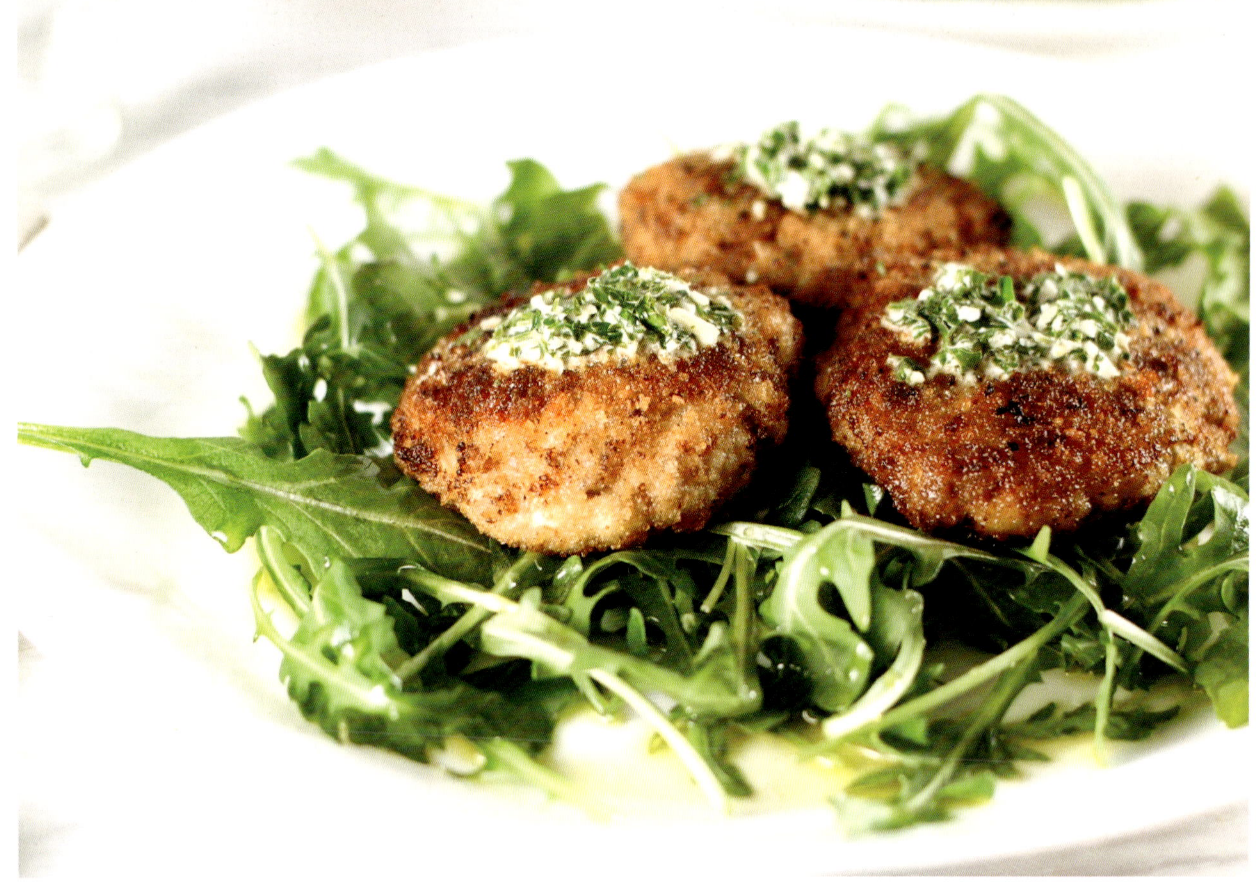

CHICKEN BUCKWHEAT PATTIES

1 cup (175g) cooked buckwheat

500g chicken mince

½ cup (60g) breadcrumbs (you can use almond flour for a lower-carb option)

½ small onion, finely chopped

2 cloves garlic, minced

1 egg

¼ cup (10g) chopped fresh parsley

1 tsp dried thyme

1 tsp paprika

½ tsp salt

¼ tsp pepper

2 tbsps olive oil

Rocket leaves to serve

STEPS

Preheat oven to 180°C.

1. In a large mixing bowl, combine the cooked buckwheat, chicken mince, breadcrumbs, onion, minced garlic, egg, chopped parsley, dried thyme, paprika, salt and pepper. Mix well until all the ingredients are evenly incorporated.
2. Take a handful of the mixture and shape it into a patty using your hands. Repeat with the remaining mixture to make all the patties.
3. Heat olive oil in a medium-sized frying pan and cook patties until they are cooked through and golden brown.
4. Once cooked, transfer the patties to a plate lined with paper towel to absorb any excess oil.
5. Serve immediately on a bed of rocket.

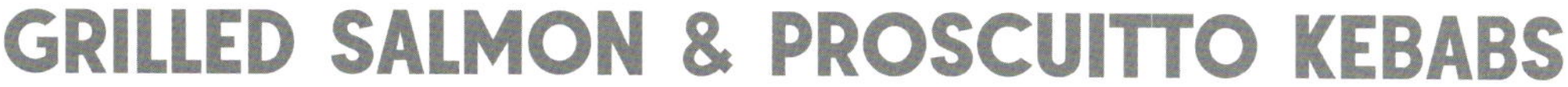

GRILLED SALMON & PROSCUITTO KEBABS

SERVES 4 | PREP + COOK TIME: 20 MINS | GLUTEN FREE | DAIRY FREE |

2 tbsps Dijon mustard
2-3 limes, cut into wedges, one half juiced
¼ tsp chilli flakes (or more to taste)
¼ tsp minced garlic
¼ tsp ground cumin
Splash of apple cider vinegar
750g salmon fillets, cut into 2cm cubes
8-10 slices of prosciutto, cut into strips
Olive oil for brushing
½ tbsp black sesame seeds, crushed
½ tbsp white sesame seeds, crushed
Fresh parsley leaves to garnish

STEPS

Heat grill to medium.

1. Whisk together mustard, lime juice, chilli flakes, garlic, cumin and vinegar in a small bowl and set aside.
2. Thread 12 metal or soaked wooden skewers, starting with a salmon cube, followed by a folded slice of prosciutto and then a lime wedge. Continue until the skewer is full, beginning and ending with salmon.
3. Brush with olive oil then liberally coat with spice mixture. Sprinkle with crushed black and white sesame seeds.
4. Grill, turning from time to time, until fish is opaque (about 5 minutes). Garnish with fresh parsley leaves.

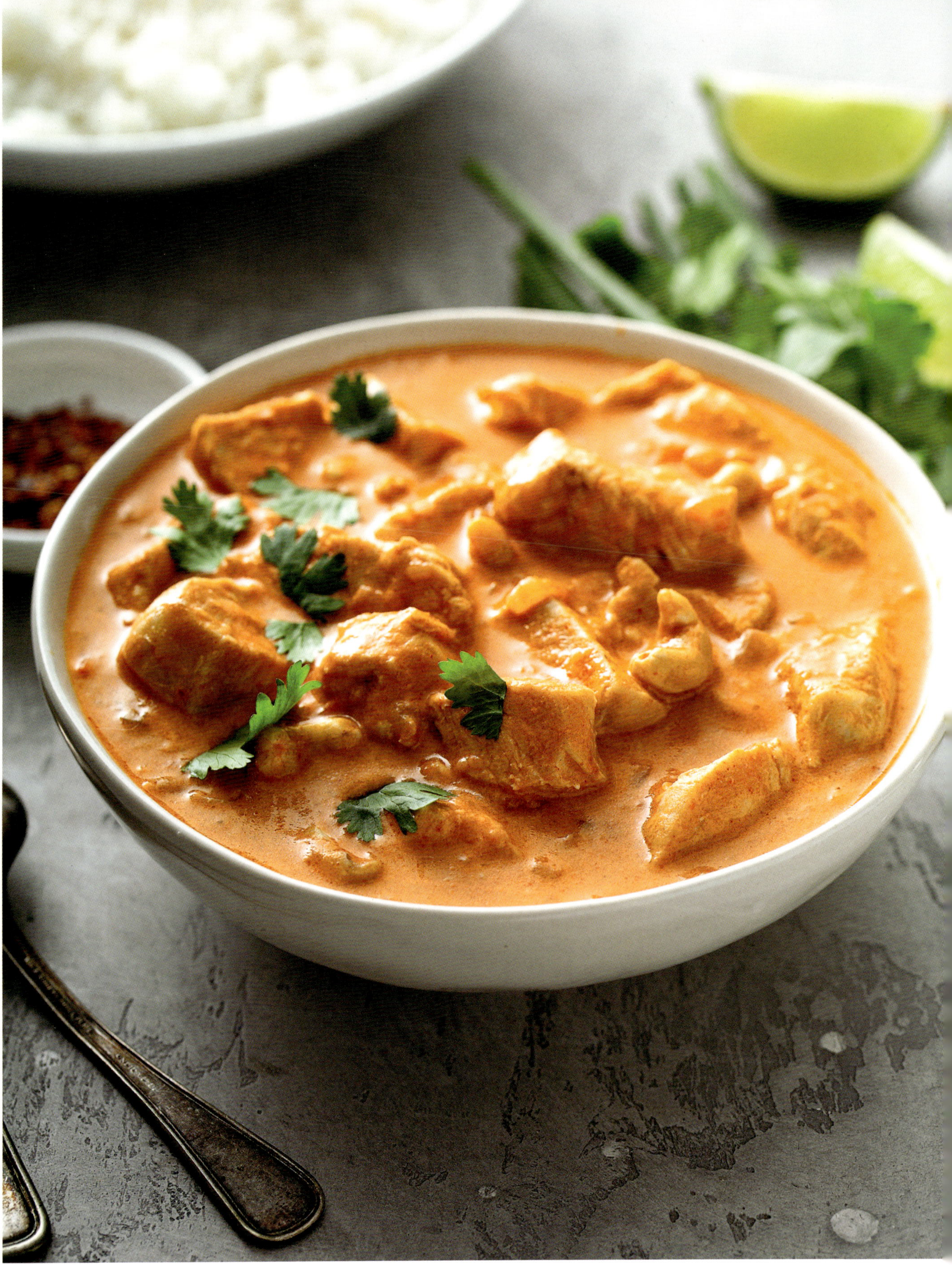

CHICKEN & CASHEW RED CURRY

1 tbsp coconut oil

2 tbsps Thai red curry paste

700g chicken breast or thigh fillets, diced

1 x 400ml can coconut cream

Juice of 2 limes

¼ cup (10g) fresh coriander leaves, roughly chopped

1 cup (125g) cashews

STEPS

1. Heat oil in a medium pan over medium heat. Add the curry paste and cook, stirring, for 1 minute until fragrant. Add the chicken and cook for 5 minutes, stirring regularly, until browned.
2. Pour in the coconut cream. Bring to a simmer, then simmer for 10 minutes, until the chicken is cooked through. Stir in the lime juice and half of the coriander. Remove from the heat.
3. Heat a dry frying pan over medium-low heat. Fry the cashews for 3-4 minutes until lightly golden.
4. Add the cashews to the curry and stir to combine.
5. Scatter with remaining coriander and serve immediately.

NOTE: Serve with cauliflower rice or zucchini noodles.

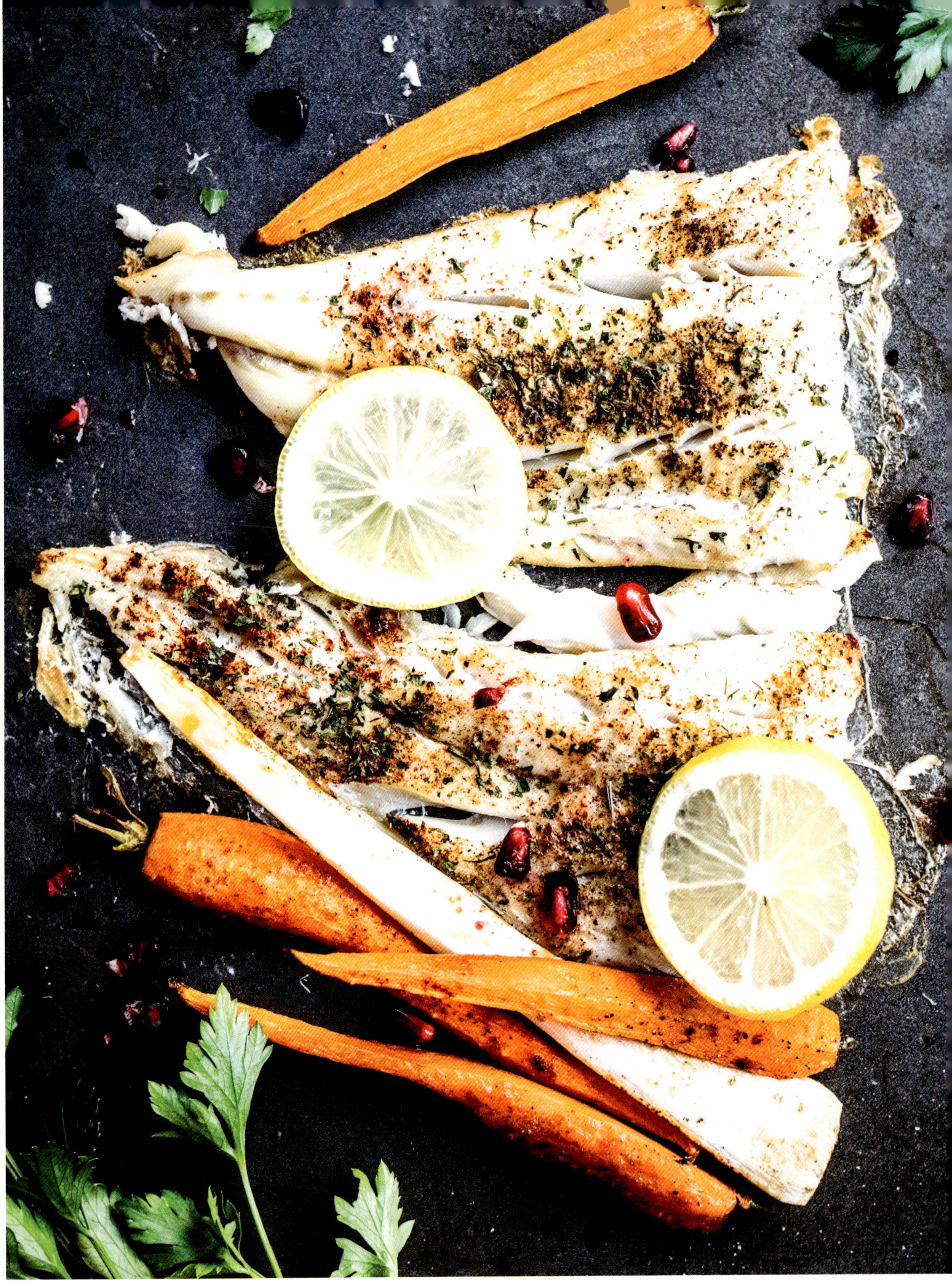

CAJUN-SPICED GRILLED FISH

½ tsps Cajun seasoning

1 tsp finely chopped parsley

Salt and pepper to taste

2 x 175g boneless firm white fish fillets

1 tsp olive oil

1 tsp lemon juice + lemon slices to serve

STEPS

1. Sprinkle Cajun seasoning, parsley and salt and pepper over both sides of the fish. Gently rub onto surface with fingertips.
2. Heat a large nonstick frying pan over medium-low heat, add olive oil and heat gently. Place fish fillets into the pan and cook for 3-4 minutes each side or until just cooked through.
3. While the fish is still in the pan pour over lemon juice. Remove fish from pan and let rest for a minute or two before serving.
4. Serve with lemon slices.

SERVES 2 | PREP + COOK TIME: 20 MINS | GLUTEN FREE | DAIRY FREE |

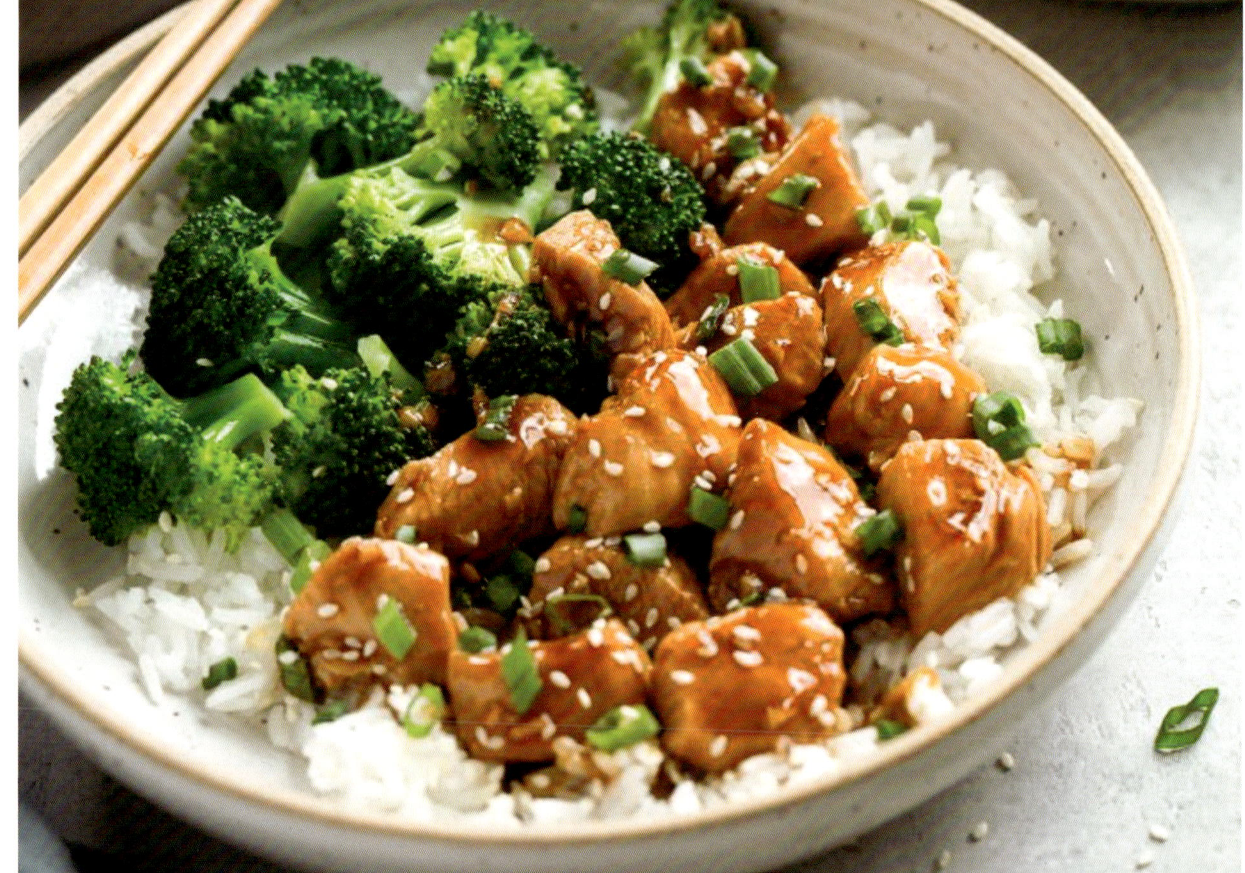

TERIYAKI CHICKEN & BROCCOLI

3 cups (225g) broccoli florets

1 tbsp oil

3 cloves garlic, crushed

2 spring onions, cut into 1cm slices

600g chicken thigh fillets, cut into bite-sized chunks

1 large red chilli, deseeded, finely chopped

⅓ cup (90ml) tamari

½ tsp stevia

1 tbsp apple cider vinegar

Salt and pepper to taste

2½ tbsps sesame seeds

STEPS

1. Boil the broccoli in a pot of salted water for 2 minutes, then rinse in cold water. Set aside.
2. Heat the oil in a large wok over medium heat. Fry the garlic and half the spring onions for 1 minute.
3. Increase the heat to high and add the chicken and stir-fry for 6 minutes until browned. Mix through the chilli, tamari, stevia, vinegar and a couple of grinds of salt and pepper for 2 minutes.
4. Spoon chicken evenly among bowls. Serve with the broccoli and garnish with sesame seeds and sliced spring onions.

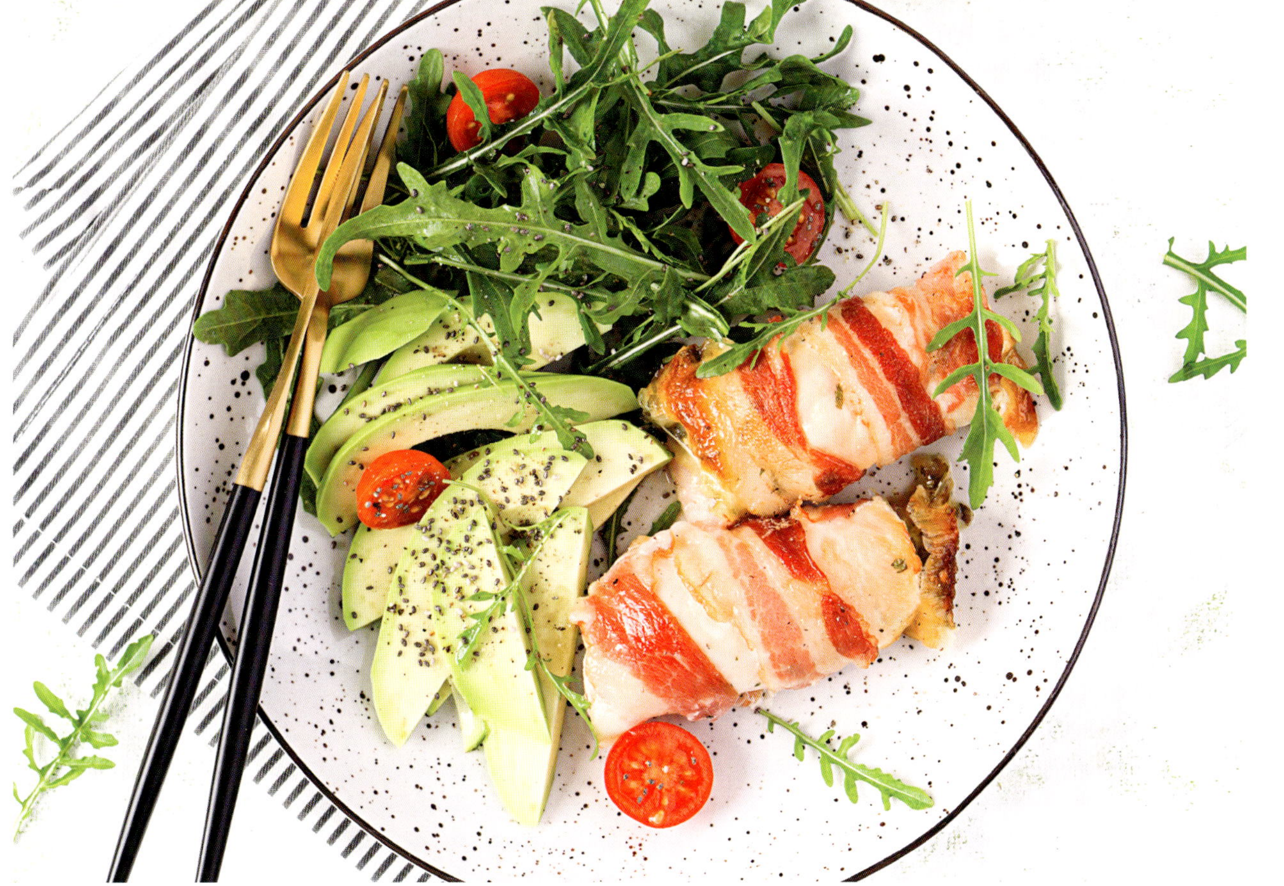

SERVES 4 | PREP + COOK TIME: 30 MINS | GLUTEN FREE | DAIRY FREE |

CHICKEN WRAPPED IN BACON

1kg chicken tenderloins

1 tsp paprika

1 tsp chilli powder

1 tsp ground cumin

1 tsp onion powder

1 tsp garlic powder

Salt and pepper to taste

12 rashers streaky bacon

150g rocket

½ cup (110g) cherry tomatoes, halved

2 avocados, sliced

2 tbsps olive oil

1 tbsp lemon juice

1 tsp chia seeds, to garnish (optional)

STEPS

Preheat oven to 200°C.

1. Place the chicken tenders in a large mixing bowl.
2. Add the paprika, chilli powder, cumin, onion powder and garlic powder to the bowl. Season lightly with salt and pepper. Toss to combine.
3. Wrap each piece of chicken in a strip of bacon, and place them on a wire rack in a roasting tin. Bake for 20-22 minutes until the chicken is cooked through and the bacon begins to crisp. Remove from the oven.
4. Divide the rocket and tomatoes evenly between four plates. Place half a sliced avocado on each plate. Drizzle the salad with olive oil and lemon juice and season with salt and pepper. Add the bacon-wrapped chicken to each plate and serve. Garnish with chia seeds if desired.

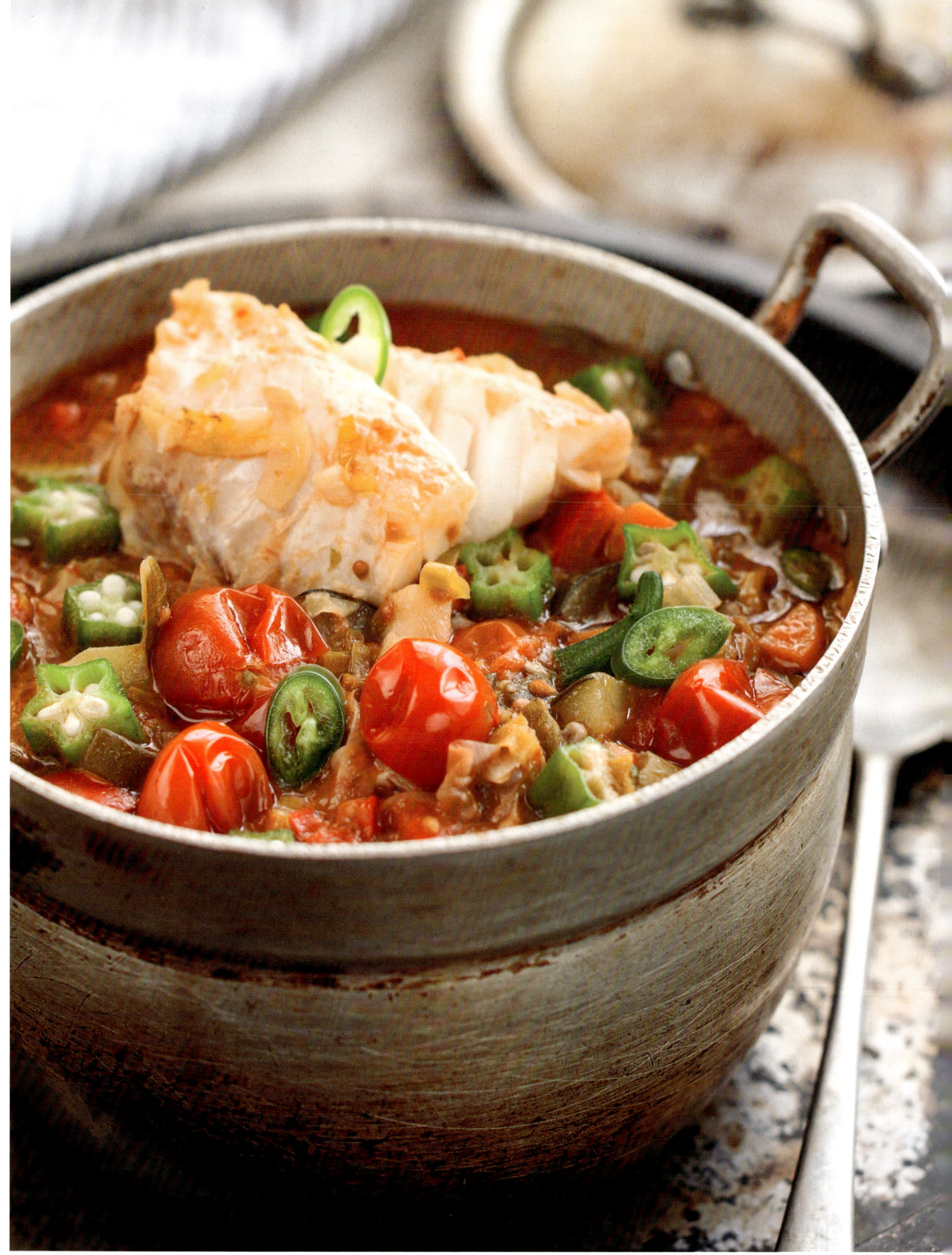

FISH STEW

2 tbsps olive oil

1 onion, finely diced

2 cloves garlic, crushed

2 stalks celery, diced

1 capsicum, diced

½ cup (125ml) dry white wine

2 cups (500ml) chicken stock

Juice of ½ lemon

1 tsp oregano

1 tsp dried thyme

Salt and pepper to taste

1 x 400g can crushed tomatoes

1 x 400g can cherry tomatoes

500g firm white fish (such as snapper or barramundi), cut into 2cm pieces

Sliced okra and green chillies to garnish (optional)

STEPS

1. Heat olive oil in a large pot over medium-high heat. Add onion and cook 6-8 minutes until fragrant, stirring often. Add in garlic, celery and capsicum. Reduce to medium heat and cook 5 minutes more.

2. Add wine, stock, lemon juice, oregano, thyme, salt and pepper. Stir and cook for 2-3 minutes then stir in both tins of tomatoes and cook for a further 10 minutes more uncovered so all the flavours can develop.

3. Add the fish pieces and stir gently into the stew, bring to the boil, then reduce heat and simmer for 5 minutes or until fish is tender and flaky.

4. Remove from heat, stir in some extra salt and pepper and garnish with sliced okra and green chillies if desired.

SERVES 4 | PREP + COOK TIME: 50 MINS | GLUTEN FREE | DAIRY FREE |

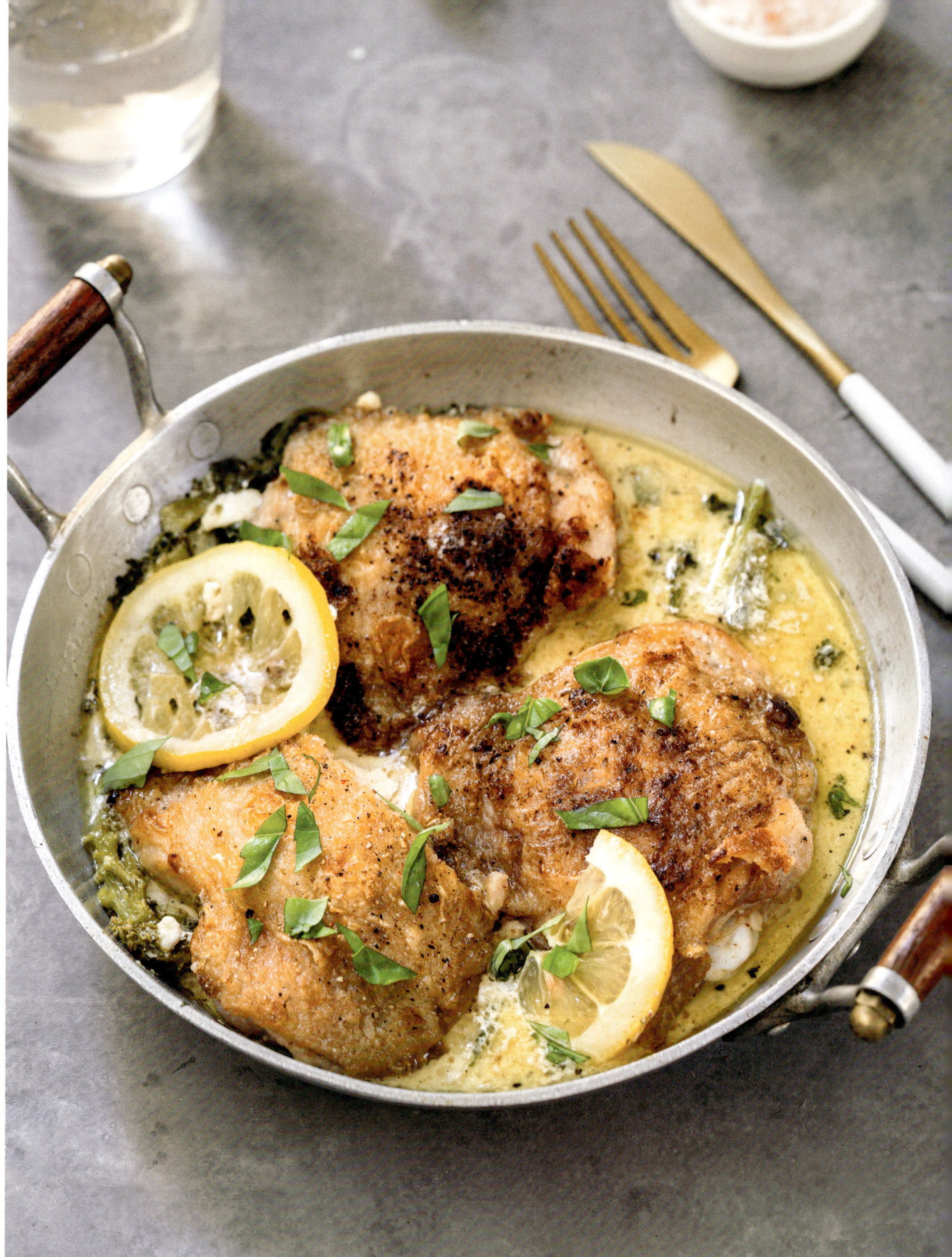

CREAMY LEMON & PARMESAN CHICKEN

4 skin-on chicken thighs
Salt and pepper to taste
1 tbsp olive oil
2 tbsps unsalted butter
4 cloves garlic, crushed
1 leek, sliced (white part only)
1 cup (250ml) chicken stock
1 tsp dried thyme
1 tsp dried rosemary
1 cup (75g) broccoli florets
1 cup (250ml) cream
2 tbsps lemon juice
½ cup (50g) grated Parmesan cheese
Fresh parsley, chopped, to serve
Lemon slices to serve

STEPS

1. Season the chicken thighs with salt and pepper on both sides.
2. Heat the olive oil and butter in an ovenproof pan or heavy-based saucepan over medium-high heat. Place the chicken thighs in the pan, skin-side down, and cook for 5-6 minutes until the skin is crispy and golden brown. Flip the chicken thighs and cook for an additional 2-3 minutes on the other side. Remove the chicken thighs from the pan and set them aside on a plate.
3. In the same pan over a medium heat add the garlic and leek and saute for about 1 minute until fragrant. Pour in the chicken stock and scrape the bottom of the pan to release any browned bits. Add the dried thyme, dried rosemary, broccoli florets and cream and stir well to combine.
4. Bring the mixture to a simmer and cook for about 5 minutes until it thickens slightly. Stir in the lemon juice and grated Parmesan cheese until melted and smooth. Return the chicken thighs to the pan, spooning the creamy sauce over them, and gently simmer for an additional 5-7 minutes or until the chicken is cooked through.
5. Serve with fresh parsley and lemon slices.

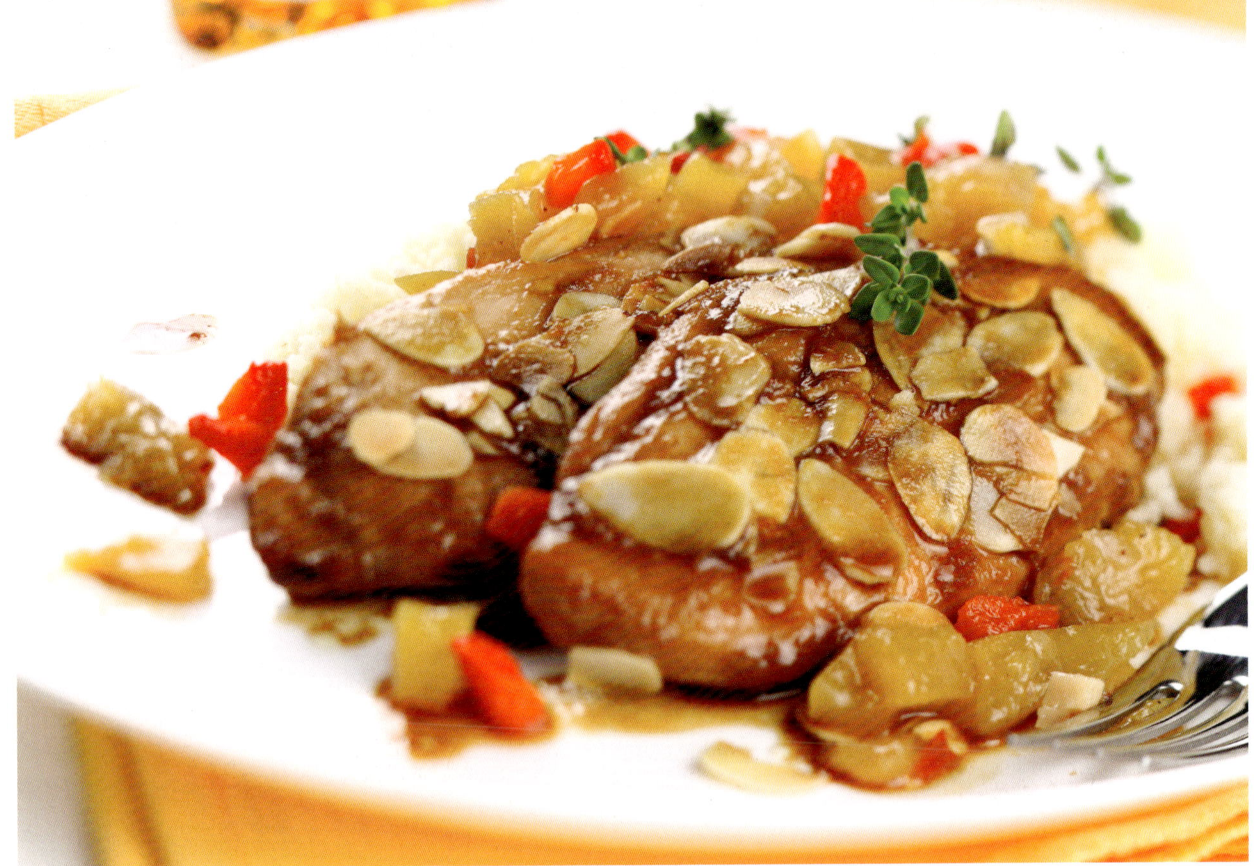

APRICOT & ALMOND BAKED CHICKEN

4 tbsps olive oil

1 tbsp Dijon mustard

1 tsp dried thyme

2 cloves garlic, crushed

1 banana chilli, deseeded and chopped

½ cup (60g) slivered almonds

½ cup (95g) dried apricots, chopped

Salt and pepper to taste

4 skinless chicken breasts

STEPS

Preheat oven to 180°C.

1. In a medium bowl, mix together the olive oil, Dijon mustard, dried thyme, garlic, chilli, almonds, chopped apricots, salt and pepper.
2. Place the chicken breasts in a greased or lined baking dish and pour over the apricot mixture, making sure the chicken breasts are well coated.
3. Bake the chicken in the preheated oven for about 25-30 minutes or until the chicken is cooked through and no longer pink in the centre.
4. Remove the chicken from the oven and let it rest for a few minutes before serving.

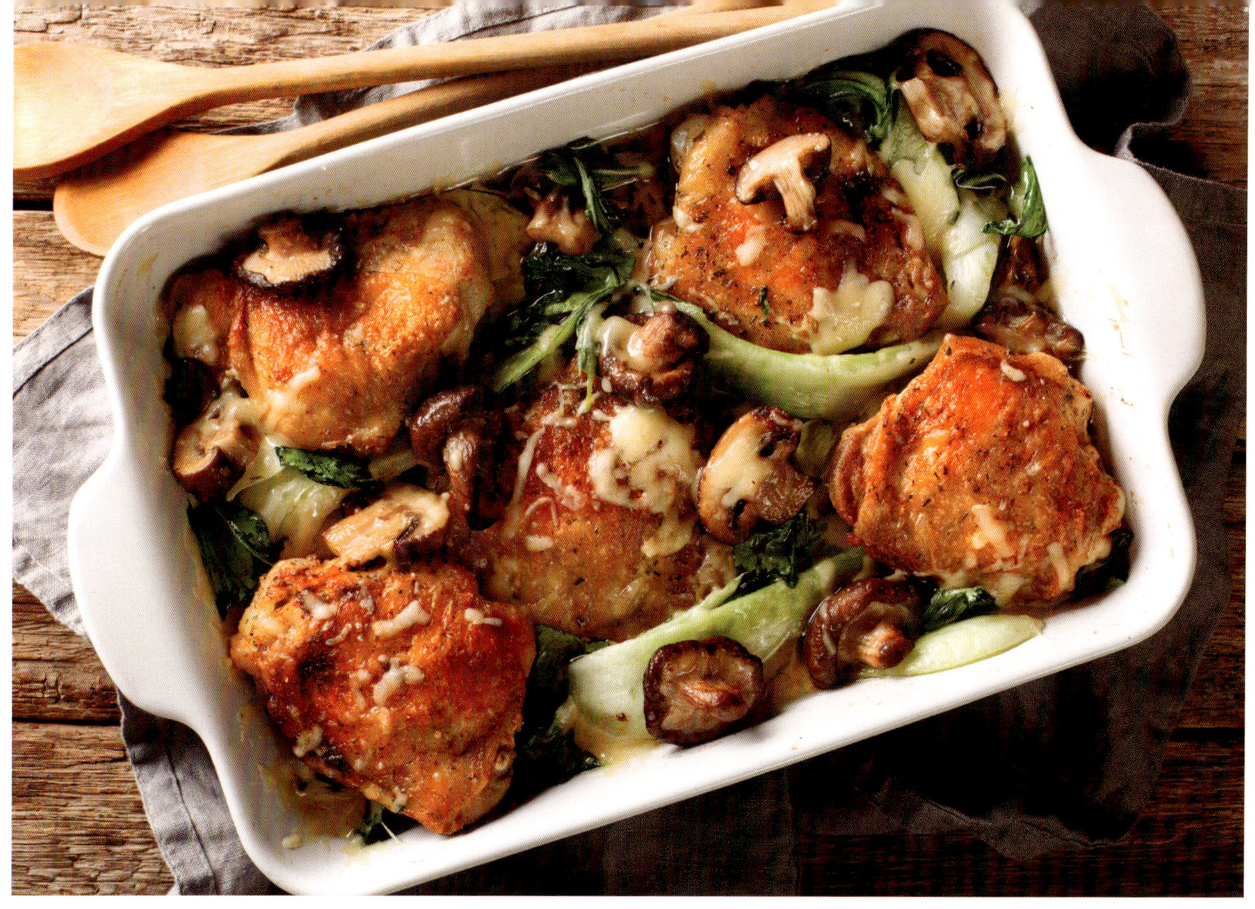

CHEESY CHICKEN WITH BOK CHOY

2 tbsps olive oil

3 large cloves garlic, crushed

1 large onion, finely chopped

1.3kg skin-on chicken thighs

350g shiitake mushrooms

2 bunches baby bok choy, ends trimmed

1 cup (125g) grated Cheddar cheese

STEPS

Preheat oven to 180°C.

1. Heat the oil in a large, deep-sided frying pan over medium heat. Fry the garlic and onion for 3 minutes. Add the chicken thighs in batches, skin-side down, for 4 minutes until the skin is crispy, then cook on the other side for 2 minutes. Remove from the pan and place in a large casserole dish, skin-side up.
2. Fry the mushrooms for 2 minutes with the onion and garlic, then turn off the heat.
3. Arrange the bok choy around the chicken pieces and then scatter the mushroom and onion over the top.
4. Scatter the cheese over the top and bake for 20 minutes until the cheese is melted and golden.

SERVES 4 | PREP + COOK TIME: 35 MINS + MARINATING | GLUTEN FREE

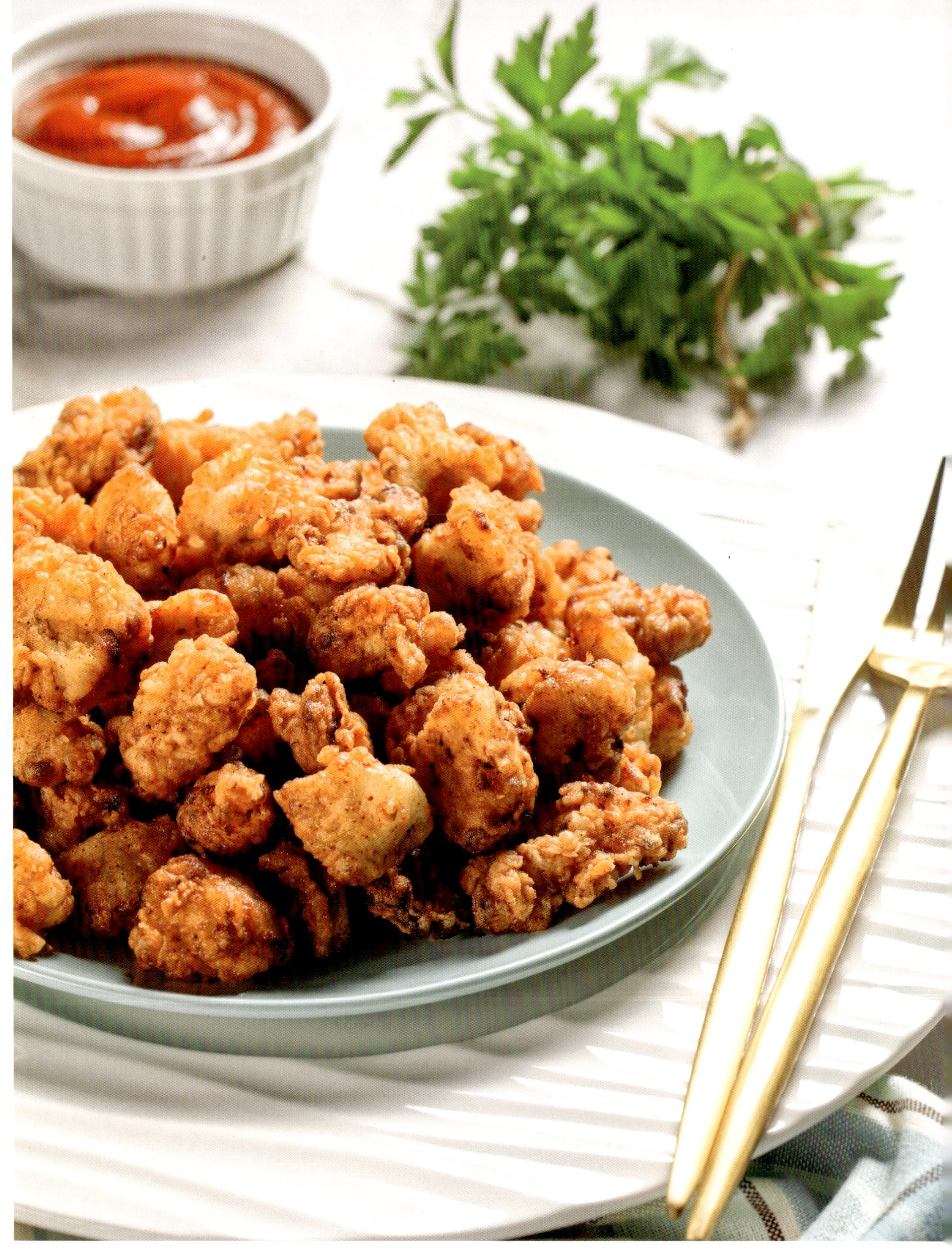

POPCORN CHICKEN

500g boneless, skinless chicken breasts, cut into bite-sized pieces

1 cup (250ml) buttermilk

¼ cup (25g) coconut flour

¼ tsp salt

⅛ tsp pepper

1 large egg

2 cups (150g) crushed pork rinds (see tip)

1 tsp onion powder

½ tsp garlic powder

½ tsp smoked paprika

STEPS

1. Place the chicken in a large bowl. Pour over the buttermilk and toss to coat. Cover and refrigerate for 24 hours.
2. Preheat the oven to 220°C. Line a baking tray with greaseproof paper.
3. Prepare three shallow dishes. In the first, combine the coconut flour, salt and pepper. Crack the egg into the second dish and beat lightly with a fork. In the third dish, mix together the pork rinds, onion powder, garlic powder and paprika.
4. Dredge the chicken first in the coconut flour, then dip in egg wash, and finally coat in the pork rind breading. Place coated chicken pieces on the prepared baking tray.
5. Transfer to the oven and bake for 20 minutes, until golden brown and crispy.

TIP: Crushed pork rinds are available to buy online or at health food stores. If you can't find them, buy a packet of pork crackle from the supermarket and crush with a rolling pin. Be sure to check the salt content and reduce the amount of salt you add accordingly.

SERVES 4 | PREP + COOK TIME: 35 MINS + MARINATING | GLUTEN FREE |

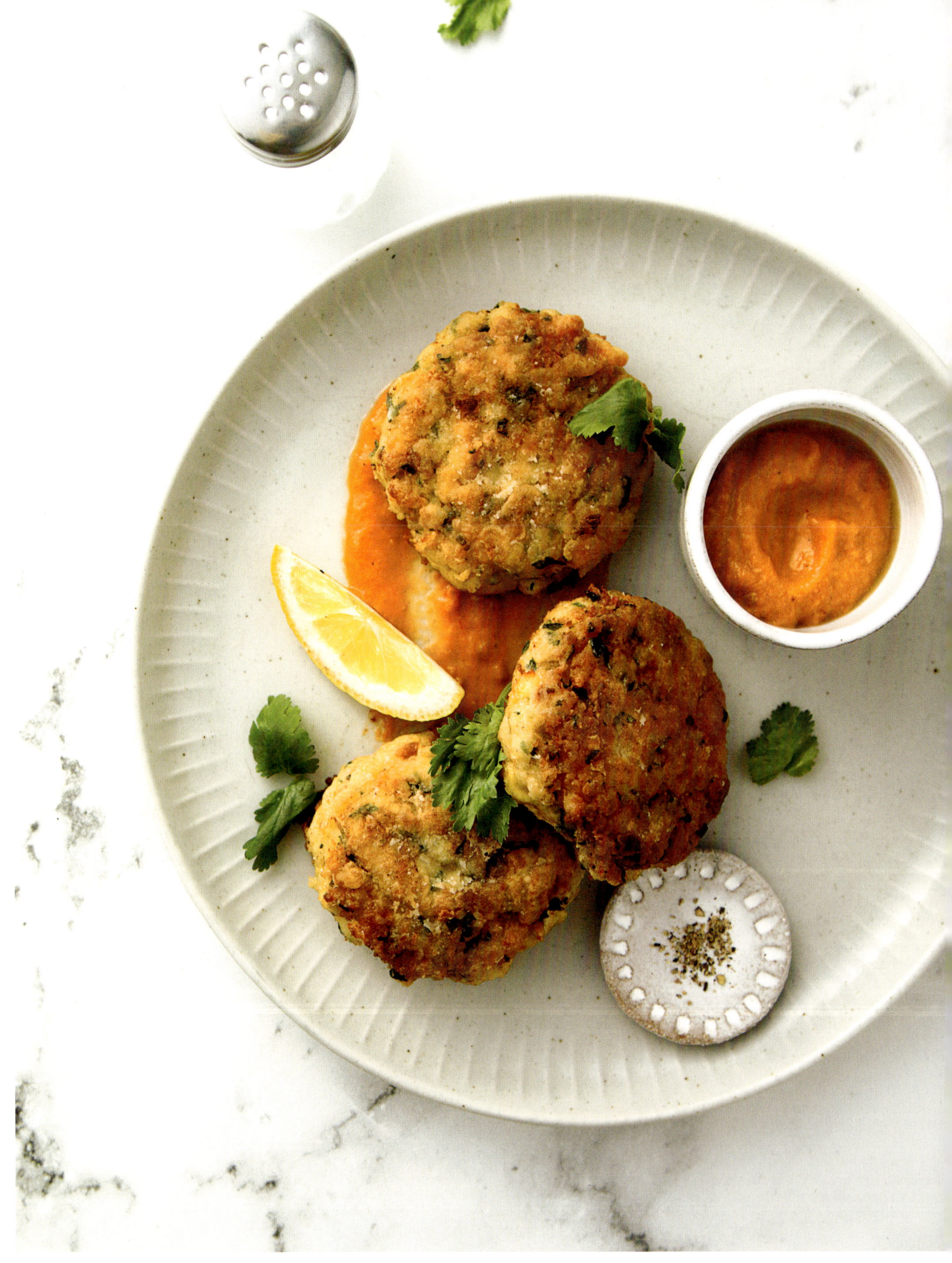

FISHCAKES WITH HOMEMADE TOMATO SAUCE

500g firm white fish fillets (such as barramundi or ling), finely diced

½ cup (60g) almond meal

½ a small brown onion, finely chopped

2 tbsps chopped fresh parsley + extra to garnish

2 tbsps mayonnaise

1 tbsp Dijon mustard

1 clove garlic, minced

1 tsp lemon zest

½ tsp salt

¼ tsp pepper

2 tbsps olive oil

Lemon wedges to serve

TOMATO SAUCE

1 tbsp olive oil

½ small brown onion, finely chopped

1 clove garlic, minced

1 x 400g can crushed tomatoes

1 tbsp tomato paste

1 tsp dried oregano

½ tsp sugar

Salt and pepper to taste

STEPS

1. To a medium-sized bowl, add chopped fish, almond meal, finely chopped onion, chopped fresh parsley, mayonnaise, Dijon mustard, minced garlic, lemon zest, salt, and pepper. Mix well until all the ingredients are well combined.

2. Shape the mixture into fish cakes, about 4-5cm in diameter and 2cm thick. You should get approximately six to eight fishcakes, depending on the size.

3. Heat the olive oil in a large frying pan over medium heat. Add the fish cakes and cook for about 4-5 minutes on each side, or until golden brown and cooked through. Remove from the pan and set aside.

4. To prepare the tomato sauce, in a separate saucepan, heat olive oil over medium heat. Add the onion and garlic, and saute until the onion is translucent and the garlic is fragrant. Add the crushed tomatoes, tomato paste, dried oregano and sugar to the saucepan. Stir well to combine. Simmer the sauce for 10-15 minutes, allowing the flavours incorporate well. Add salt and pepper to taste.

5. To serve, divide fishcakes onto plates and serve with tomato sauce, fresh parsley and lemon wedges.

SERVES 4 | PREP + COOK TIME: 45 MINS | GLUTEN FREE | DAIRY FREE |

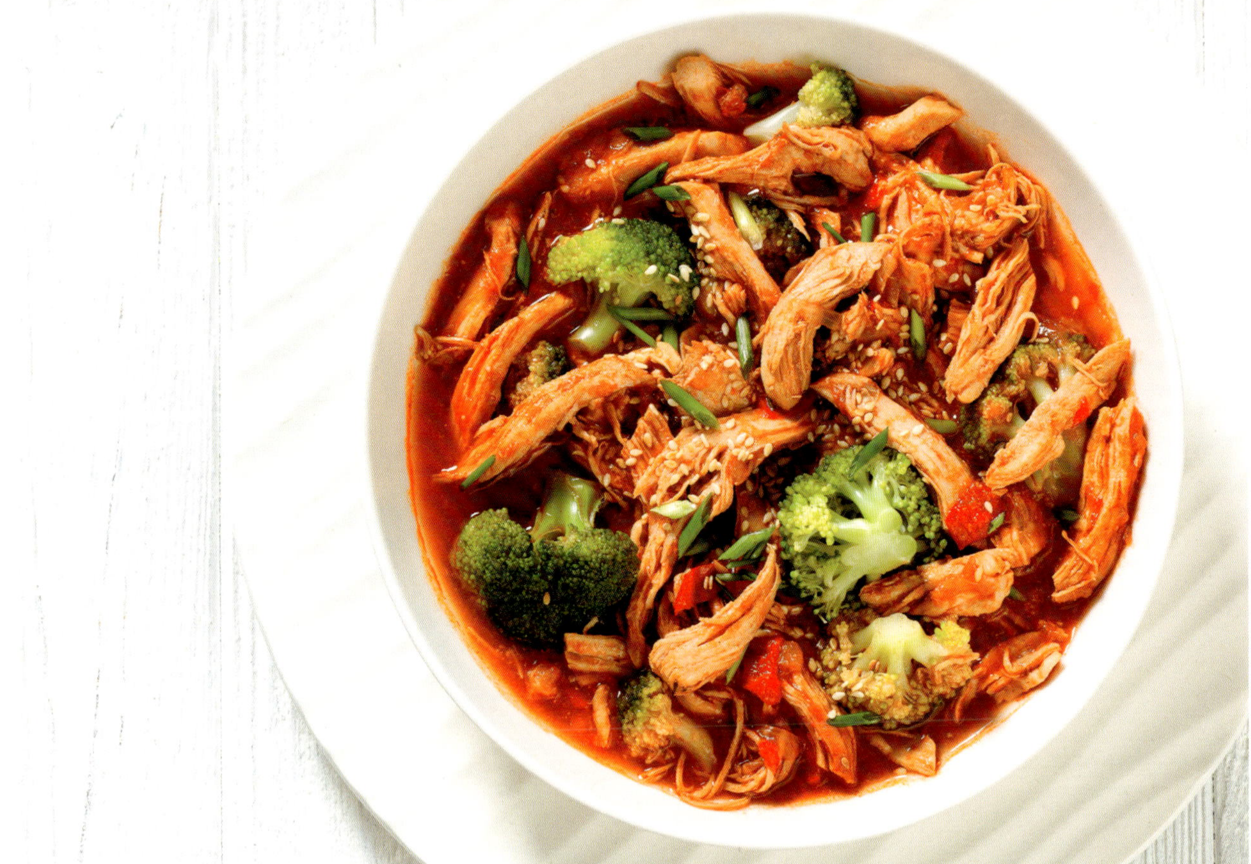

SERVES 4 | PREP + COOK TIME: 5 HOURS 20 MINS | GLUTEN FREE | DAIRY FREE |

TOMATO CHICKEN & BROCCOLI

600g skinless chicken breasts
Salt and pepper to taste
1 onion, diced
1 capsicum, diced
2 cloves garlic, crushed
1 x 400g can crushed tomatoes
1 cup (250ml) chicken stock
1 tsp dried basil
1 tsp dried oregano
½ tsp paprika
¼ tsp chilli flakes (optional)
2 cups (150g) broccoli florets
Sliced spring onions fto garnish

STEPS

1. Season chicken with salt and pepper. Add chicken, onion, capsicum, garlic, crushed tomatoes, chicken stock, basil, oregano, paprika and chilli flakes (if using) to a slow cooker. Stir well to combine.
2. Cover and slow cook for 4-5 hours on low heat or 2-3 hours on high heat, until the chicken is tender and easily shreds. Remove the chicken breasts from the slow cooker and use two forks to shred the meat.
3. Return the shredded chicken to the slow cooker and add the broccoli florets. Stir to combine. Continue cooking for an additional 15-20 minutes, or until the broccoli is tender. Taste the stew and adjust the seasoning with additional salt and pepper if needed.
4. Garnish with sliced spring onions.

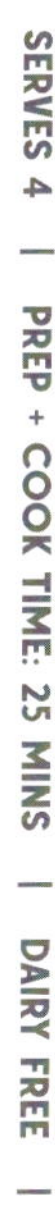

PEANUT CHICKEN STIR-FRY

2 tbsps soy sauce
2 tbsps hoisin sauce
2 tbsps peanut butter
2 tbsps lime juice
1 tbsp sesame oil
2 cloves garlic, crushed
1 tsp grated ginger
2 tbsps vegetable oil
2 skinless chicken breasts, thinly sliced
2 cups (60g) baby spinach
¼ cup (30g) unsalted peanuts, chopped
Spring onions, sliced, to garnish
Red chillies, sliced, to garnish

STEPS

1. In a bowl, whisk together the soy sauce, hoisin sauce, peanut butter, lime juice, sesame oil, crushed garlic and grated ginger. Set the sauce aside.
2. Heat the vegetable oil in a large frying pan or wok over medium-high heat. Add the sliced chicken to the pan and stir-fry for a minute or two then add the prepared stir-fry sauce. Toss the chicken in the pan to coat well.
3. Continue cooking for an additional 2-3 minutes until the sauce has heated through and thickened slightly then add the spinach and peanuts and toss well.
4. Divide among bowls and garnish with spring onions and sliced red chillies.

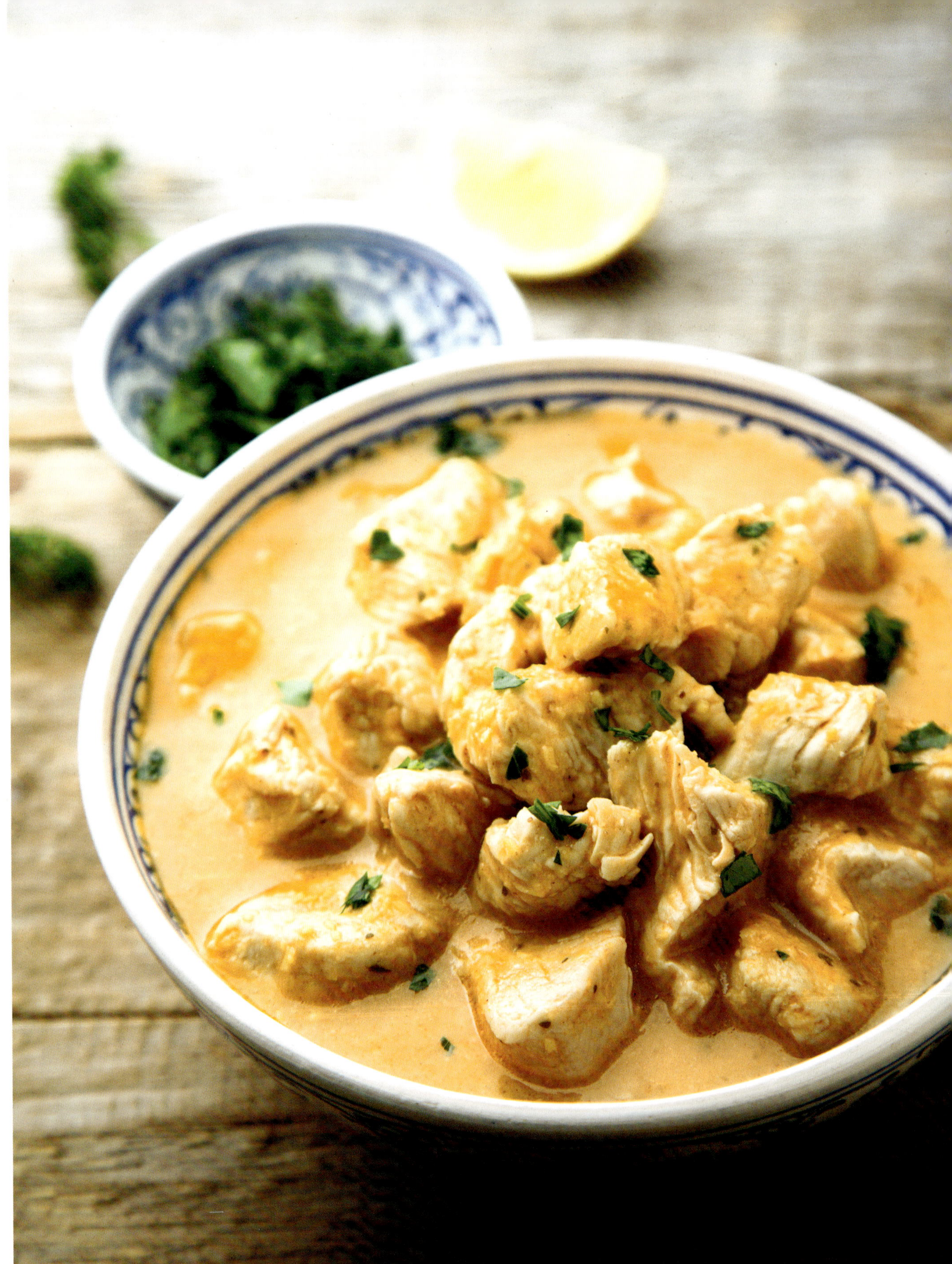

SPICY COCONUT CHICKEN

⅓ cup (100ml) coconut milk

⅓ cup (100ml) coconut cream

2 cups (500ml) chicken stock

2 tbsps lime juice

2 tsps fish sauce

1 green chilli, deseeded and finely chopped

1 tsp chilli sauce

2 tbsps shredded fresh basil

500g chicken breast, cut into 3cm cubes

Salt and pepper to taste

Lemon wedges to serve

STEPS

1. Heat the coconut milk, coconut cream, stock, lime juice, fish sauce, chilli and chilli sauce in a large pot until boiling.
2. Reduce the heat to a simmer, add half the basil and the chicken. Cover and simmer for 15 minutes.
3. Adjust taste with salt and pepper.
4. Serve with lemon wedges and garnished with the rest of the basil.

SERVES 2 | PREP + COOK TIME: 30 MINS | GLUTEN FREE | DAIRY FREE |

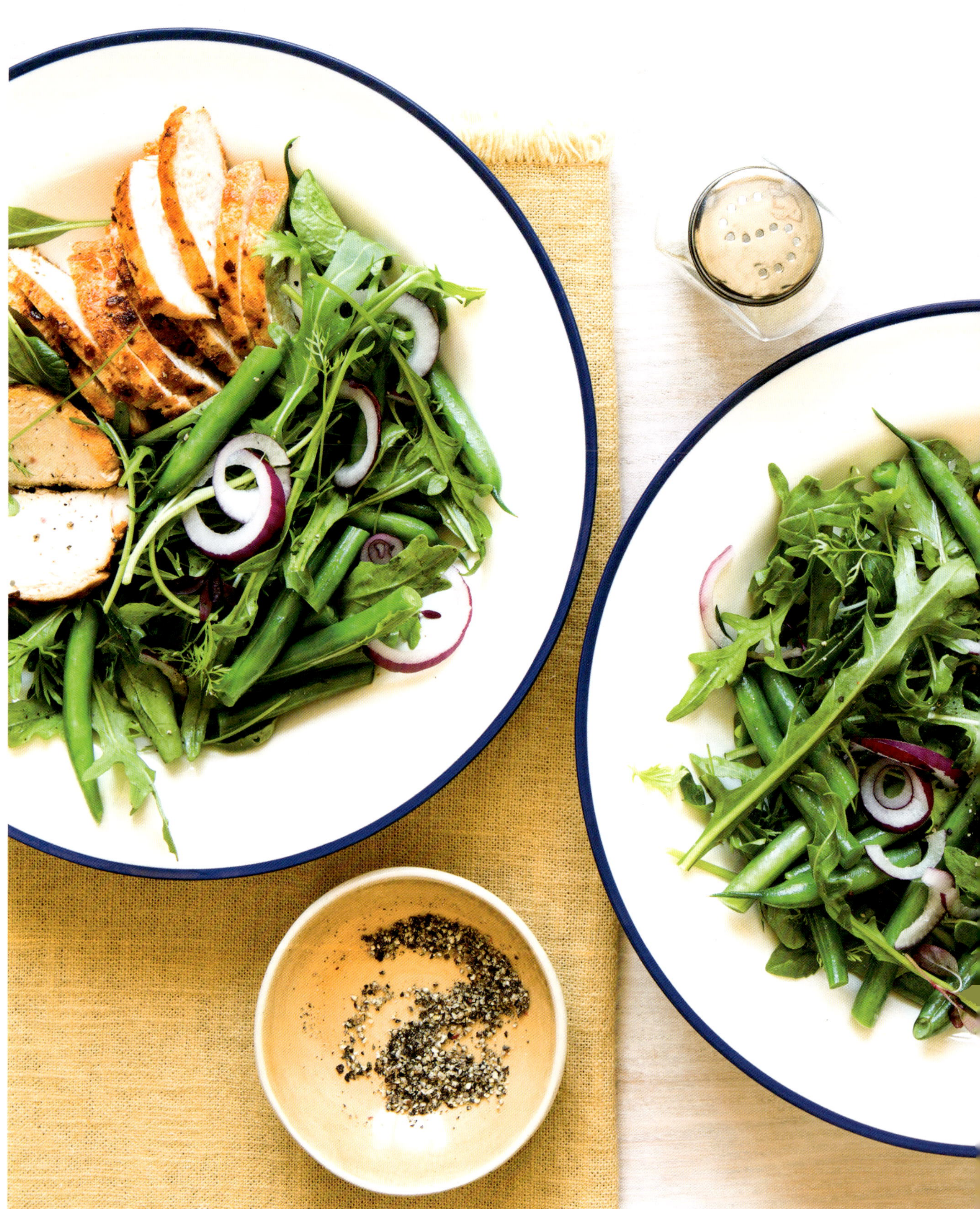

MARINATED CHICKEN WITH GREEN SALAD

CHICKEN

½ tsp paprika

½ tsp garlic powder

½ tsp onion powder

1 tbsp olive oil

Salt and pepper to taste

2 chicken breasts

SALAD

200g rocket leaves

1 cup (150g) green beans, halved

½ small red onion, finely sliced

Juice of ½ lemon

1 tbsp olive oil

Salt and pepper to taste

STEPS

Preheat oven to 180°C.

1. In a medium-sized bowl, add paprika, garlic powder, onion powder, olive oil, salt and pepper and whisk until well combined. Add the chicken breast and let sit for 15 minutes.
2. Place marinated chicken breasts on a lined baking tray and bake for 15-20 minutes or until chicken is cooked through.
3. For the salad, place the rocket leaves, green beans and onion in a serving bowl and toss to combine. Pour over lemon juice and olive oil and season with salt and pepper. Toss one more time making sure all the ingredients are well coated.
4. Once the chicken is cooked, remove from the oven and let rest for a minute or two, then slice thinly. Serve warm with salad on the side.

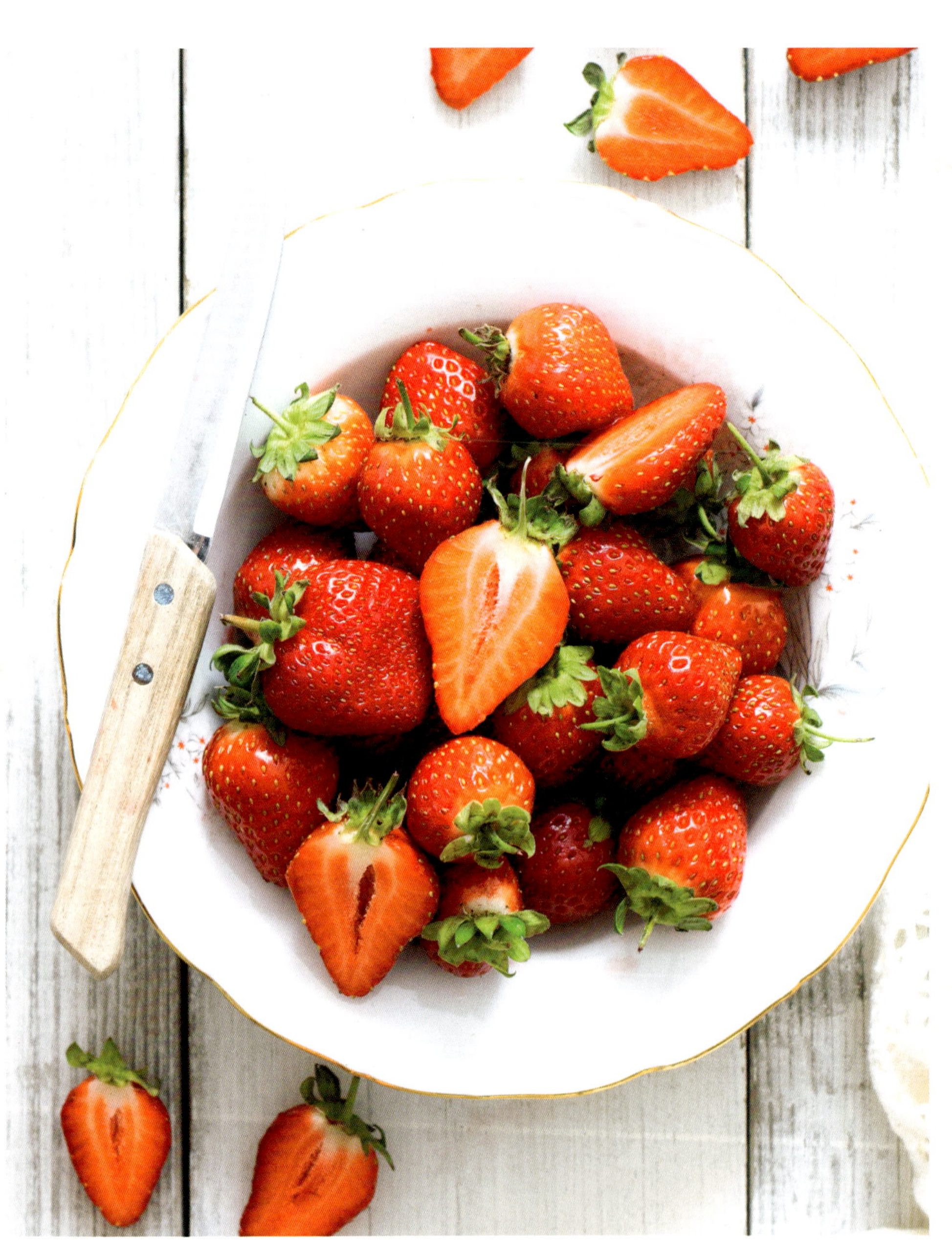

DESSERTS & TREATS

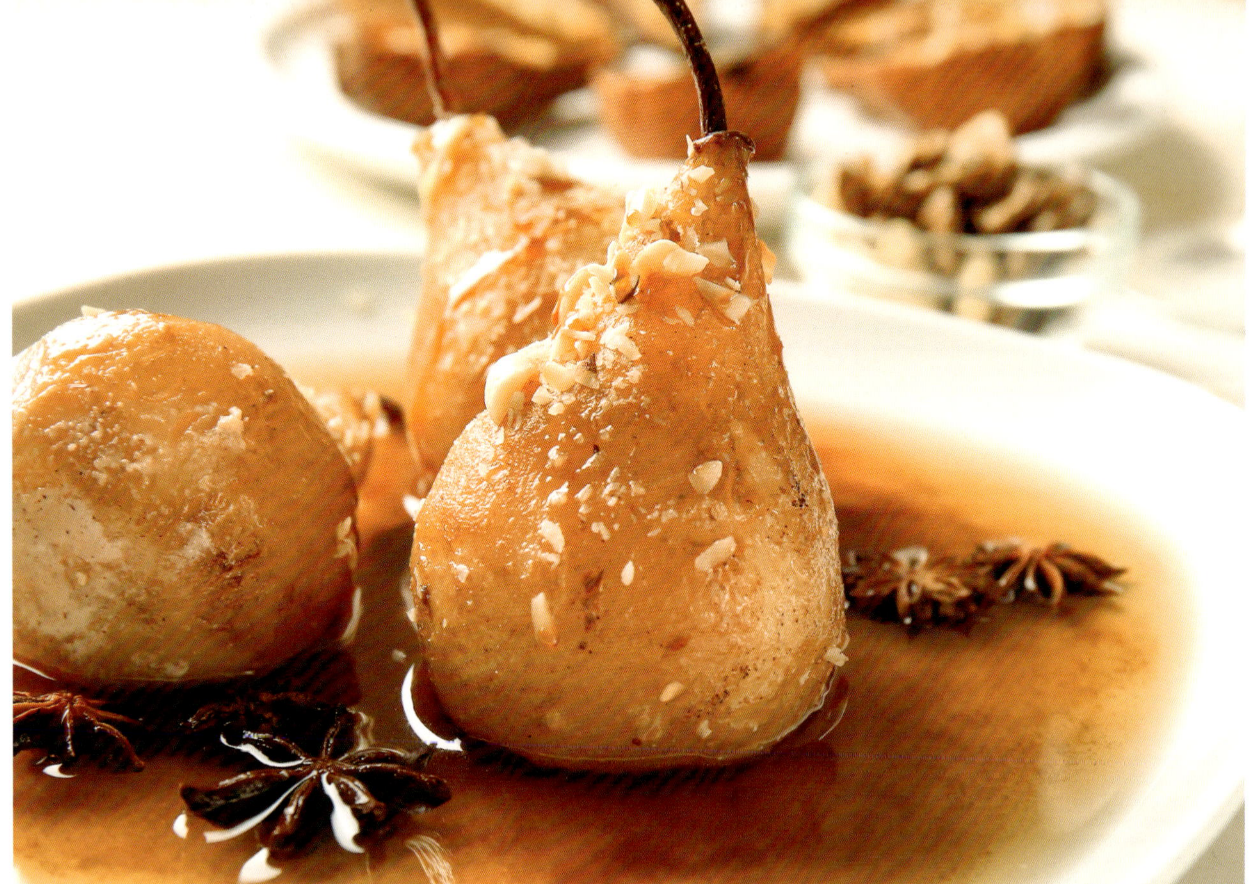

SPICED PEARS

4 firm, medium-sized Beurre Bosc pears

¼ cup (60ml) apple juice

¼ cup (60ml) water

2 tbsps honey

1 tbsp butter

1 tbsp coconut oil

1 cinnamon stick

2 star anise

¼ cup (30g) blanched almonds, crushed

STEPS

Preheat the oven to 200°C.

1. Peel the pears, keeping the stems intact, and place in a medium-sized, deep-sided baking dish.
2. Place the juice, water, honey, butter, coconut oil, cinnamon stick and star anise in a small saucepan and heat until simmering.
3. Pour the sauce over the pears.
4. Bake in the oven for 35 minutes. Remove the cinnamon and star anise.
5. Allow pears to sit for 5 minutes, then place each pear in a serving bowl, drizzle with the extra sauce and serve garnished with crushed almonds.

SERVES 6 | PREP + COOK TIME: 15 MINS + CHILLING | VEG | GLUTEN FREE |

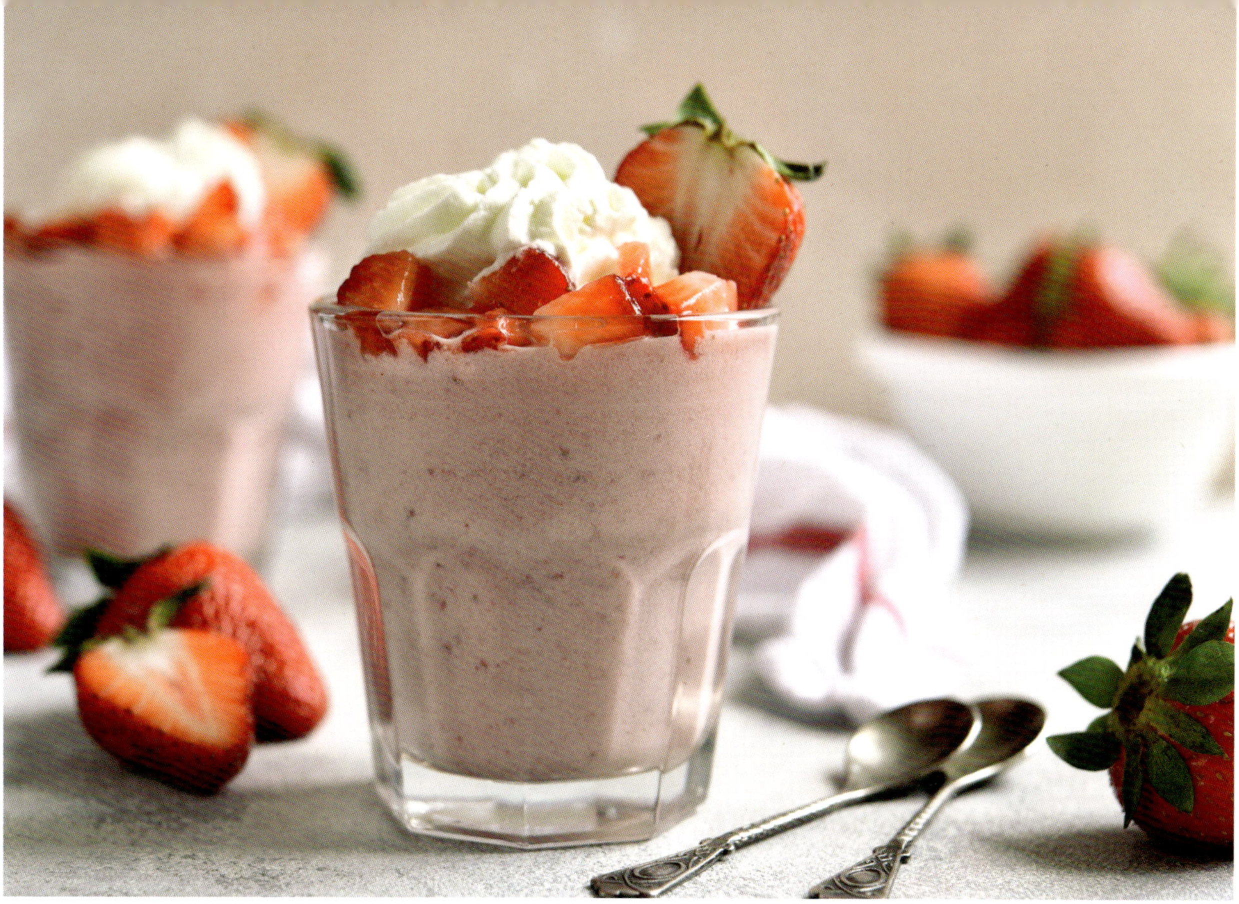

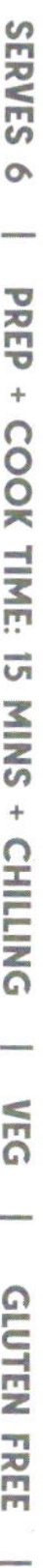

STRAWBERRY MOUSSE

2 cups (400g) chopped strawberries

½ cup (100g) monkfruit sweetener or erythritol

1½ cups (375ml) thickened cream

STEPS

1. In a high-speed blender or food processor, combine 1½ cups strawberries with the sweetener. Process until smooth.
2. In a mixing bowl, whisk 1 cup cream until stiff peaks form. Gently fold through the pureed strawberry mixture. Divide the mixture evenly between six small glasses. Refrigerate for at least 2 hours, to firm up.
3. Whip the remaining cream and pipe on top of the mousse using a piping bag with a star-shaped nozzle. Decorate with the remaining chopped strawberries to serve.

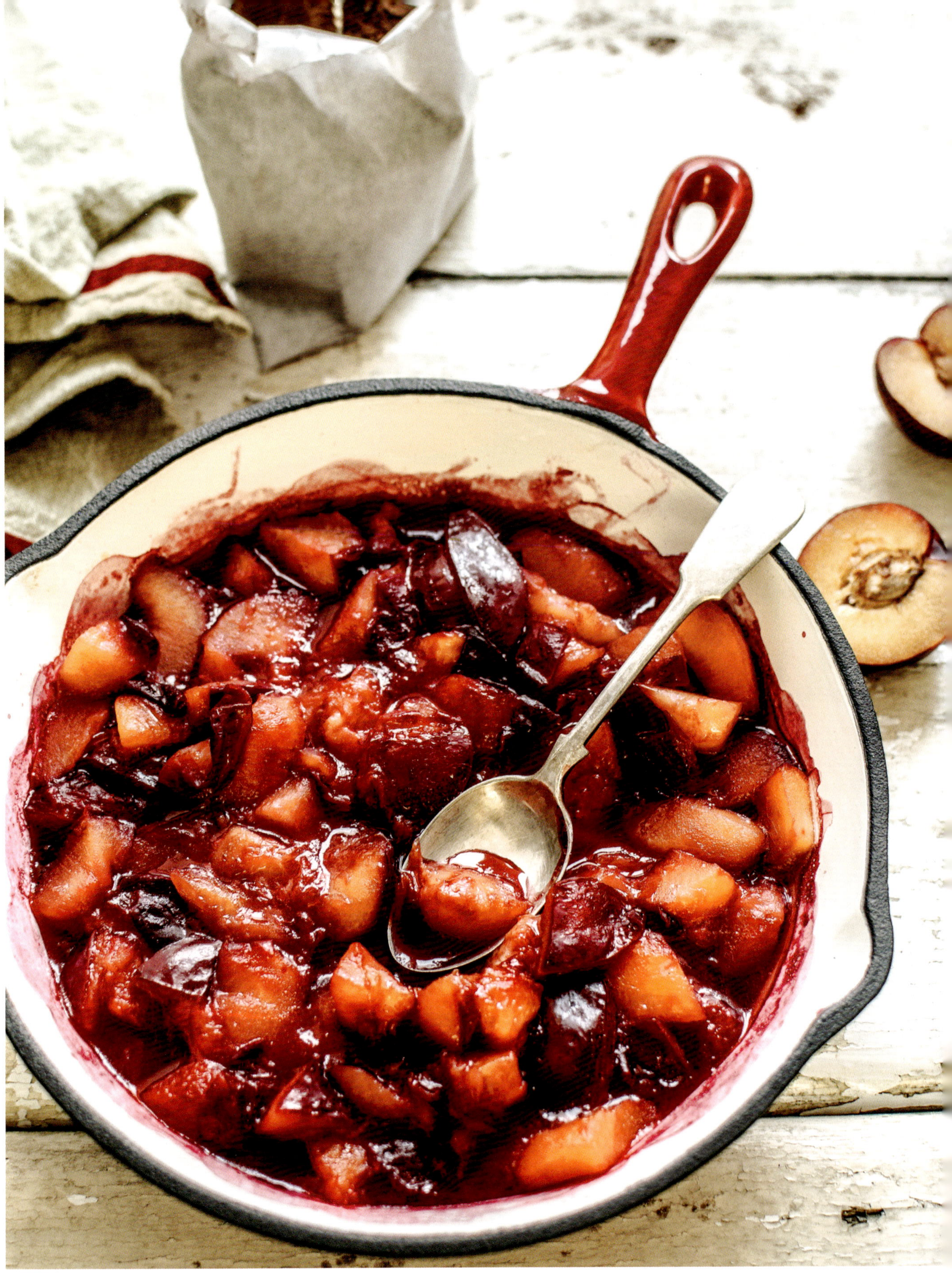

STEWED STONE FRUIT

800g peaches, stones removed, cut into small wedges

800g blood plums, stones removed, cut into small wedges

½ cup (180g) honey

Juice of ½ lemon

1 tsp cinnamon

½ tsp vanilla extract

STEPS

1. In a heavy-based shallow pan, add the prepared peaches and plums. Then add the honey, lemon juice, cinnamon and vanilla and stir gently, making sure the fruit is well coated.
2. Bring to the boil, then reduce heat to medium-low and simmer, covered, for 20-25 minutes until fruit is tender. Remove from heat, uncover and set aside to cool slightly.
3. Serve warm as a topping for oats or with natural yoghurt.

SERVES 6 | PREP + COOK TIME: 40 MINS | VEG | GLUTEN FREE | DAIRY FREE |

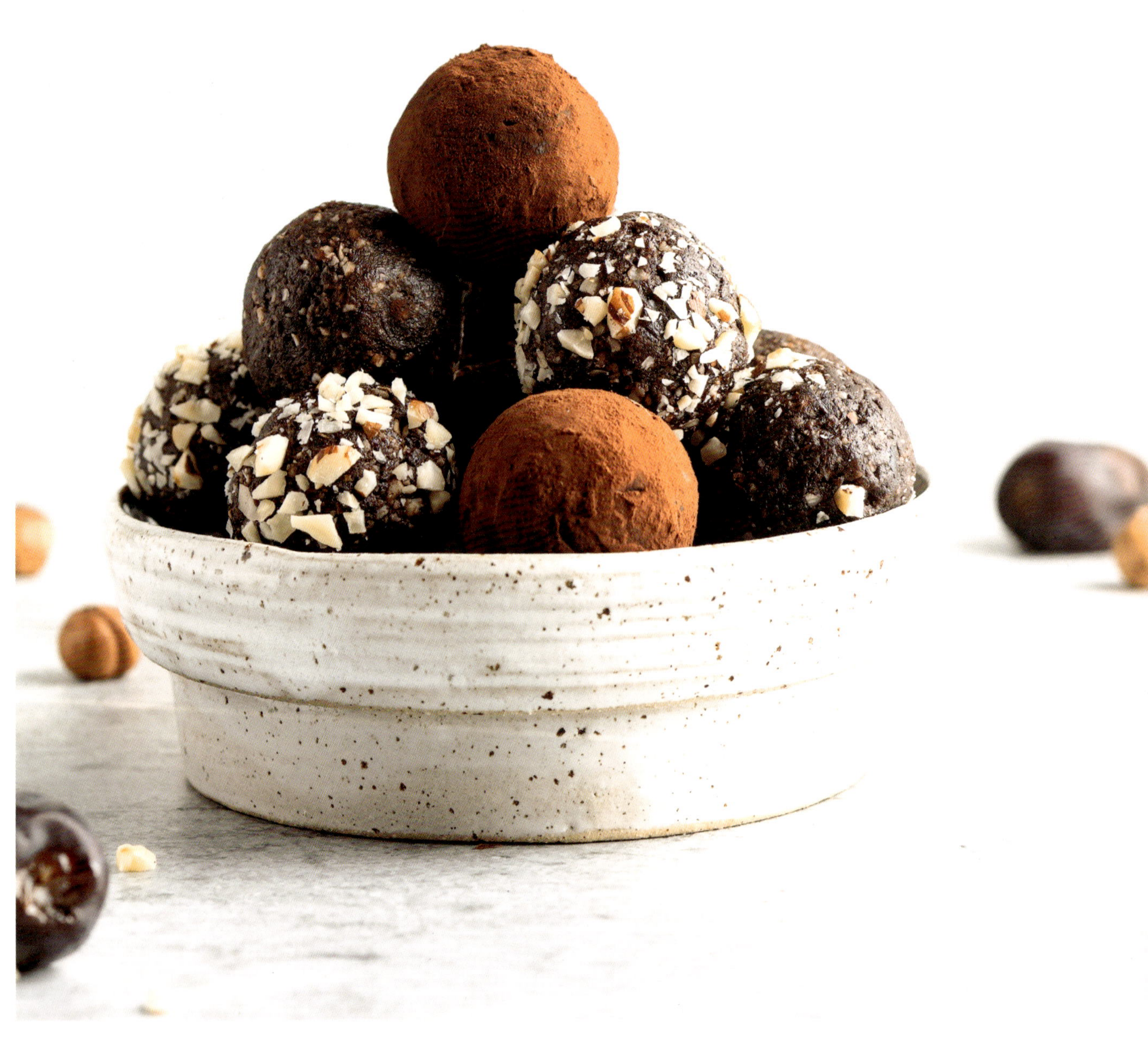

CHOCOLATE ENERGY BALLS

¾ cup (90g) unsweetened dark chocolate, roughly chopped

1 cup (115g) almonds, divided

¾ cup (90g) pistachios, divided

2 tbsps ground flaxseed

2 tbsps chia seeds

1 tbsp honey

1 cup (160g) Medjool dates, pitted

1 tbsp coconut oil

1 tbsp cacao powder, divided

STEPS

1. Add half the almonds to the food processor and pulse to crush into pieces suitable for coating the energy balls. Place in a small bowl and set aside.
2. Place the chocolate, remaining whole almonds, half the pistachios, flaxseed and chia seeds in the food processor. Blitz for 1 minute, until a breadcrumb consistency forms.
3. Add the honey, dates, coconut oil and half the cacao powder and blend for a further 1 minute until a dough forms.
4. Using your hands, form the mixture into little balls.
5. Place the crushed almond onto a shallow bowl or plate, and in a separate bowl or plate place the remaining cocoa. Roll half the balls in the crushed almonds and the rest in the cocoa powder.

NOTE: Place in the refrigerator for 1 hour to firm up before serving, and store in a sealed container in the fridge.

MAKES 20 | PREP + COOK TIME: 15 MINS + CHILLING | VEG | GLUTEN FREE | DAIRY FREE |

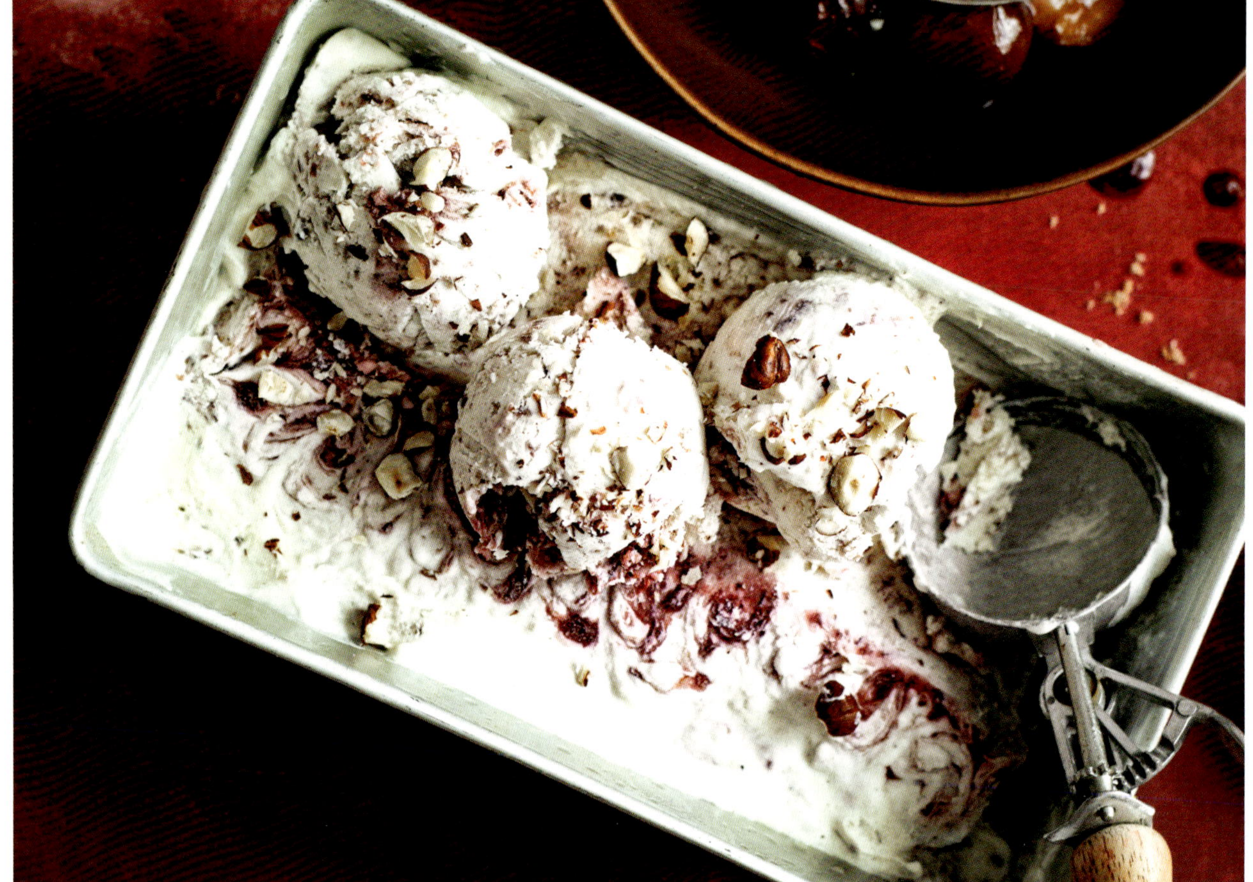

BLACKBERRY NO CHURN ICE CREAM

SERVES 4 | PREP + COOK TIME: 15 MINS + FREEZING | VEG | GLUTEN FREE | DAIRY FREE

1 x 400ml can full-fat coconut milk

1 tsp vanilla extract

½ tbsp lemon zest

¼ cup (90g) raw honey (runny)

1 cup (145g) blackberries (fresh or frozen)

¼ cup (30g) toasted almonds, roughly chopped

STEPS

1. Add coconut milk, vanilla, lemon zest and honey to a food processor and puree until ingredients are incorporated and you get a smooth mixture.
2. In a small bowl add the blackberries and mash them with a fork until they resemble a chunky jam, then set aside.
3. Transfer coconut mixture to a 24cm stainless steel loaf tin and swirl the blackberry mash into the cream mixture, incorporating well. Sprinkle the toasted almonds evenly over the top.
4. Place tin in the freezer and freeze for at least 4 hours.
5. Take ice cream out of freezer and let sit for 15-20 minutes at room temperature before serving.

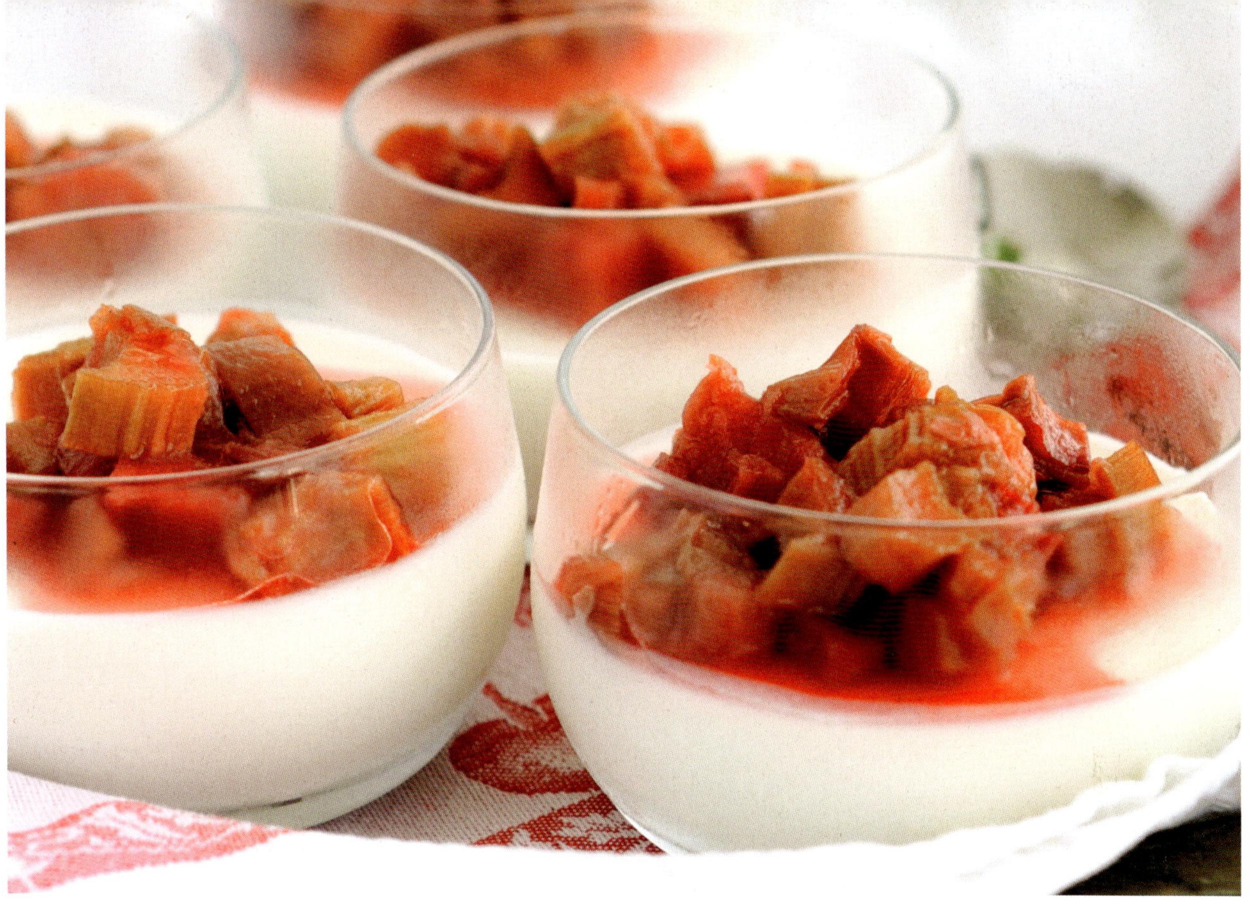

COCONUT CREAMS WITH RHUBARB

3⅓ cups (400g) rhubarb, chopped

⅓ cup (80ml) water

½ cup (95g) erythritol or monkfruit powder

15 drops liquid stevia

½ tsp vanilla bean powder or 1 tsp vanilla extract

2 sheets leaf gelatin

1 x 400ml can coconut milk

2 tbsps caster sugar or low-carb sugar substitute

1 tsp vanilla extract

STEPS

1. Place the rhubarb and water in a saucepan and bring to a boil over a medium-high heat. When it starts to simmer, lower the heat to medium and cook for 4-5 minutes until tender. Add sweeteners and vanilla. Mix well until the sweeteners dissolve.

2. For the coconut creams, place the gelatin into a bowl and cover with cold water. Leave to soak for 5 minutes or until softened.

3. Heat coconut milk and sugar in a pan. Bring to a gentle simmer, then remove from the heat. Lift the gelatin from the water and stir it into the coconut milk. Keep stirring until the gelatin has dissolved, then pour mixture into four small glass dishes or tumblers. When the creams are cool, transfer to the fridge and leave to set for around 2-4 hours.

4. Once the creams have set remove from the fridge and serve with a spoonful of rhubarb.

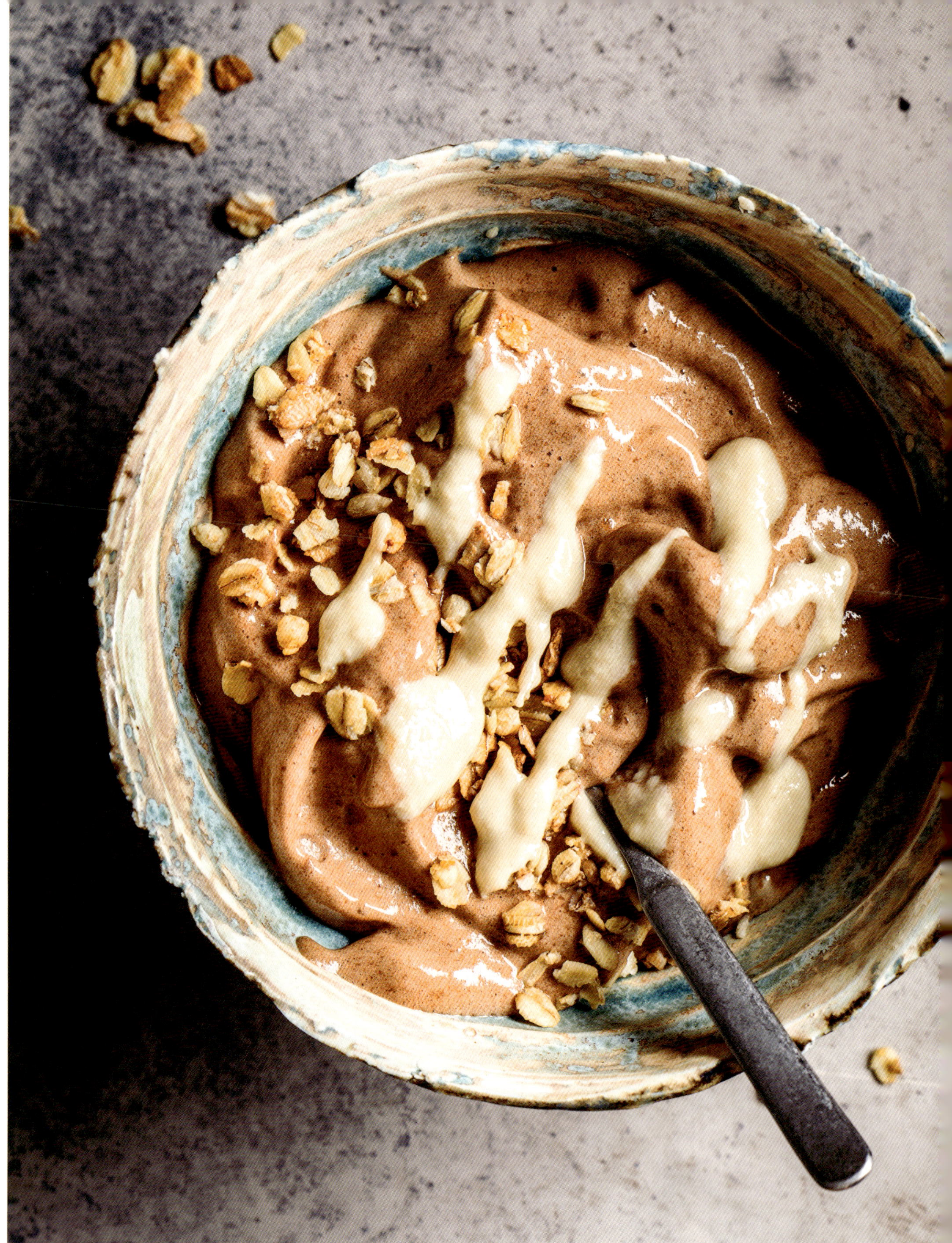

CHOCOLATE BANANA NICE CREAM

3 frozen bananas, peeled and sliced

2 tbsps unsweetened cocoa powder

1-2 tbsps honey (optional, for added sweetness)

½ tsp vanilla extract

Toppings of your choice

STEPS

1. Add the bananas, cocoa powder, honey and vanilla to a food processor or blender. Puree the mixture until smooth and creamy, scraping down the sides as needed. You may need to stop and stir the mixture a few times to ensure even blending.

2. Scoop the mixture into bowls and serve immediately.

3. Serve with your favourite toppings such as crunchy granola and tahini or fresh berries and nuts.

SERVES 2 | PREP + COOK TIME: 5 MINS | VEG | GLUTEN FREE | DAIRY FREE |

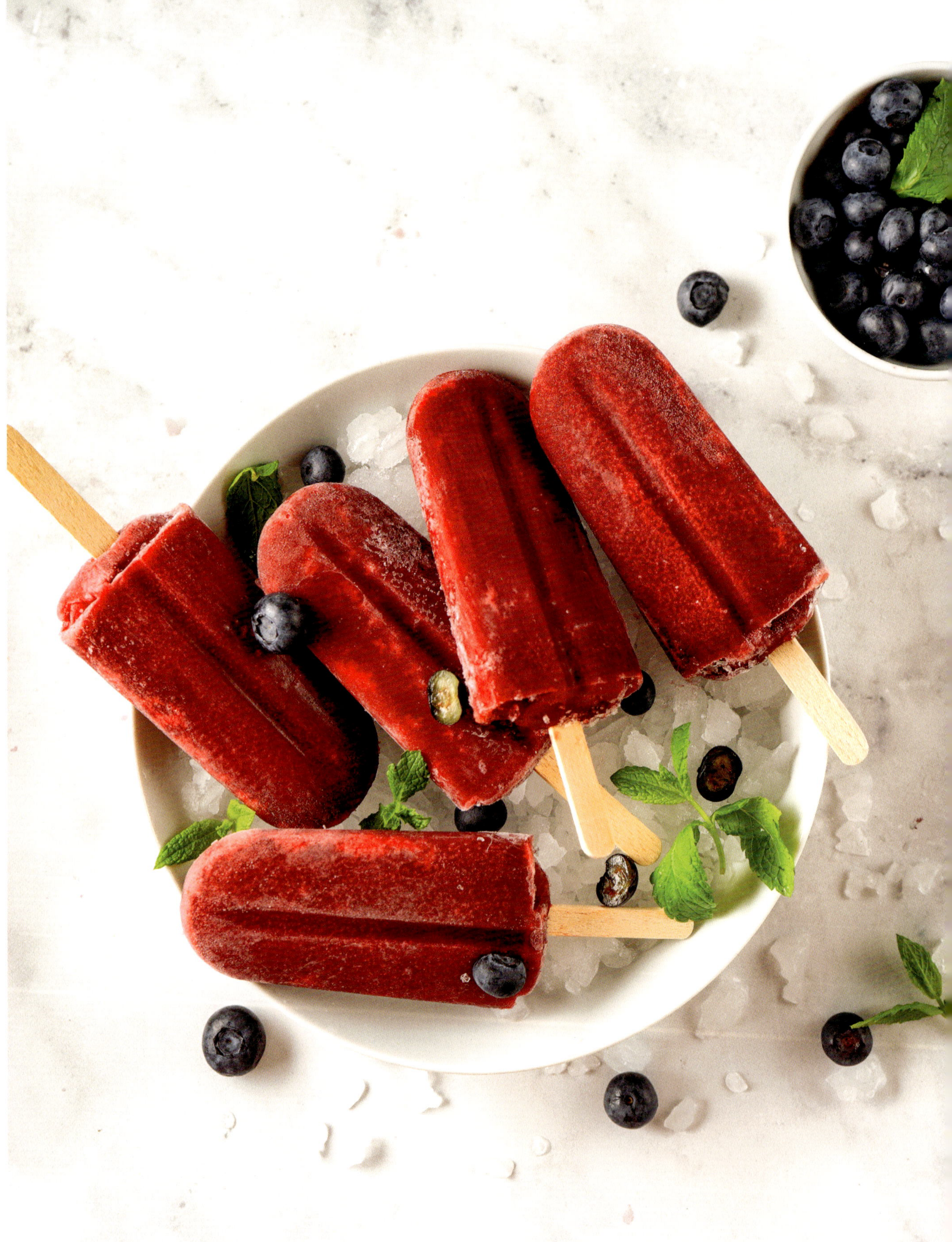

BERRY POPSICLES

2 cups (200g) blueberries (fresh or frozen)

½ cup (60g) raspberries (fresh or frozen)

1 tbsp finely chopped fresh mint

1 cup (250ml) Greek yoghurt

½ cup (125ml) water

2 tbsps honey

STEPS

1. Place the berries in a blender with the mint and blend until smooth.
2. Mix yoghurt, water and honey in a large bowl and stir through the berry mixture.
3. Fill icy-pole moulds to 3mm from the top.
4. Place a wooden stick in the middle of each mould with half sticking out.
5. Transfer to the freezer and freeze for 8 hours. Remove from moulds and eat cold.

MAKES 6 | PREP + COOK TIME: 10 MINS + FREEZING | VEG | GLUTEN FREE |

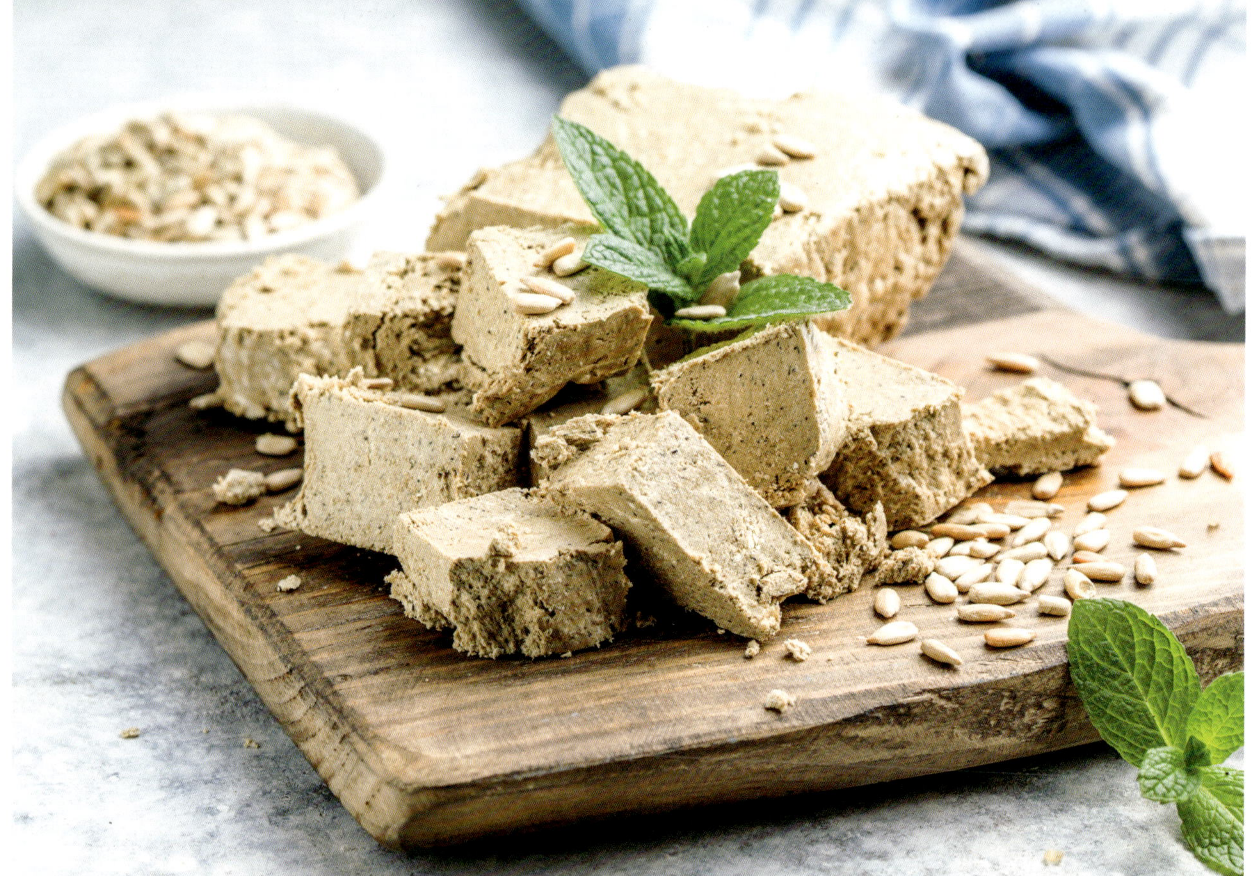

SUNFLOWER HALVA

½ cup (100g) erythritol
3 tsps lemon juice
¼ tsp xanthan gum
Pinch of salt
2 tbsps water
½ tsp vanilla extract
12 drops vanilla liquid stevia
⅔ cup (140g) tahini
¼ cup (65g) sunflower seed butter
2 tbsps coconut flour

STEPS

1. Put erythritol, lemon juice, xanthan gum, salt and water in a small saucepan, whisk and bring to the boil over medium heat. Continue to whisk for 3 minutes until the mixture thickens. Stir in vanilla extract and vanilla liquid stevia, then add the tahini, sunflower seed butter and coconut flour; fold through with a spatula.
2. Line a 15 x 10cm container with greaseproof paper.
3. Pour the mixture into the prepared container. Press down evenly with a spatula. Allow to cool to room temperature before transferring to the fridge to chill for 24 hours.
4. Remove the halva from its container and cut into slices. Store in the fridge in an airtight container.

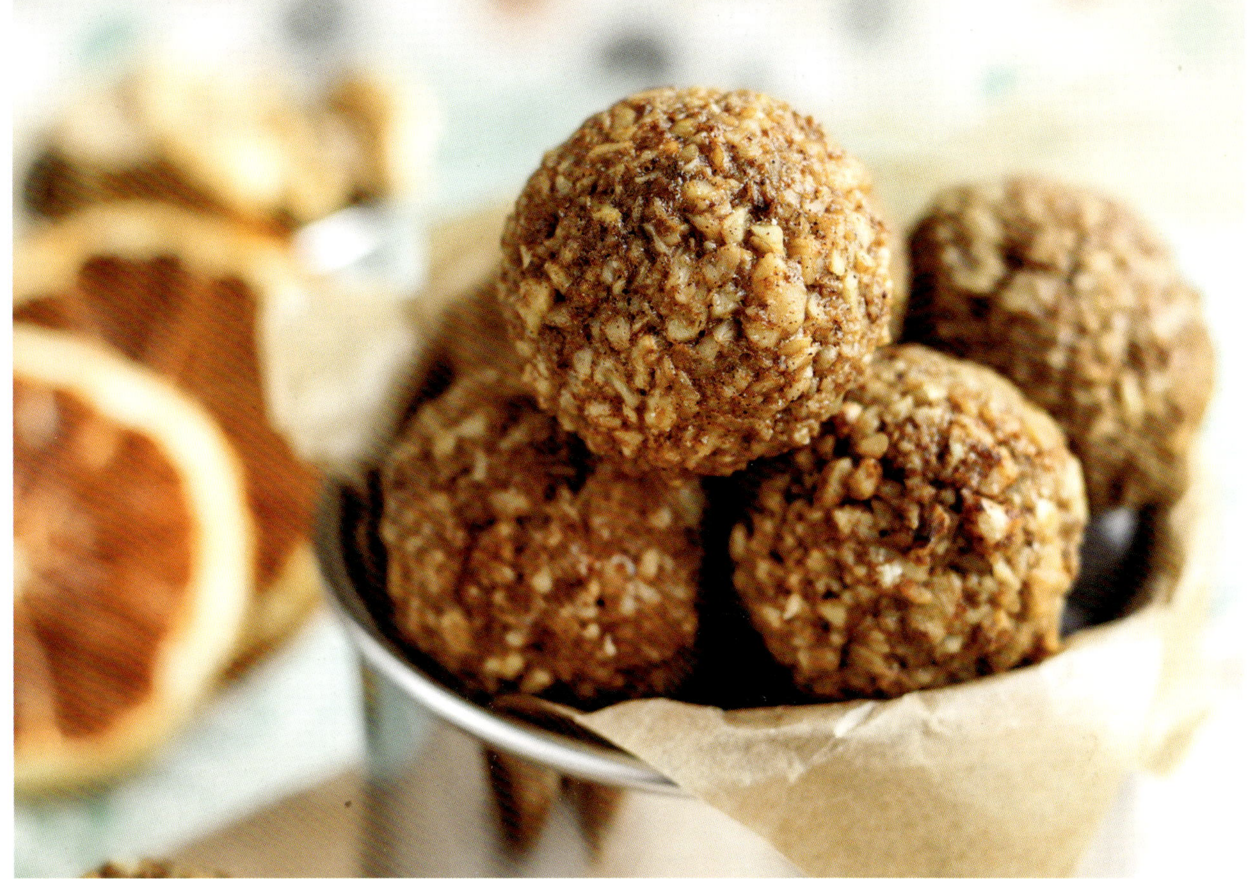

WALNUT ORANGE BALLS

1 egg

2 heaped tbsps powdered monkfruit sweetener

1 tsp cinnamon

1 tsp orange zest

1½ cups (180g) coarsely ground walnuts

STEPS

Preheat oven to 180°C.

1. Beat the egg with the sweetener, cinnamon and orange zest.
2. Add the walnuts and mix well.
3. Form the mixture into walnut-sized balls and place on a baking tray lined with greaseproof paper.
4. Bake for 10 minutes or until nicely browned.

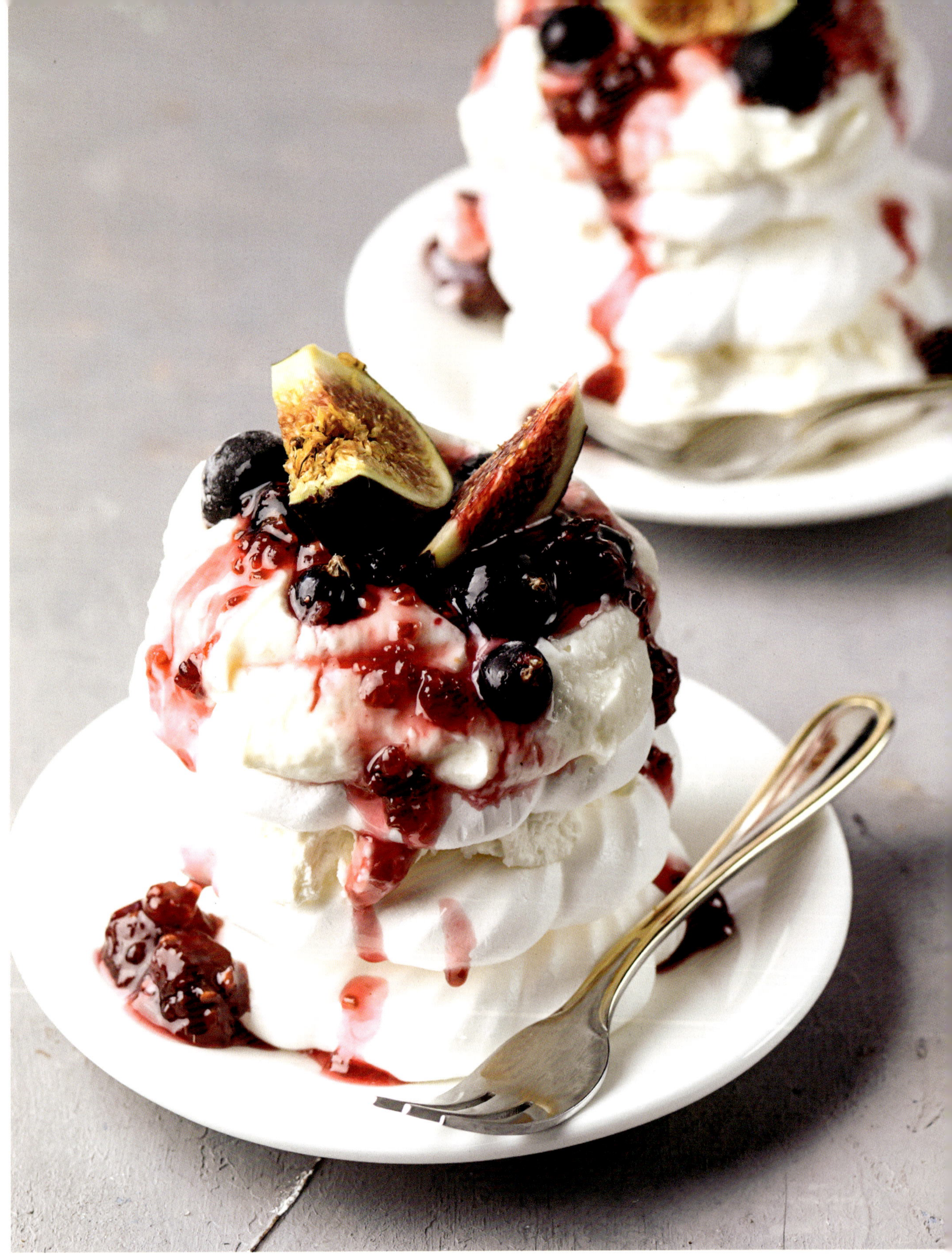

MINI PAVLOVAS

4 egg whites

½ cup (80g) powdered erythritol or another low-calorie sweetener

1 tsp white vinegar

1 tsp cornflour

½ tsp vanilla extract

1 cup (250ml) double cream

4 figs, quartered

1 cup (100g) blueberries

STEPS

Preheat oven to 120°C.

1. In a mixing bowl, whisk the egg whites on medium speed until soft peaks form. Gradually add the powdered erythritol, a spoonful at a time, while continuing to whisk until stiff peaks form and the mixture is glossy.
2. In a separate small bowl, whisk together the white vinegar and cornflour until smooth. Add the vinegar mixture and vanilla extract to the whipped egg whites. Gently fold them in until fully incorporated.
3. Spoon or pipe the meringue mixture onto a lined baking tray, creating mini pavlova nests. Make an indent in the centre of each nest to hold the toppings.
4. Bake in the preheated oven for about 60-70 minutes or until the pavlovas are crisp and dry on the outside. The centres should still be slightly soft. Turn off the oven and leave the pavlovas inside to cool completely with the oven door slightly ajar. This helps prevent them from cracking.
5. Once the pavlovas have cooled, layer them with fresh double cream, them finish them with figs and blueberries.

MAKES 8 | PREP + COOK TIME: 1 HOUR + 15 MINS | VEG | GLUTEN FREE |

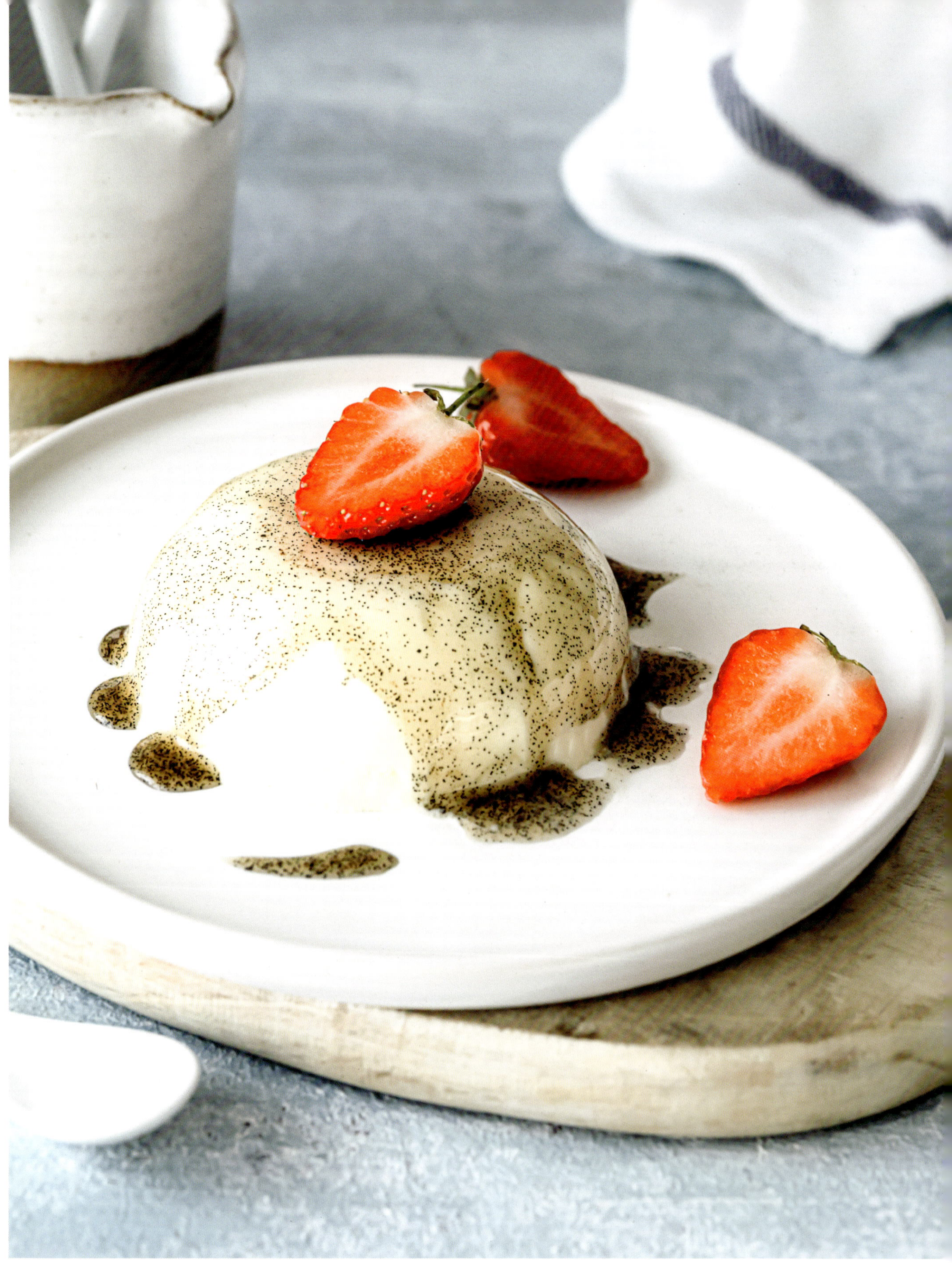

VANILLA PANNA COTTA

2 tsps powdered gelatin

2 tbsps cold water

2 cups (500ml) double cream

1 tbsp vanilla extract

1 tbsp erythritol

VANILLA SYRUP

1 tsp vanilla paste (seeds in)

¼ cup (60ml) water

2 tbsps sugar or low-carb sugar substitute

STEPS

1. In a small bowl mix the gelatin with the cold water. Set aside.
2. To make the vanilla syrup add vanilla paste, water and sugar to a small saucepan on a low heat and simmer for 5 minutes or until syrup thickens nicely. Set aside.
3. In a separate bowl add cream, vanilla extract and erythritol and bring to a boil over medium heat. Reduce the heat to medium-low and let simmer for 2 minutes or until the cream begins to thicken.
4. Remove the cream from the heat and add the gelatin. Whisk until the gelatin dissolves completely.
5. Pour into serving glasses. Allow to cool completely before covering with plastic wrap and placing in the fridge for 2-3 hours or overnight. When ready to serve add a spoonful of vanilla syrup and scatter fresh strawberries on top.

SERVES 4 | PREP + COOK TIME: 20 MINS + COOLING AND CHILLING | GLUTEN FREE |

CHOCOLATE BROWNIES

1 cup (200g) mashed ripe bananas (about 2 medium-sized bananas)

¼ cup (65g) natural nut butter (such as almond butter or peanut butter)

¼ cup (90g) honey or maple syrup

¼ cup (40g) unsweetened apple sauce

¼ cup (30g) unsweetened cocoa powder

½ cup (50g) almond flour

¼ tsp bicarbonate of soda

¼ tsp salt

½ cup (60g) fresh or frozen raspberries

¼ cup (30g) grated dark chocolate

STEPS

Preheat oven to 180°C.

1. In a mixing bowl, combine the mashed bananas, nut butter, honey or maple syrup and apple sauce. Mix well until smooth.
2. Add the cocoa powder, almond flour, bicarb and salt to the bowl. Stir until all the dry ingredients are fully incorporated into the batter.
3. Pour the brownie batter into a lined 20cm baking tin and spread it evenly.
4. Scatter the raspberries over the top and gently press them down to penetrate the batter.
5. Transfer to the preheated oven and bake for about 20-25 minutes. Remove from the oven and while still warm sprinkle the grated chocolate over the top, then once cooled cut into even squares.

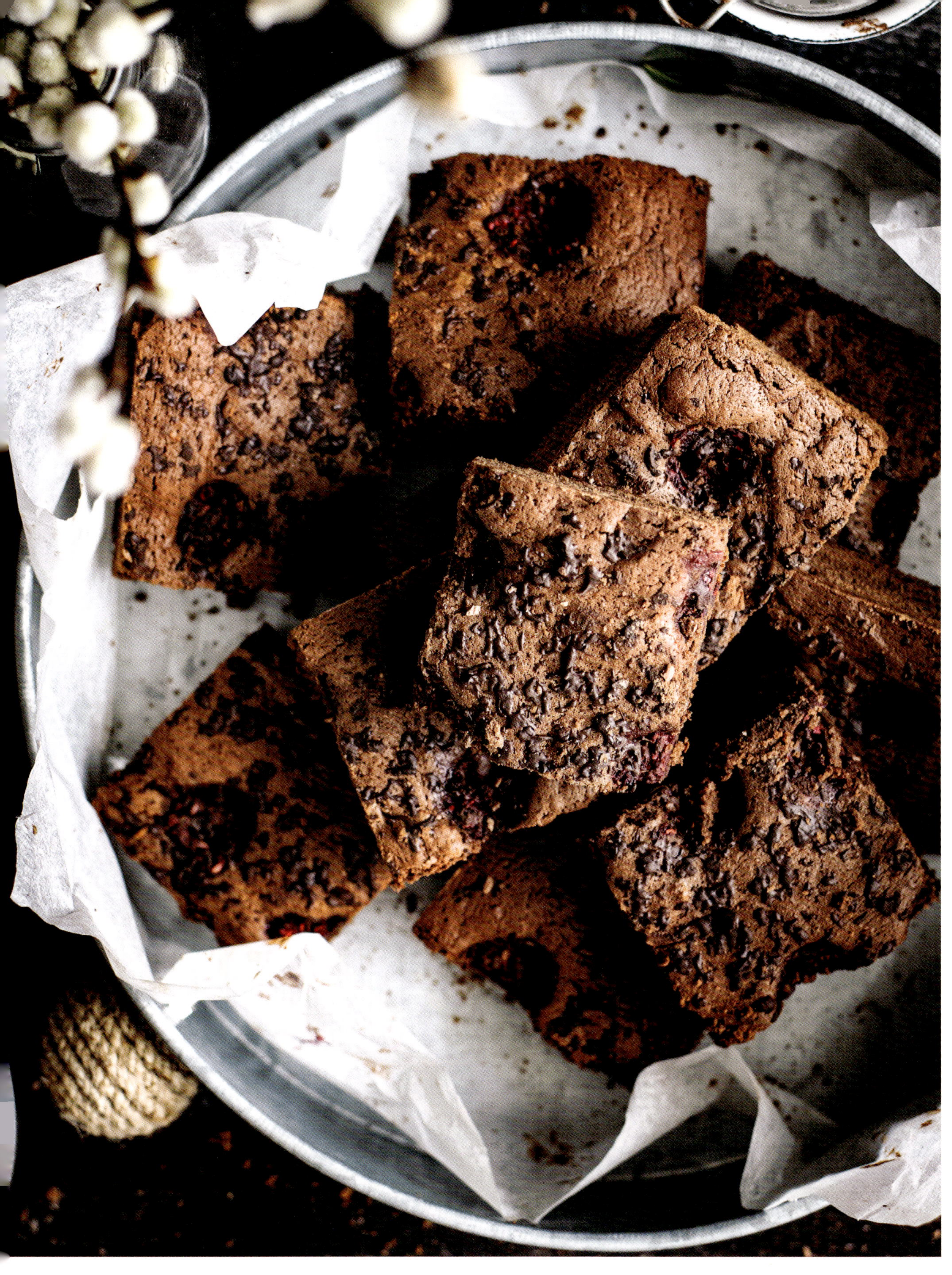

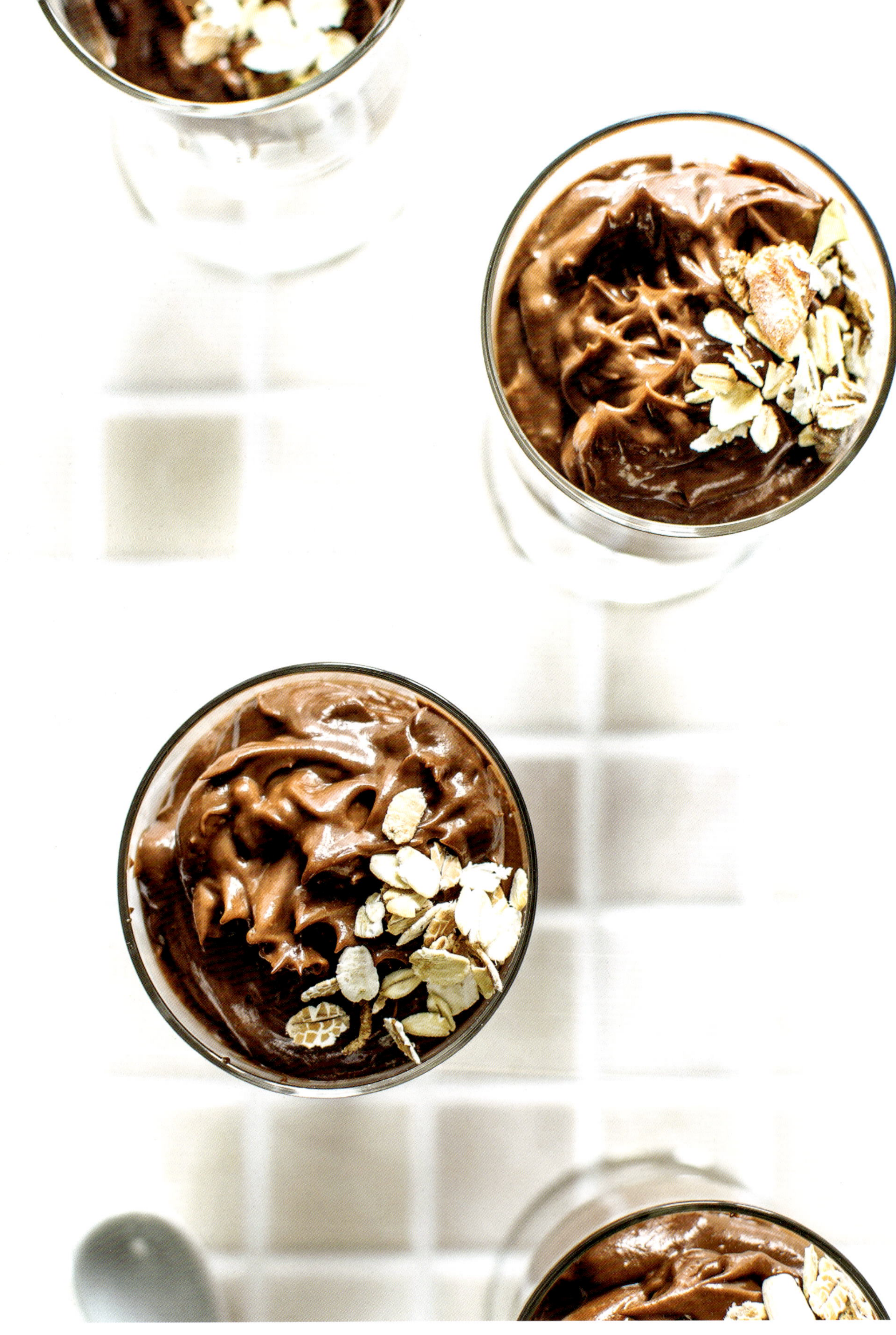

CHOCOLATE AVOCADO MOUSSE

2 ripe avocados

¼ cup (30g) cocoa powder

¼ cup (80g) honey

¼ cup (60ml) almond milk or any non-dairy milk

1 tsp vanilla extract

Pinch of salt

Toasted oats to garnish (optional)

STEPS

1. Cut the avocados in half, remove the seeds, and scoop out the flesh into a blender or food processor.
2. Add the cocoa powder, honey, almond milk, vanilla and salt to the blender or food processor.
3. Blend or process the ingredients until smooth and creamy, scraping down the sides as needed to ensure everything is well combined.
4. Taste the mixture and adjust the sweetness if desired by adding more honey.
5. Once the mousse is smooth and sweetened to your liking, transfer it to individual serving bowls or glasses. Cover with plastic wrap and refrigerate for at least 1-2 hours to chill and firm up. Sprinkle with toasted oats or topping of your choice.

SERVES 2 | PREP + COOK TIME: 10 MINS + CHILLING | VEG | GLUTEN FREE | DAIRY FREE |

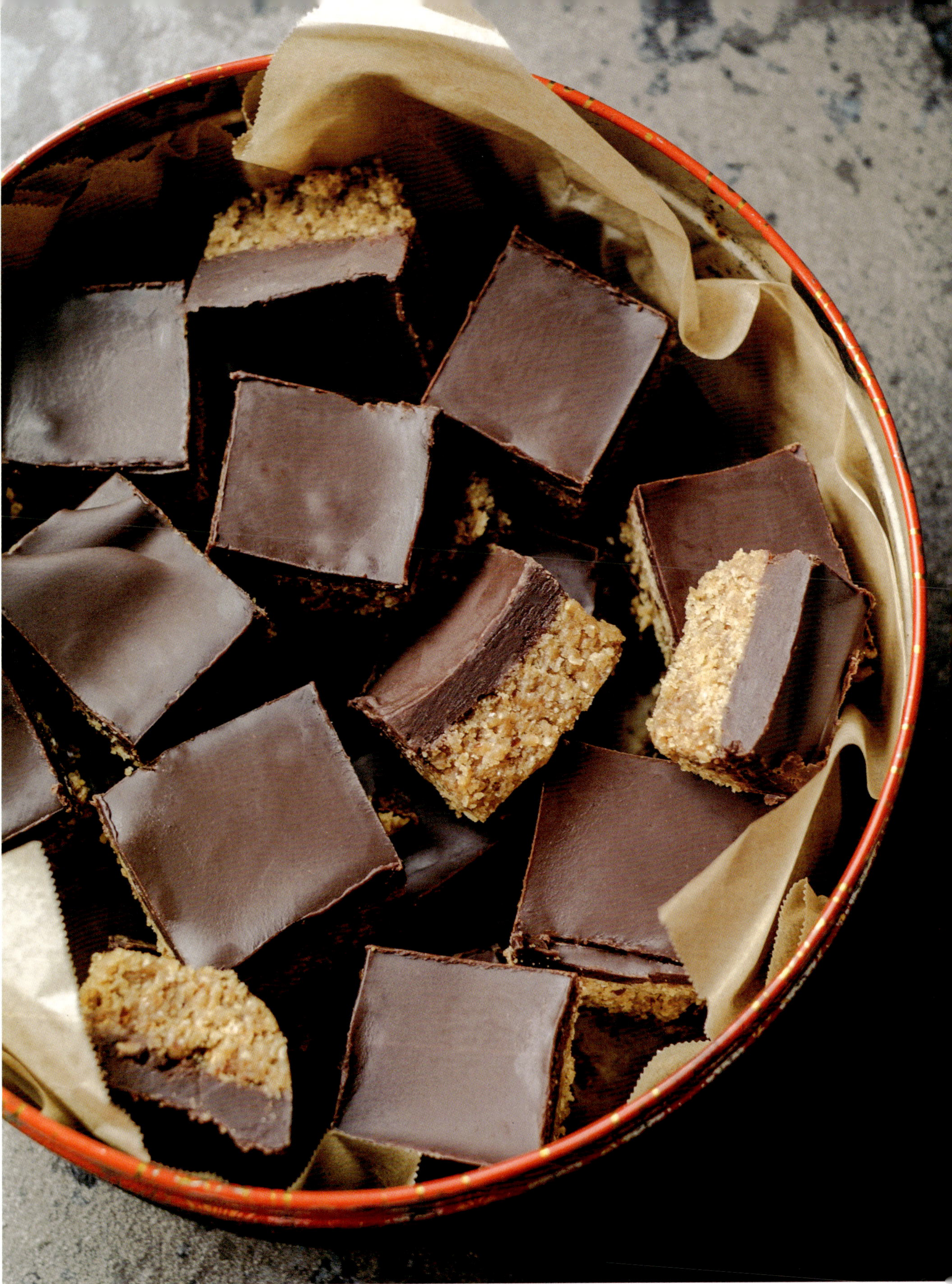

ALMOND CHOC SQUARES

1¼ cups (310g) almond butter

1 cup (100g) almond flour

1 tbsp ground flaxseed

½ cup (155g) honey

1 tsp vanilla

Pinch of salt

1½ cups (235g) sugar-free dark chocolate chips

1 tbsp coconut oil

STEPS

1. In a medium bowl mix together almond butter, almond flour, flaxseed, honey, vanilla and salt and mix until well combined.
2. Spread the almond butter mixture in a lined square baking tin, pressing down to make a nice even layer.
3. In a small saucepan boil some water over a gentle heat and then add a heatproof bowl on top of the saucepan. Add the chocolate chips and coconut oil to the bowl and stir occasionally until you have a smooth, velvety chocolate mixture.
4. Pour chocolate mixture over the almond layer evenly and then cover and place in the fridge for at least 2-3 hours (or overnight) until the chocolate has hardened and almond layer has set.
5. When ready to serve, let the tin sit at room temperature for about 10 minutes before slicing into squares, to avoid cracking the chocolate. Place in an airtight container and keep stored in the fridge.

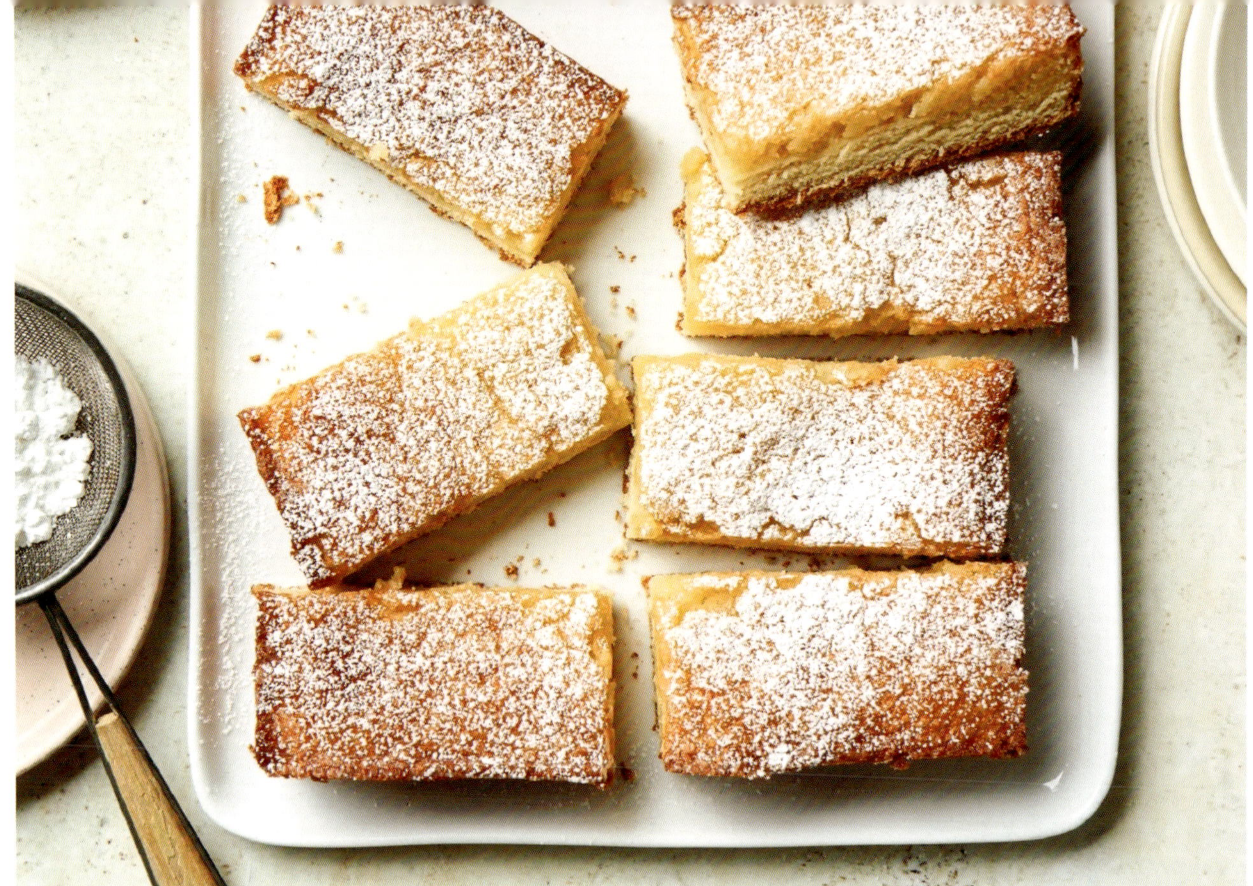

SOFT BUTTER CAKE

125g salted butter, softened

250g cream cheese, softened

1½ cups (300g) monkfruit sweetener

2 eggs

1 tsp vanilla

2½ cups (300g) almond meal

¼ cup (40g) powdered erythritol

1 tbsp baking powder

TOPPING

125g salted butter, melted

Powdered erythritol, to serve

STEPS

Preheat oven to 175°C.

1. Cream together the butter, cream cheese and monkfruit sweetener with an electric mixer. Add in the eggs and vanilla and mix to combine. Add in almond meal, powdered erythritol and baking powder. Mix to incorporate.
2. Spread batter in a greased and lined baking tin. Drizzle the melted butter over the cake.
3. Bake for 30-32 minutes until the cake is just golden and no longer looks wet on top. Do not over-bake to ensure a soft centre to the cake.
4. Dust with more powdered sweetener before slicing and serving.

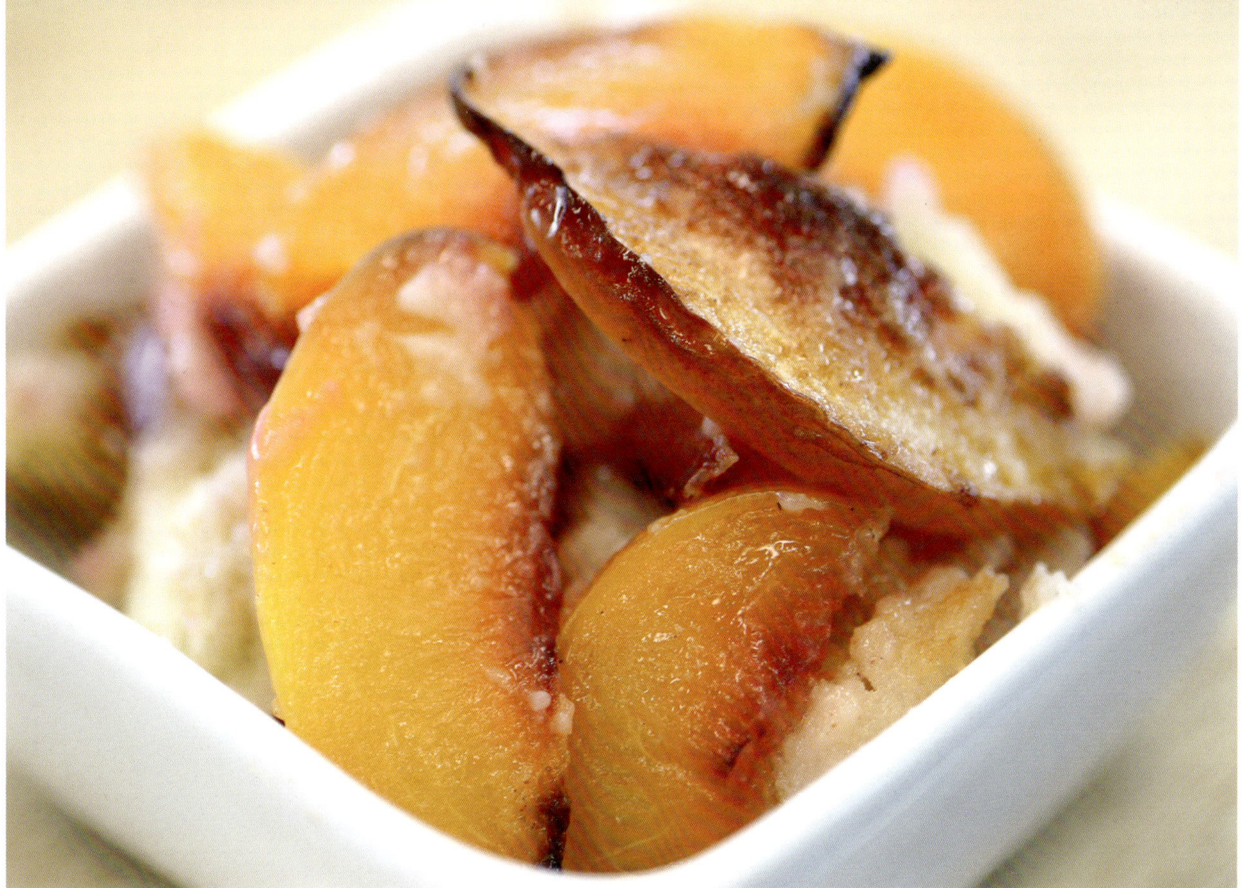

NECTARINE COBBLER

2 medium nectarines, stones removed and sliced

¼ cup (55g) sugar or substitute (such as erythritol or stevia)

1¼ cups (125g) almond flour

1 tsp bicarbonate of soda

¼ tsp cinnamon

1 tsp vanilla extract

4 tbsps butter, melted

STEPS

Preheat the oven to 180°C.

1. Add the sliced nectarines to the bottom of a well-greased medium baking dish, and sprinkle with 2 tablespoons of the sugar. Stir to combine.
2. In a mixing bowl, add the almond flour, bicarb, cinnamon, vanilla and butter and stir to combine.
3. Layer the almond mixture over the peaches in the baking dish.
4. Bake for 30 minutes, then let slightly cool before serving.

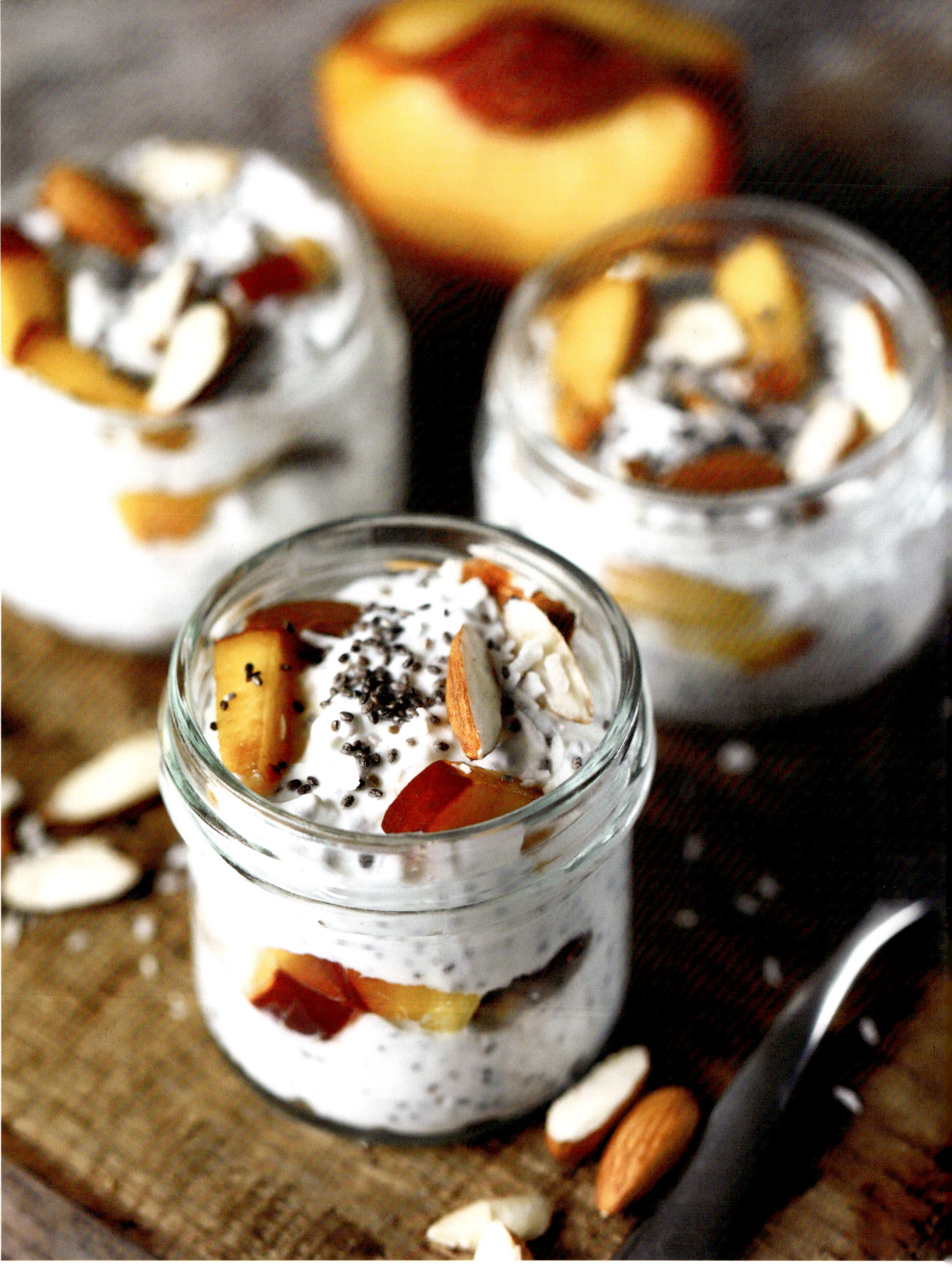

CHIA & FRUIT PARFAIT

4 tbsps chia seeds + ½ tsp for serving

1 tbsp honey

1 tsp vanilla extract

1 cup (125ml) Greek yoghurt

2 peaches, stones removed, sliced into small pieces

¼ cup (30g) almonds, chopped

STEPS

1. Add chia seeds, honey, vanilla and Greek yoghurt to a medium-sized bowl and mix well to combine.
2. Transfer to the fridge for at least 1 hour or preferably overnight.
3. To serve, layer the yoghurt and sliced peaches in a small glass or serving jar. Repeat once and finish with the yoghurt.
4. Top with extra peach slices, chia seeds and chopped almonds.

SERVES 6 | PREP + COOK TIME: 20 MINS + CHILLING | VEG | GLUTEN FREE |

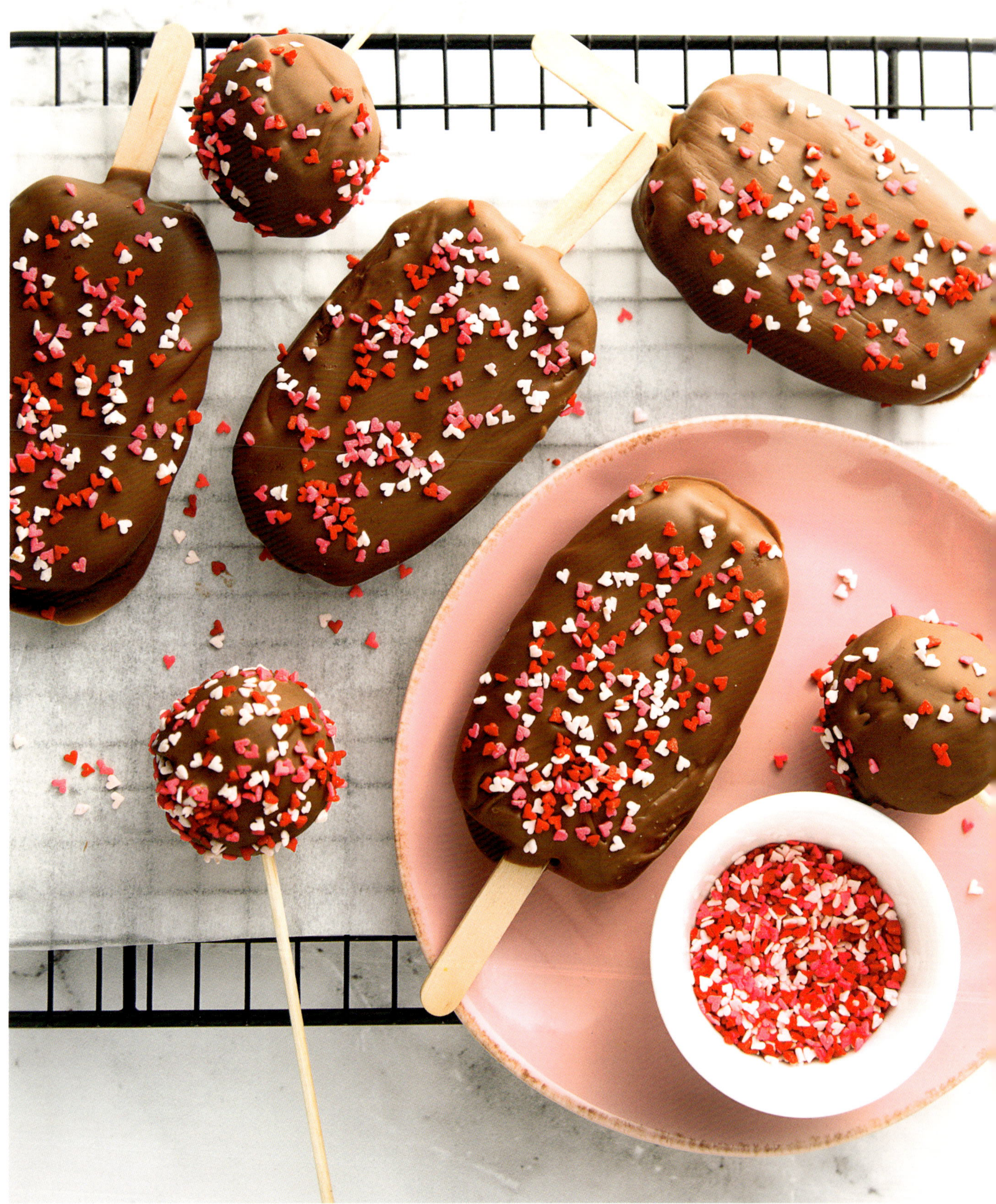

GLUTEN-FREE CAKESICLES

1 box low-carb, gluten-free chocolate cake mix of choice

3¼ cups (500g) sugar-free dark chocolate chips

2 tbsps coconut oil

Sugar-free cake decorations

ICING

125g unsalted butter, softened

125g cream cheese, softened

1½ tsps vanilla extract

⅓ cup (55g) powdered erythritol or powdered low-carb sweetener of choice

2 tbsps cocoa powder

⅛ tsp salt

STEPS

1. Prepare cake according to package instructions. Allow cake to cool completely.
2. To make the icing, cream together butter and cream cheese with an electric mixer until light and fluffy. Add vanilla and mix to combine. Sift in the powdered sweetener, cocoa powder and salt. Mix on low speed until well incorporated.
3. Crumble cooled cake into a large bowl. Add icing and use your hands to combine with the cake crumbs.
4. Add cake mixture filling to popsicle moulds then press a popsicle stick up the centre of your cakesicle. Chill for 15 minutes.
5. Melt chocolate chips and coconut oil in a heatproof bowl over a pan of simmering water. Stir until smooth and remove from heat. Remove cakesicles from their moulds and dip in the melted chocolate. Place flat onto a lined baking tray, then top cakesicles with sugar-free decorations. Place in the freezer for a further 15 minutes before serving.

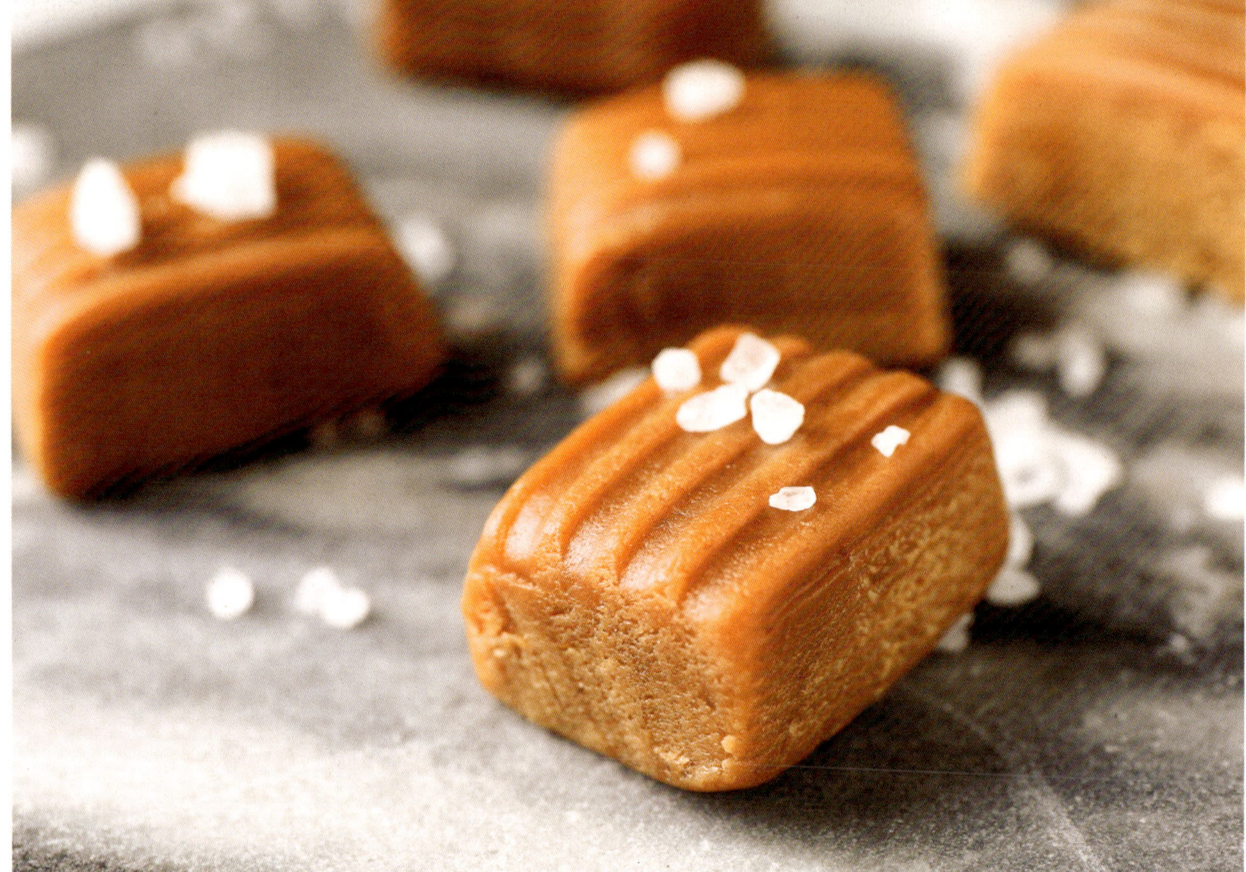

SALTED CARAMELS

1 cup (190g) dates, pitted and soaked for 10 minutes

1 cup (125g) raw cashews

¼ cup (65g) almond butter

¼ cup (60ml) coconut oil, melted

2 tbsps honey

1 tsp vanilla extract

Pinch of salt

STEPS

1. In a food processor, combine the soaked dates, cashews, almond butter, coconut oil, honey, vanilla and salt. Process until the mixture becomes smooth and creamy. You may need to scrape down the sides of the food processor a few times to ensure everything is well blended.
2. Line a square baking dish with baking paper and transfer the mixture into the dish and spread it out evenly.
3. Place the dish in the freezer and let it set for at least 2 hours, or until firm.
4. Once the fudge has hardened, remove it from the freezer and let it sit at room temperature for a few minutes to soften slightly. Cut it into small rectangles and press a fork into each piece to create an indent then sprinkle with extra salt.

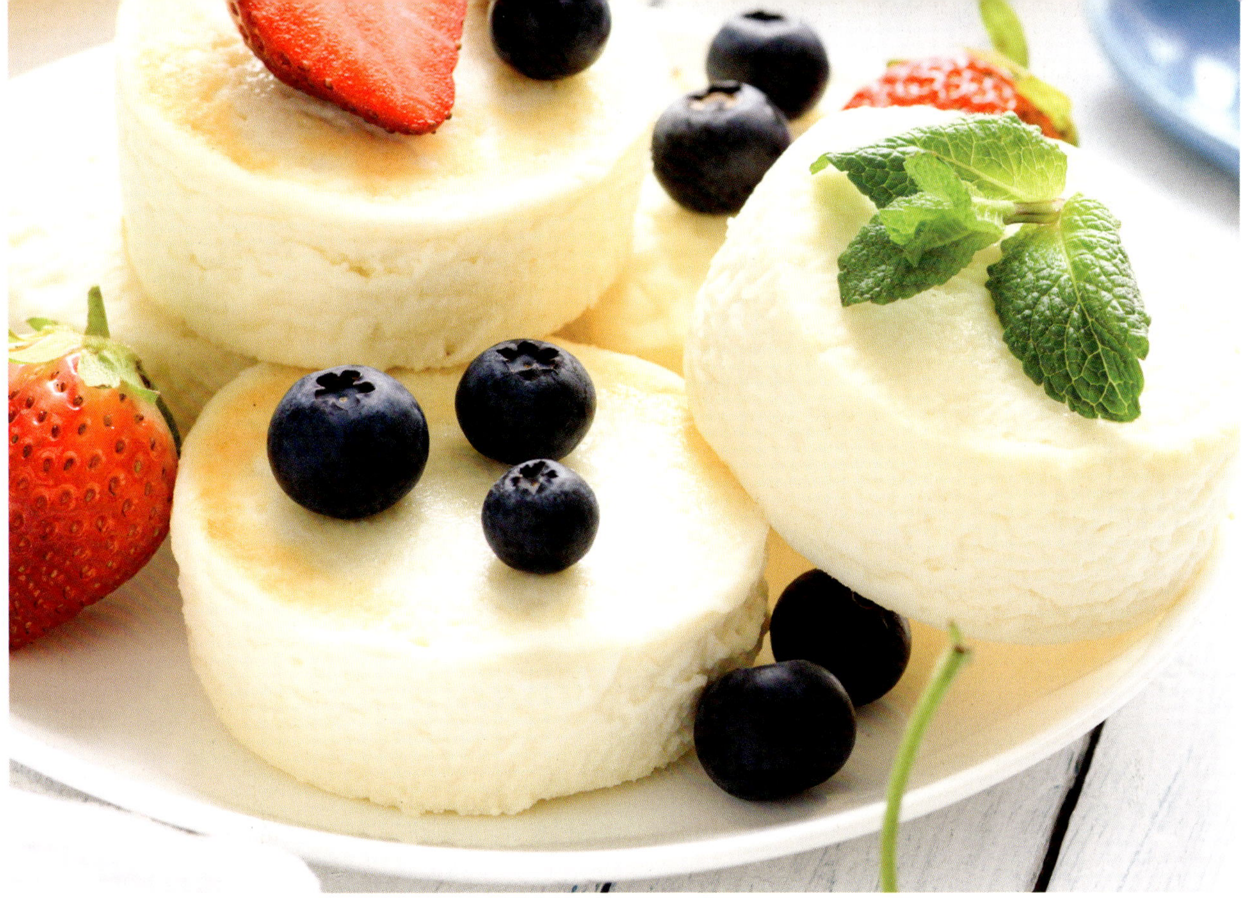

MINI CHEESECAKES

225g cream cheese, softened

¼ cup (60g) sour cream

¼ cup (60g) plain Greek yoghurt

¼ cup (55g) sugar or sugar substitute (such as erythritol or stevia)

2 large eggs

1 tsp vanilla extract

Fresh berries or sugar-free fruit compote for topping (optional)

STEPS

Preheat oven to 170°C.

1. In a mixing bowl, combine cream cheese, sour cream, Greek yoghurt and sugar or sugar substitute. Use an electric mixer to blend the ingredients together until smooth and creamy.
2. Add the eggs, one at a time, mixing well after each addition. Stir in the vanilla and continue mixing until the batter is well combined and velvety.
3. Divide evenly among lined mini cheesecake tins or a muffin tin, filling each about three-quarters full.
4. Bake in oven for 20-25 minutes, or until set and slightly golden around the edges. They should still have a slight jiggle in the centre.
5. Remove from the oven and let cool in the tin for about 10 minutes. Transfer to a wire rack to cool completely. Then refrigerate for at least 2 hours, or overnight, to allow them to set and firm up.

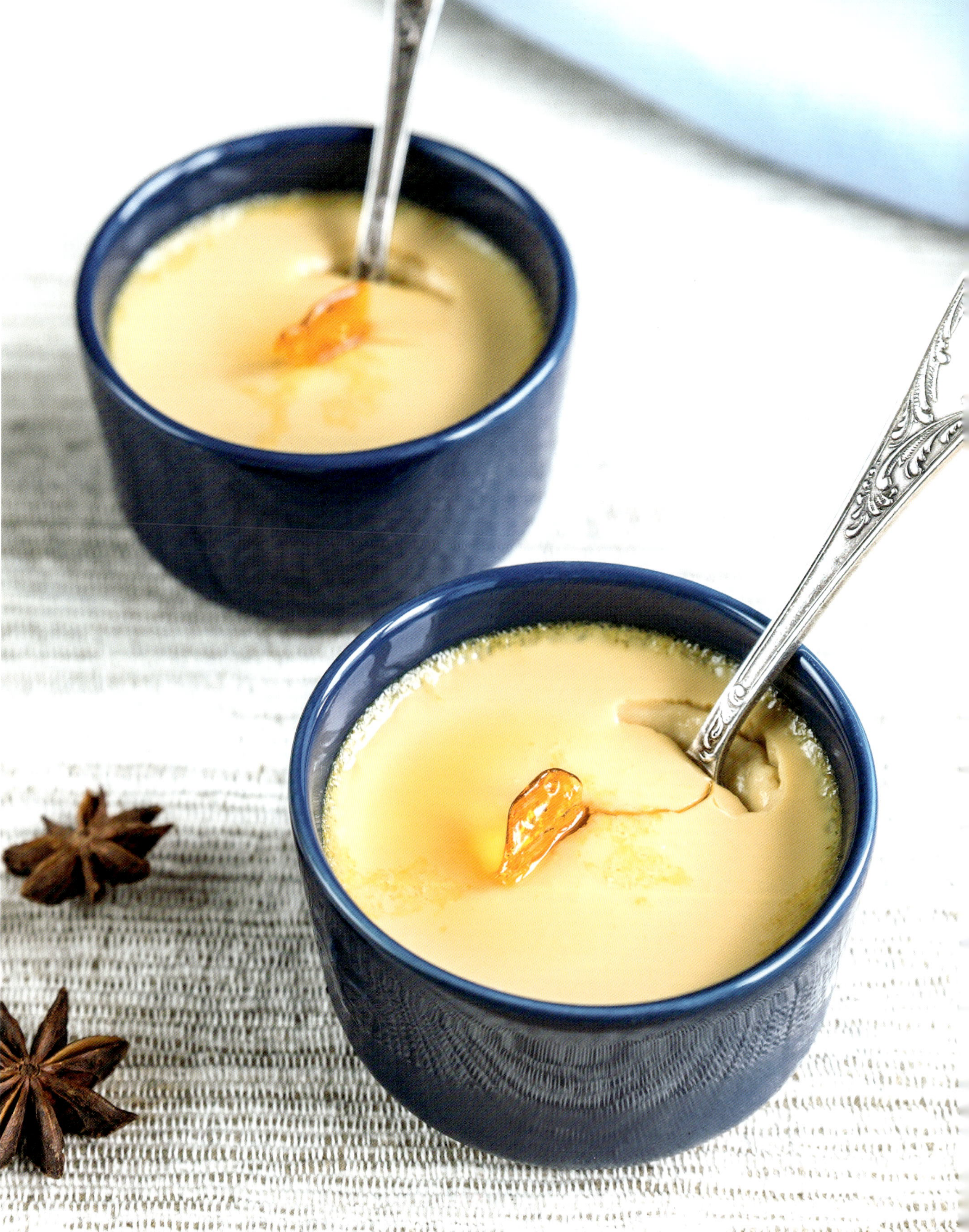

BAKED CUSTARD

3 large eggs

2 tbsps sugar or low-carb sweetener

2 tsps vanilla essence

1 cup (250ml) thickened cream

1 cup (250ml) unsweetened almond milk

¼ tsp allspice

STEPS

Preheat oven to 150°C.

1. Place the eggs and sweetener in a large bowl and whisk together for 5 minutes, until pale and creamy. Add vanilla, cream, almond milk and allspice a little at a time, whisking continuously.
2. Grease four ramekins and divide the mixture between them. Place into a roasting dish and pour in enough hot water to go halfway up the sides of the ramekins. Bake for 1 hour until the custard is set with a slight wobble in the centre.
3. Leave to cool for 15 minutes before serving.

SERVES 4 | PREP + COOK TIME: 1 HOUR 30 MINS | VEG | GLUTEN FREE |

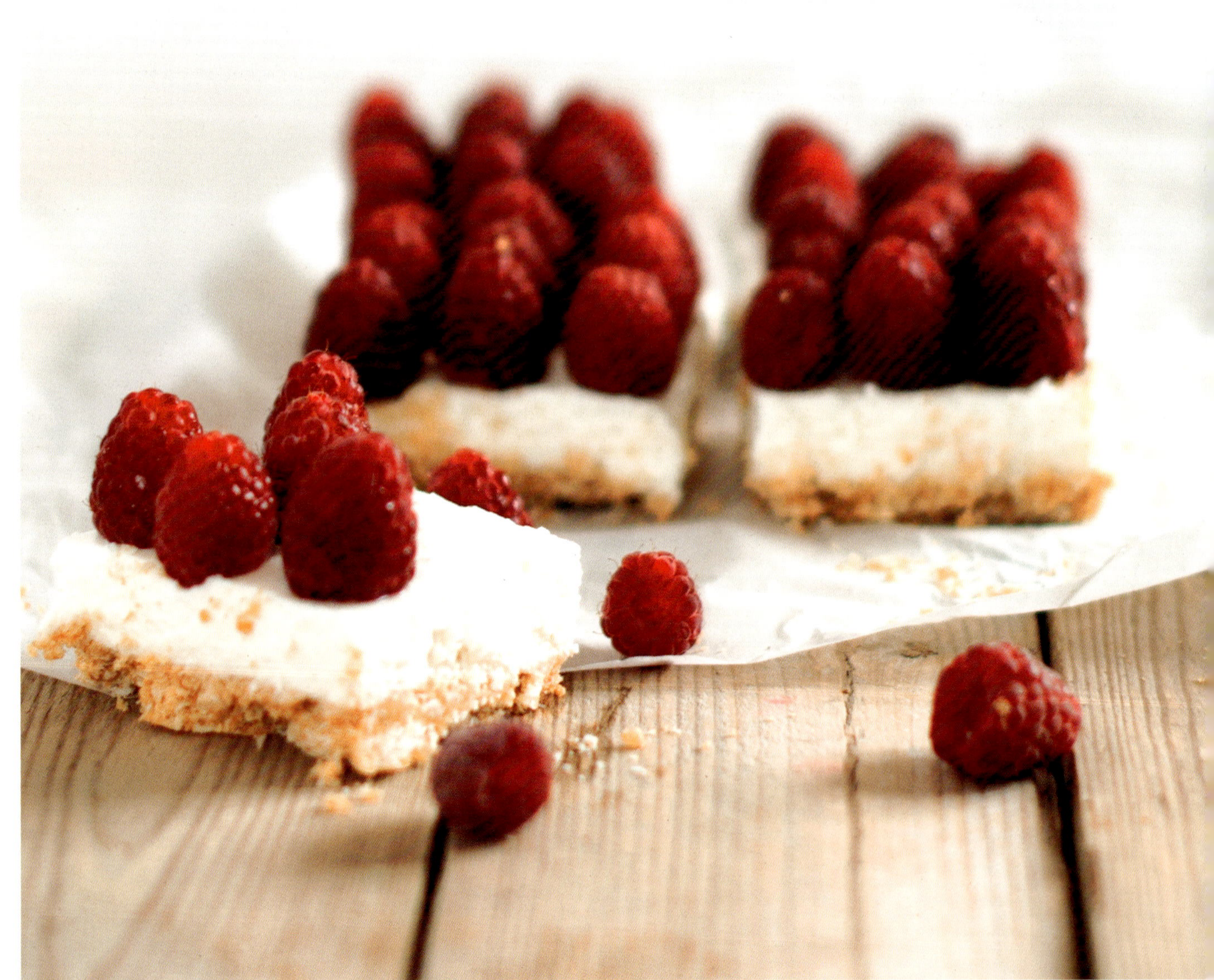

RAW COCONUT SLICE WITH RASPBERRIES

CRUST

2 cups (250g) raw almonds, pecans or walnuts

1 cup (175g) soft Medjool dates

1 cup (90g) desiccated coconut

1 tsp salt

FILLING

3 cups (375g) raw cashews, soaked

3 lemons, juiced

2 tsps vanilla extract

⅓ cup (160ml) coconut oil, melted

⅓ cup (115g) raw honey

TOPPING

2 cups (250g) raspberries (fresh or frozen)

STEPS

1. To make the crust, place the nuts, dates, coconut and salt in a food processor and process until the ingredients hold together and nuts and dates have been chopped to the desired consistency.

2. Scrape the mixture into a square or rectangle springform tin and press mixture down to form a flat layer. Place in the fridge while you complete the next step.

3. Place the filling ingredients in the bowl of a clean food processor or high-speed blender and process on the highest speed for 3-5 minutes until very smooth.

4. Pour the mixture onto the prepared base. Place raspberries on top of the filling. Transfer to the freezer for 4-6 hours until solid.

5. Remove from the freezer 30 minutes before eating. Use a very sharp knife warmed under the hot tap to cut.

NOTE: Store in the freezer.

SERVES 8 | PREP + COOK TIME: 30 MINS + FREEZING | VEG | GLUTEN FREE | DAIRY FREE |

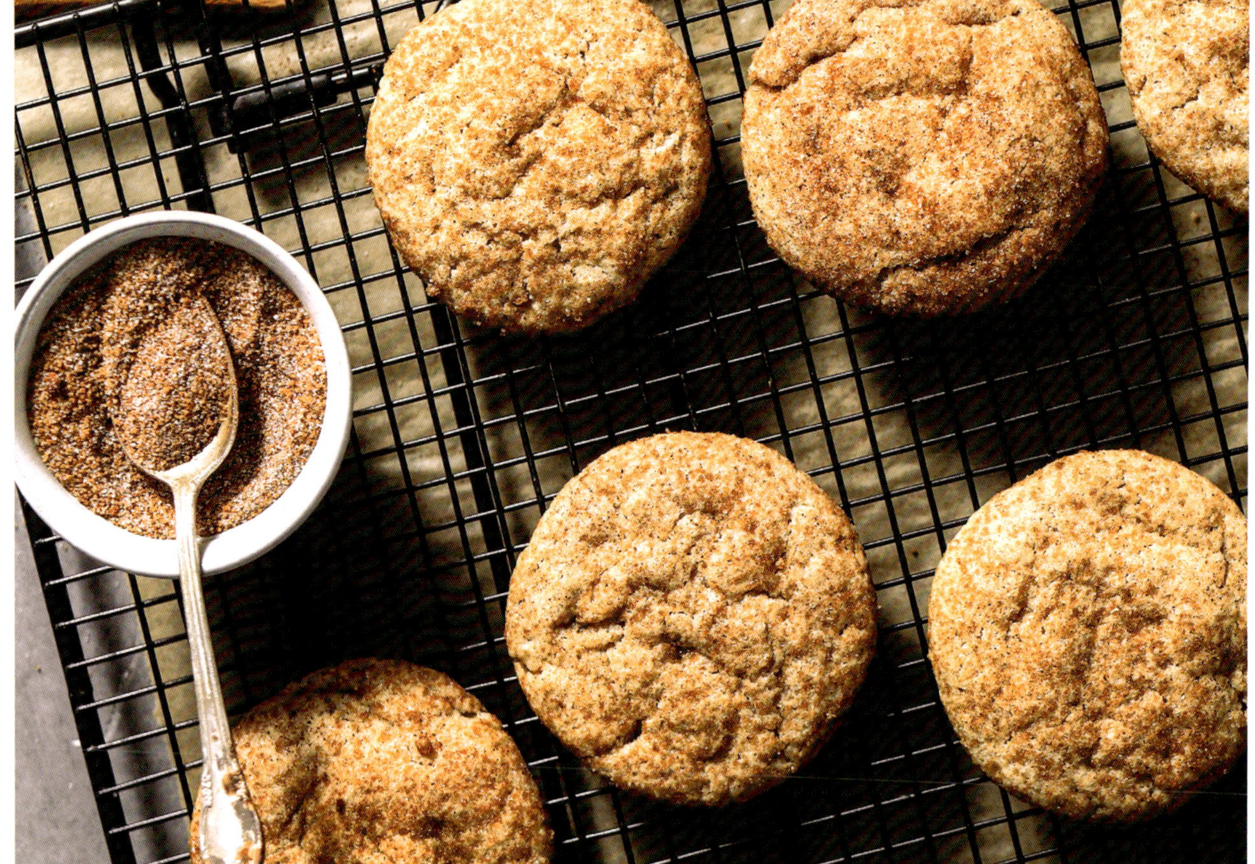

CINNAMON COOKIES

2 cups (200g) almond flour

¼ cup (25g) coconut flour

½ cup (110g) sugar or substitute (such as erythritol or stevia)

1 tsp cinnamon

½ tsp baking powder

¼ tsp salt

115g unsalted butter, melted

1 large egg

1 tsp vanilla extract

STEPS

Preheat oven to 180°C.

1. In a large bowl, whisk together the almond flour, coconut flour, sugar or substitute, cinnamon, baking powder and salt.
2. Add the melted butter, egg and vanilla to the dry ingredients. Mix until well combined, forming a dough. If the dough feels too wet, you can add a little more almond flour to achieve the desired consistency.
3. Roll tablespoon-sized portions of the dough into balls and place them on a lined baking tray. Flatten each ball slightly with the palm of your hand and sprinkle with extra sugar and cinnamon.
4. Bake the cookies in the preheated oven for 10-12 minutes, or until the edges are golden brown.

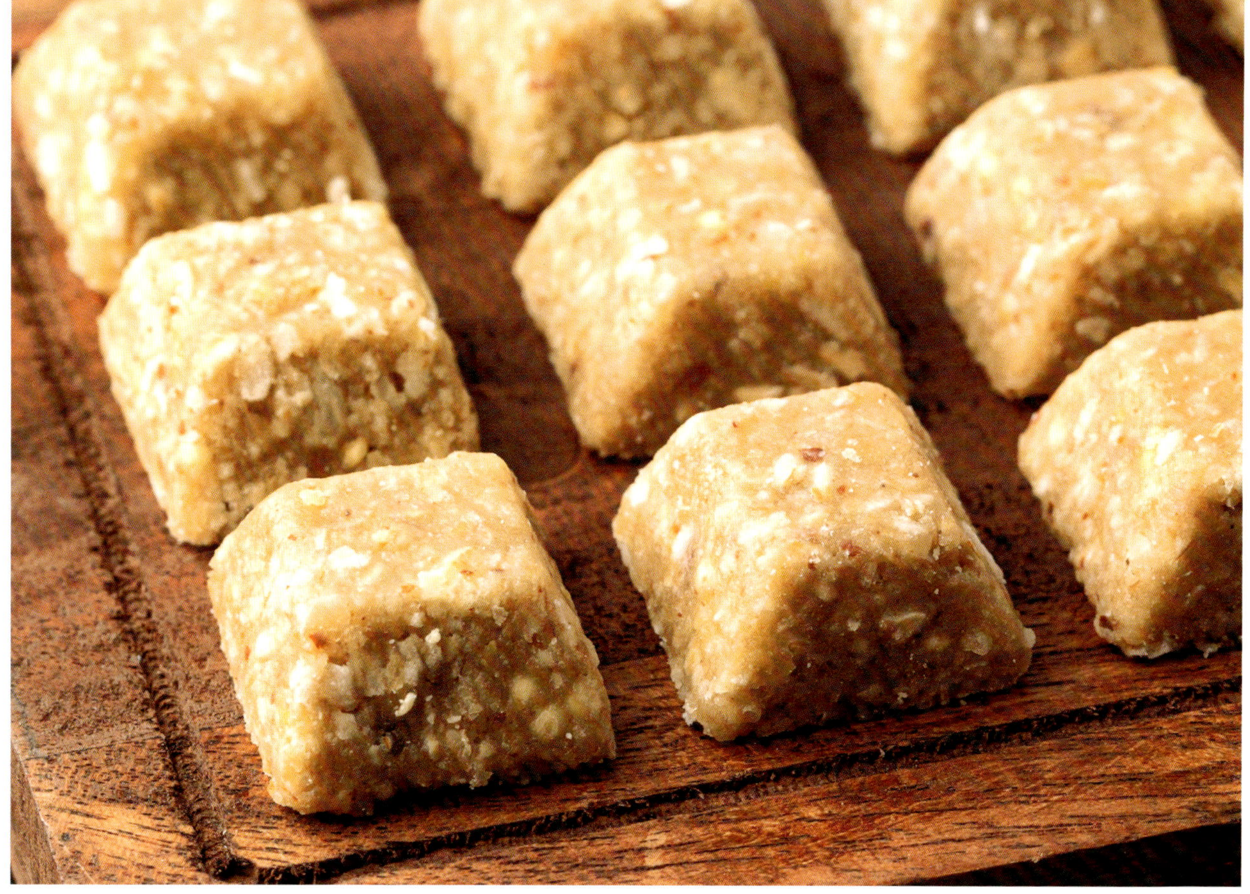

SERVES 4 | PREP + COOK TIME: 10 MINS + CHILLING | VEG | DAIRY FREE |

VANILLA & OATMEAL BITES

1¼ cups (110g) oats

½ cup (125g) peanut butter

¼ cup (80g) honey

¼ tsp vanilla

¼ tsp cinnamon

STEPS

1. In a medium bowl, combine oats, peanut butter, honey, vanilla and cinnamon and mix until well combined.
2. Roll the mixture into 3cm balls and press into a greased ice cube tray, then refrigerate until hardened slightly, about 1 hour.
3. Remove the oat vanilla bites from the tray and place in an airtight container to store.

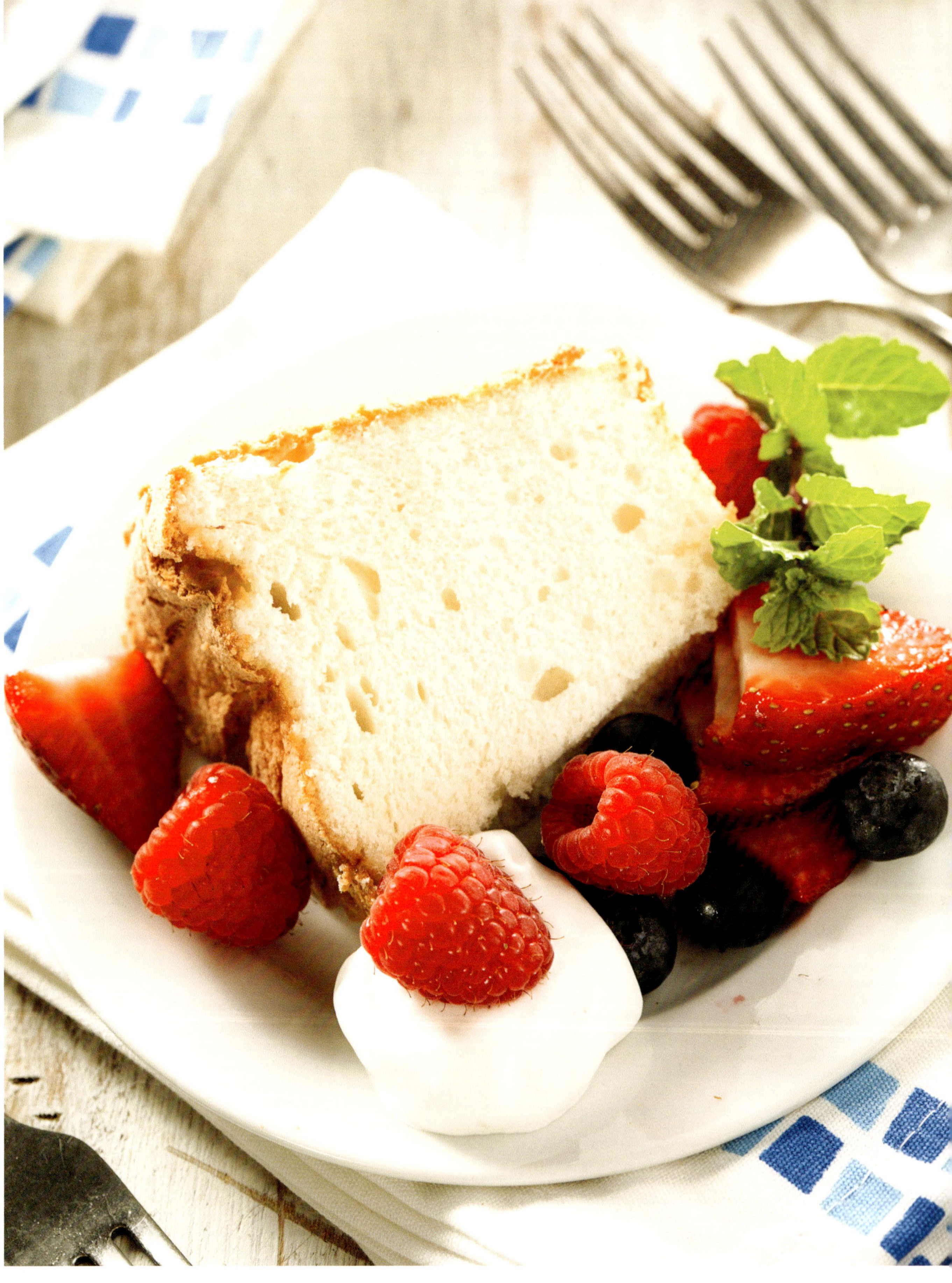

ANGEL CAKE WITH BERRIES & CREAM

6 large egg whites

½ tsp cream of tartar

½ cup (110g) sugar or substitute (such as erythritol or stevia)

½ cup (50g) almond flour

¼ cup (25g) coconut flour

½ tsp vanilla extract

1 cup (250ml) cream

1 cup (125g) mixed berries, sliced (such as strawberries, blueberries and raspberries)

Mint sprigs to garnish

STEPS

Preheat oven to 180°C.

1. In a large bowl, beat the egg whites and cream of tartar with an electric mixer until frothy. Gradually add the sugar or substitute while continuing to beat. Beat until the mixture forms stiff peaks.
2. In a separate bowl, combine the almond flour and coconut flour. Gently fold the flour mixture into the egg white mixture, being careful not to deflate the batter. Stir in the vanilla extract.
3. Pour the batter into a lined cake tin and smooth the top with a spatula. Bake for 35-40 minutes, or until the cake is lightly golden and a toothpick inserted into the centre comes out clean.
4. Remove the cake from the oven and let it cool upside down in the pan. This will prevent the cake from collapsing as it cools.
5. In a bowl whip the cream until soft peaks form and set aside. Once cake has cooled completely serve cake with fresh sliced berries, mint sprigs and dollops of whipped cream.

SERVES 6 | PREP + COOK TIME: 1 HOUR | VEG | GLUTEN FREE |

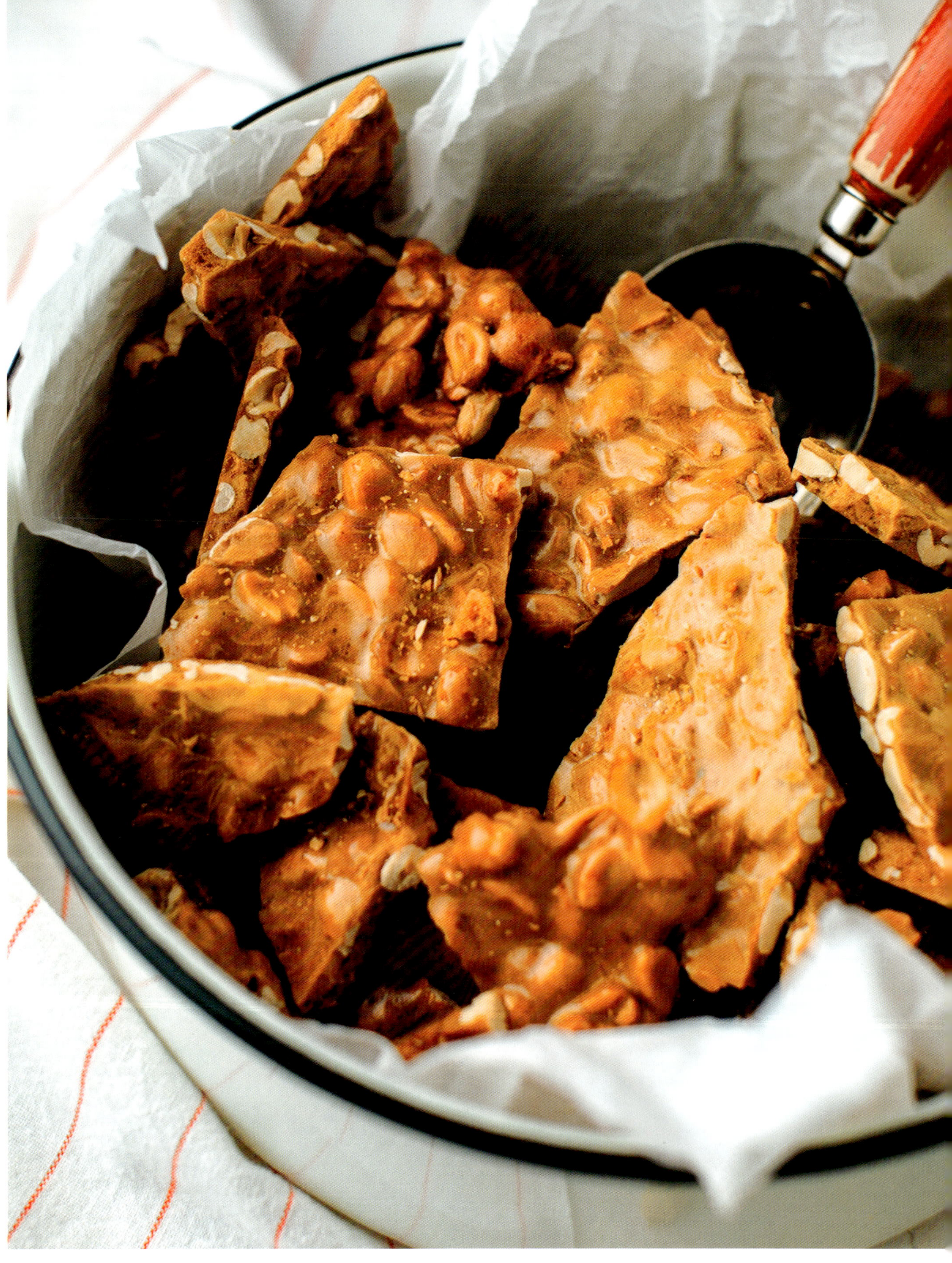

PEANUT BRITTLE

¼ cup (55g) erythritol

75g butter

1 tsp vanilla essence

¼ tsp bicarbonate of soda

1¼ cups (155g) roasted and salted peanuts

STEPS

1. Line and grease a large, flat baking tray with baking paper.
2. Place all the ingredients except the peanuts in a large saucepan over medium-high heat.
3. Keep at a simmer until the mixture turns golden brown, about 3-5 minutes.
4. Stir in the peanuts and then spread over the baking tray in a thin layer.
5. Let cool, break into bite-sized pieces and serve.

NOTE: Erythritol will work better than stevia in this recipe as it behaves more similarly to sugar.

SERVES 4 | PREP + COOK TIME: 20 MINS | VEG | GLUTEN FREE |

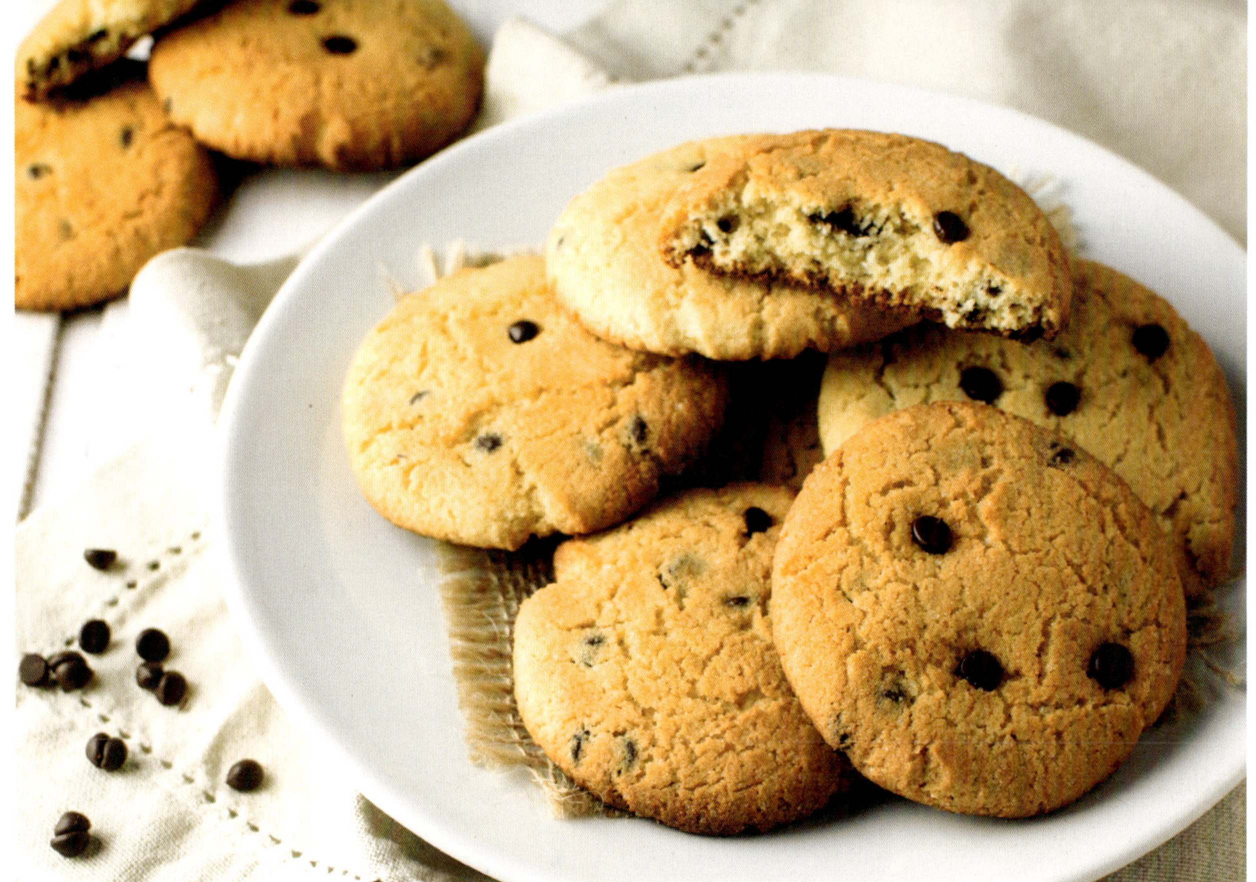

CHOC CHIP COOKIES

1 egg

1 tsp vanilla extract

2 tbsps honey

½ cup (125g) almond butter

¼ cup (60ml) coconut oil, softened

2 cups (200g) almond flour

1 tsp baking powder

½ cup (80g) sugar-free dark chocolate chips

STEPS

Preheat oven to 180°C.

1. In a medium-large bowl, whisk together egg, vanilla and honey. Add in the almond butter and coconut oil then whisk again until well combined.
2. In a separate medium bowl, mix together almond flour, baking powder and chocolate chips. Pour the mixture into wet ingredients and mix until a dough forms.
3. Roll the dough into 3cm balls then place dough balls onto a lined baking tray and bake for 10-12 minutes or until nicely browned.
4. Remove from oven then allow to cool before serving.

SERVES 16 | PREP + COOK TIME: 45 MINS + CHILLING | VEG | GLUTEN FREE | DAIRY FREE |

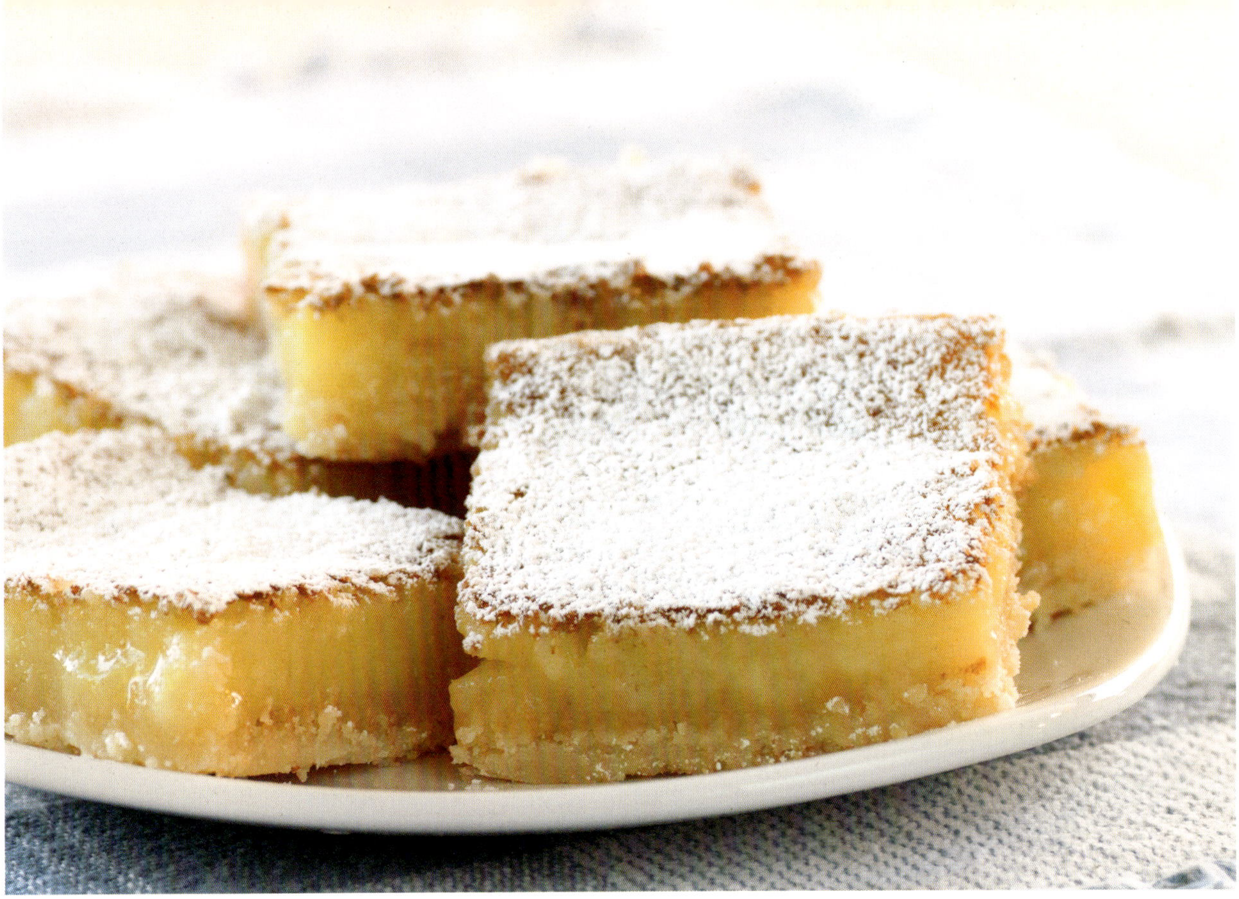

LEMON SQUARES

BASE

1 cup (100g) almond flour

¼ cup (25g) coconut flour

2 tbsps honey

2 tbsps coconut oil, melted

Pinch of salt

LEMON FILLING

½ cup (125ml) fresh lemon juice

2 tsps lemon zest

¼ cup (90g) honey

4 large eggs

2 tbsps coconut flour

¼ tsp baking powder

Pinch of salt

STEPS

Preheat oven to 180°C.

1. In a mixing bowl, combine almond flour, coconut flour, honey, coconut oil and salt. Stir well until the mixture forms a dough-like consistency.
2. Press evenly into the bottom of a lined baking dish. Bake for about 10-12 minutes, until golden brown. Remove from the oven and let it cool.
3. In a separate bowl, whisk together the lemon juice, lemon zest, honey, eggs, coconut flour, baking powder and salt until smooth.
4. Pour lemon filling over cooled base and spread out evenly. Bake in the oven for 20-25 minutes, or until filling is set and edges are lightly golden.
5. Remove from oven and let cool completely. Then refrigerate for at least 2 hours to allow the slice to set. Once chilled, cut into squares or rectangles.

DESSERTS & TREATS |

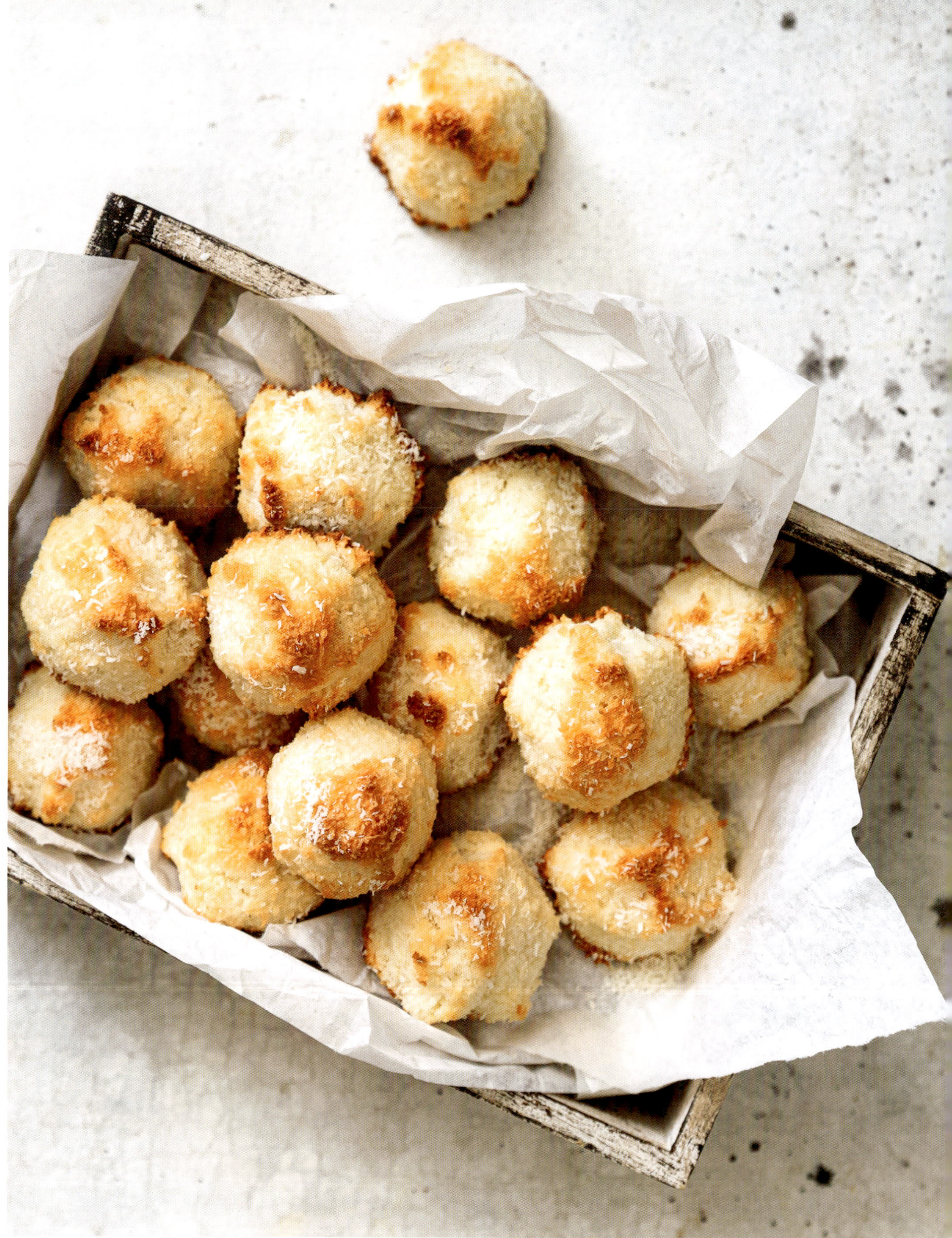

COCONUT MACAROONS

3 large egg whites, room temperature
½ tsp + a pinch of stevia
1 tbsp + 1 tsp coconut oil
½ tbsp vanilla essence
¼ cup (25g) almond flour
2 tbsps coconut flour
¾ cup (65g) shredded coconut

SERVES 4 | PREP + COOK TIME: 15 MINS | VEG | GLUTEN FREE | DAIRY FREE |

STEPS

Preheat oven to 180°C.

1. Whisk the egg whites and ½ teaspoon of stevia together until stiff peaks form.
2. In a small saucepan, gently heat all the coconut oil together with the vanilla essence. Add the flours and stir until well combined. Fold the flour mixture into the egg whites, then gently fold in the coconut.
3. Place spoonfuls of mixture onto a lined baking tray. Bake for 12 minutes or until golden. Cool to room temperature before serving.

CARROT CAKE & CREAM SANDWICH COOKIES

COOKIES

1 cup (90g) instant oats

¾ cup (90g) almond flour

1½ tsps baking powder

1½ tsps ground cinnamon

1 tsp ground ginger

1 large egg, room temperature

60g cream cheese, room temperature

1 tsp vanilla extract

½ cup (180g) honey

1 medium carrot, finely grated

FILLING

110g cream cheese

1 tbsp honey

½ tsp cinnamon

STEPS

Preheat the oven to 180°C.

1. In a medium bowl combine the oats, almond flour, baking powder, cinnamon and ginger.
2. In a separate bowl, whisk the egg and cream cheese until smooth then add in the vanilla and honey and mix well to combine. Add the flour mixture to the wet ingredients and stir to incorporate. Fold in the grated carrot.
3. Using an ice cream scoop, add dollops of cookie dough onto a lined baking tray, making sure to leave space in between them. Flatten the dough to create even shapes. Bake for 12-15 minutes, then allow the cookies to cool on a wire rack.
4. To make the filling, in a medium bowl add the cream cheese, honey and cinnamon and using an electric beater mix until the mixture becomes light and fluffy.
5. Spoon a teaspoon of the mixture onto one of the cooled cookies then add another one on top, sandwiching the filling. Repeat with the remainder of the cookies.

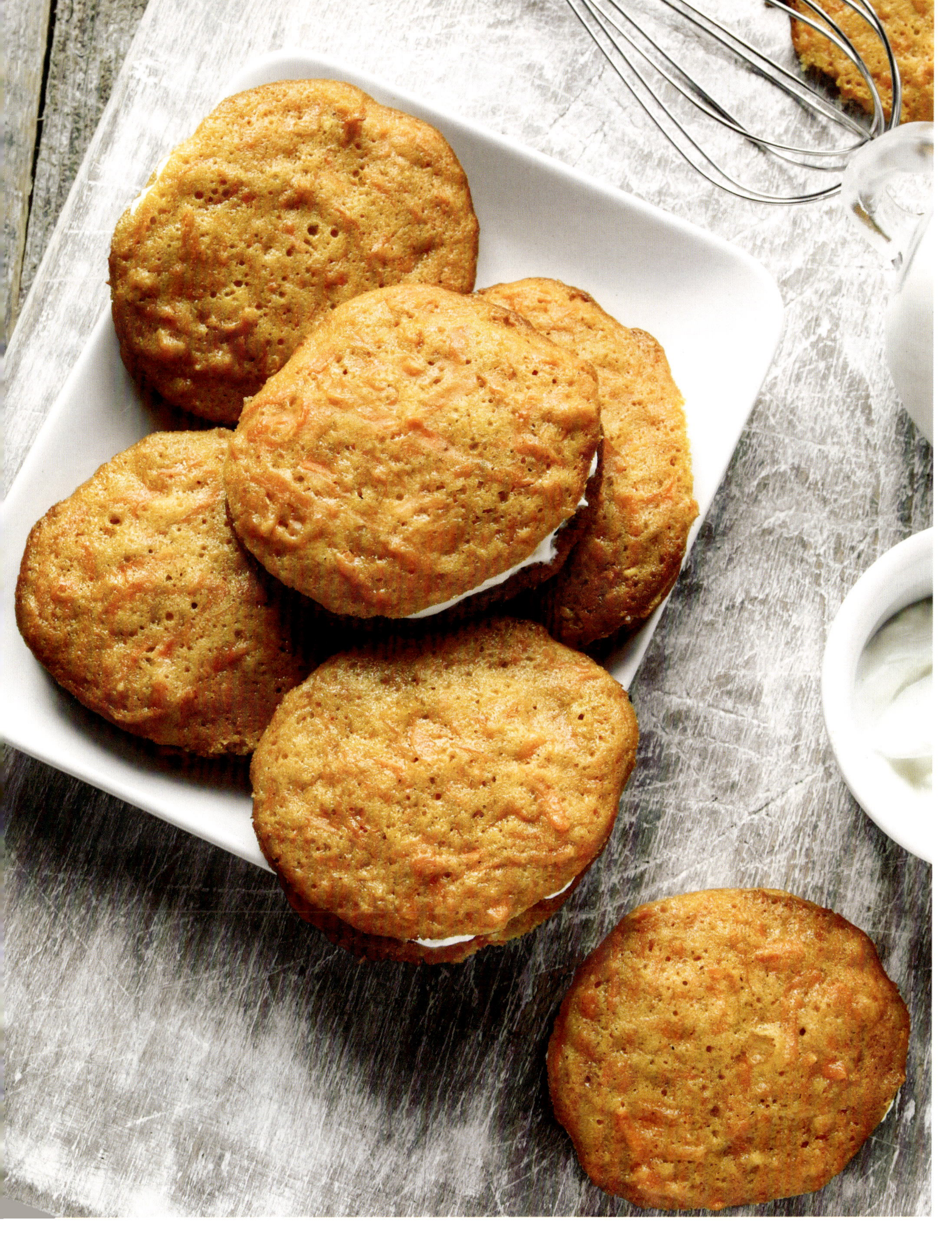

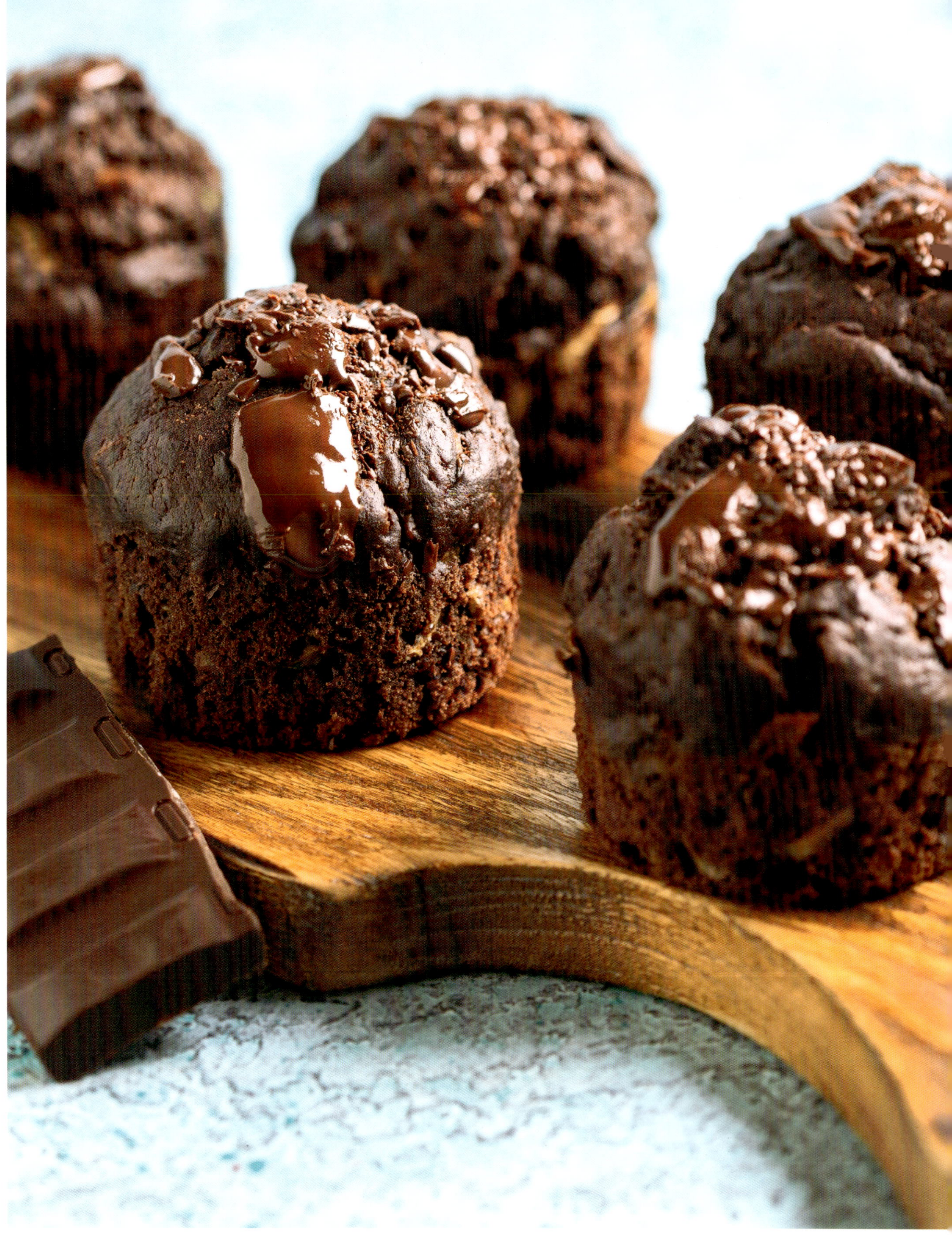

LOW-CARB CHOCOLATE MUFFINS

1 cup (120g) almond meal

½ cup (60g) unsweetened cocoa powder

½ cup (100g) erythritol

1½ tsps baking powder

1 tsp vanilla extract

3 large eggs

⅔ cup (160ml) double cream

85g butter, melted

½ cup (80g) sugar-free chocolate chips + extra, melted, to serve

STEPS

Preheat oven to 175°C.

1. In a large bowl, combine almond meal, cocoa powder, erythritol and baking powder.
2. Add the vanilla extract, eggs and cream. Mix well. Add the melted butter and chocolate chips. Stir to combine.
3. Line a muffin tin with paper or silicone liners. Spoon the mixture into the muffin tin.
4. Transfer to oven and bake for 20 minutes until puffed up and springy.
5. Allow to cool in the muffin tin, then top with a little extra melted chocolate to serve.

SERVES 4 | PREP + COOK TIME: 40 MINS | VEG | GLUTEN FREE |

INDEX

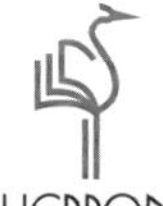

HERRON
First Published in 2023 by Herron Book Distributors Pty Ltd
14 Manton St
Morningside
QLD 4170
www.herronbooks.com

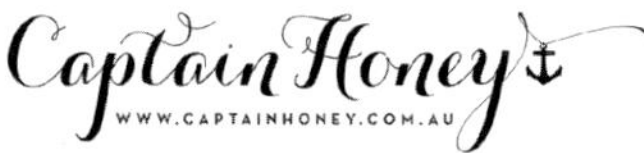

Custom book production by Captain Honey Pty Ltd
12 Station St
Bangalow
NSW 2479
www.captainhoney.com.au

Cataloguing-in-Publication. A catalogue record for this book is available from the National Library of Australia

ISBN 978-1-922944-33-7

Printed and bound in China.

5 4 3 2 1 23 24 25 26 27

NOTES FOR THE READER

All reasonable efforts have been made to ensure the accuracy of the content in this book. Information in this book is not intended as a substitute for medical advice. The author and publisher cannot and do not accept any legal duty of care or responsibility in relation to the content in this book, and disclaim any liabilities relating to its use.